Praise for Previous Editions

"Keene has written a comprehensive handbook to serve as a road map for others, from diagnosis through treatment."

— *Library Journal*,
starred review and chosen for "Nursing Your Children's Health Collection"

⁕ ⁕ ⁕ ⁕ ⁕

"This most complete parent guide available covers not only detailed and precise medical information about leukemia and the various treatment options, but also day-to-day practical advice. . . . Parents who read this book will have the opportunity to ensure that, as much as possible, they can give their child the very best opportunity to be 'truly cured.'"

— F. Leonard Johnson, MD,
Chief, Division of Pediatric Hematology/Oncology Oregon Health Sciences University

⁕ ⁕ ⁕ ⁕ ⁕

"This wonderful book is an informative addition to the House library, and one we will recommend whole-heartedly. By providing this resource to the children and families staying here, you enable them to find a bit of hope and peace of mind in a time of great difficulty and confusion."

— Peggy Enright, House Director,
Boston Ronald McDonald House

⁕ ⁕ ⁕ ⁕ ⁕

"As the mother of a two-time survivor of ALL—yes it can recur, in my daughter's case after a 14-year remission—I can vouch that the road to cure is bumpy, filled with life-threatening complications and requiring aggressive in-hospital care. A valuable resource to help parents and children regain their equilibrium after diagnosis and during the two to three years of treatment."

— Patricia Dane Rogers,
The Washington Post

⁕ ⁕ ⁕ ⁕ ⁕

"Highly recommended. In this new edition, Keene provides updates on treatment including bone marrow transplants, chemotherapy drugs, and methods of dealing with side effects. . . . Poignant and supportive."

— Alan Rees,
Consumer Health, A Majors Report

⁕ ⁕ ⁕ ⁕ ⁕

"Of all the many kinds of help we had (and we had lots) Childhood Leukemia was the single best gift we received. It was the gift of knowledge, so we could ask intelligent questions about our daughter's care. It was the gift of security, allowing us to foresee much of what was coming, and giving us the tools we needed to cope. And it was the gift of hope, for we could see that many children do, indeed, get through this trying time, and come through the grueling treatment intact."

— Kim Warren,
mother of a child with leukemia

⁕ ⁕ ⁕ ⁕ ⁕

"The great value of Nancy Keene's exceptional book is that it puts the facts and explanations into understandable terms while acknowledging and dealing with the emotional aspects as only parents who have had similar experience can."

— Mark L. Greenberg, MD,
Medical Director, Pediatric Oncology Group of Ontario

Childhood Leukemia

A Guide for Families, Friends & Caregivers

Fifth Edition

Nancy Keene

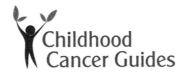

Childhood
Cancer Guides

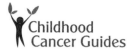
Childhood
Cancer Guides

Childhood Leukemia: A Guide for Families, Friends & Caregivers, 5th Edition, by Nancy Keene

ISBN 978-1-941089-040

Library of Congress Cataloging-in-Publication Data

Names: Keene, Nancy, author.
Title: Childhood leukemia : a guide for families, friends & caregivers /
   Nancy Keene.
Description: Fifth edition. | Bellingham, WA : Childhood Cancer Guides,
   [2018] | Includes index.
Identifiers: LCCN 2017031837 (print) | LCCN 2017032121 (ebook) | ISBN
   9781941089064 (pdf) | ISBN 9781941089071 (mobi) | ISBN 9781941089118
   (ebook) | ISBN 9781941089040 (pbk. : alk. paper)
Subjects: LCSH: Childhood Leukemia.
Classification: LCC RJ416.L4 (ebook) | LCC RJ416.L4 K44 2018 (print) | DDC
   618.92/99419--dc23
LC record available at *https://lccn.loc.gov/2017031837*

 This book is printed on acid-free, recycled paper. Childhood Cancer Guides is committed to using paper with the highest recycled content available consistent with high quality.

In memory of
Bill and Doris Keene

Table of Contents

Appendices

Introduction

*"We are all in the same boat, in a stormy sea,
and we owe each other a terrible loyalty."*

— G. K. Chesterton

MY LIFE ABRUPTLY CHANGED on Valentine's Day, 1992, when my 3-year-old daughter was diagnosed with acute lymphoblastic leukemia (high risk). At the time, I was the full-time mother of two young daughters. I understand that nothing prepares a parent for the utter devastation of having a child diagnosed with cancer. My family has walked the path from that life-changing moment through information gathering, treatment, and survivorship. We know that fear and worry are lessened by having accurate information and through hearing the stories of other children and families who have walked the path before us. We are honored to share with you what hundreds of parents and healthcare providers have learned to try to ease your journey down this hard road.

What This Book Offers

This book is not autobiographical. Instead, I wanted to blend basic technical information in easy-to-understand language with stories and advice from many parents and children. I wanted to provide the insights and experiences of parents who have all felt the hope, helplessness, anger, humor, longing, panic, ignorance, warmth, and anguish of their children's cancer treatment. I wanted parents to know how other children react to treatment and to offer tips to make the experience easier.

Obtaining a basic understanding of topics such as medical terminology, common side effects of treatment, and how to interpret laboratory results can help improve quality of life for the whole family. Learning how to develop a partnership with your child's medical team can vastly increase your family's peace of mind. Hearing parents describe their emotional ups and downs, how they coped, and how they molded their family life around hospitalizations is a tremendous comfort. And knowing there are other parents out there who hold their breath with each test hoping for good news can help you feel less alone. My hope is that parents who read this book will find understandable medical information, obtain advice that eases their daily life, and feel empowered to be strong advocates for their children.

The stories and suggestions in this book are absolutely true, although some names have been changed to protect children's privacy. Every word has been spoken by the parent of a child with cancer, a sibling of a child with cancer, or a childhood cancer survivor. There are no composites—just the actual words of people who wanted to share what they learned with families of children newly diagnosed with leukemia.

How This Book Is Organized

This book is organized sequentially in an attempt to parallel most families' journeys through treatment. We all start with diagnosis, then learn about leukemia and its treatment, try to cope with procedures, adjust to medical personnel, and deal with family and friends. We all seek out various methods of support and struggle with the strong feelings felt by our child with cancer, our other children, and ourselves. We also try to work with our child's school to provide the richest and most appropriate education for our ill child.

Because it is tremendously hard to focus on learning new things when you are emotionally battered and extremely tired, I tried to keep each chapter short. The first time I introduce a medical term, I define it in the text. Because both boys and girls get cancer, I did not adopt the common convention of using only masculine personal pronouns (e.g., he, him). Instead, I alternated personal pronouns (e.g., she, he) within chapters. This may seem awkward as you read, but it prevents half of the parents from feeling that the text does not apply to their child.

All the medical information contained in this fifth edition of *Childhood Leukemia* is current as of 2017. As treatment is constantly evolving and improving, there will inevitably be changes. For example, researchers are currently studying new targeted medications and genetically determined responses to specific drugs that may dramatically improve treatments. You will learn in this book how to discover the newest and most appropriate treatments for your child. However, this book should not be used as a substitute for professional medical care.

Three appendices are included: Appendix A, *Blood Tests and What They Mean*; Appendix B, *Resource Organizations*; and Appendix C, *Books, Websites, and Support Groups*.

How to Use This Book

While conducting research for this book, I was repeatedly told by parents to "write the truth." Because the "truth" varies for each person, more than 170 parents, children with leukemia, and their siblings share portions of their experiences. This book is full of these snapshots in time, some of which may be hard to read, especially by families of newly diagnosed children. Here are suggestions for positive ways to use the information contained in this book:

- Consider reading only the sections that apply to the present or the immediate future.

- Realize that only a fraction of the problems that parents describe will affect your child. Every child is different; each one sails smoothly through some portions of treatment but encounters difficulties during others.

- Take any concerns or questions that arise to your child's oncologist and/or nurse practitioner for answers. The more you learn, the better you can advocate for your child.

- Share this book with family and friends. Usually, they desperately want to help and just don't know how. This book not only explains the disease and treatments but also offers dozens of concrete suggestions for helpful things family and friends can do.

Best wishes for a smooth journey through treatment and a bright future for your entire family.

Acknowledgments

This book is truly a collaborative effort—without the help of many, it would simply not exist. My heartfelt thanks to my family and friends who supported and encouraged me while I wrote all five editions of this book. Special thanks to my first editor, Linda Lamb, whose creative instinct and gentle guidance shaped this book from its inception; to Sarah Farmer (editor), Susan Jarmolowski (graphic designer), and Alison Leake (copy editor) for their expertise, attention to detail, and unfailing good cheer. Tremendous thanks to the Momcology and ACOR (Association of Online Resources) support groups who introduced me to dozens of families currently in treatment. We all know it takes a village. I deeply appreciate all of you for helping make this a comprehensive, up-to-date resource for families of children with leukemia and those who love them. We are also grateful to Genentech and several other generous donors who wish to remain anonymous for providing funding to support publication of this book.

All five editions of this book are true collaborations between families of children with leukemia and medical professionals. Many well-known and respected members of the pediatric oncology community, members of national organizations, and parents carved time out of their busy schedules to review chapters, make invaluable suggestions, and catch errors. I especially appreciate the patient and thoughtful responses to my many emails and phone calls. Thank you: Peter C. Adamson, MD; Kristin Bradley, MD; Nancy Bunin, MD; Colleen Callahan, MSN, CRNP; Bruce Camitta, MD; William Carroll, MD; Barbara Clark, MD; Lynne Conlon, PhD; Max Coppes, MD, PhD; Elizabeth Cummings, MSN, CPNP-AC; Kenneth B. DeSantes, MD; Connie DiDomenico, CRNP; Brian J. Druker, MD; Debra Ethier, RTT; Patty Feist, MS; Daniel Fiduccia, BA; Kerry Frank, MSEd; Debra Friedman, MD; Mark Greenberg, MD; Joanne M. Hilden, MD; Wendy Hobbie, RN, MSN, PNT; JoAnne Holt, MA; F. Leonard Johnson, MD; Anne Kazak, PhD; Marie Lappin; Susan J. Leclair, MS, CLS (NCA);

Laurie D. Leigh, MA; Ellen M. Levy, MSN, CRNP; Mignon Lee-Cheun Loh, MD; Grace Ann Monaco, JD; Ann Newman, RN; Mark Newman, MD; Katie Oranges, MSN, CRNP, CPHON; Stephanie Powell, MSN, PCNS-BC, CPON; Joanne Quillen, MSN, PNP-BC; Mary Relling, PharmD; Mary Riecke, pharmacist; Susan Shurin, MD; Shannon J. Snow, JD, RN; Sheryl Lozowski Sullivan, MPH; Heidi Suni, MSW; and David Unger, MD.

More than words can express, I am deeply grateful to the parents, children with cancer, and their siblings, who generously opened their hearts while sharing their experiences with me. To all of you whose words form the heart and soul of this book, thank you: Brenda Andrews; Robin B.; Jan Barber; Barbara Bradley; Jocelyne Brent; Betty Bright; Sue Brooks; Ann Olson Brown; Nancy and Ernie Bullard; Amy C; Michelle Caldwell; Kari Carbon; Edie Cardwell; Paulette Carles; Ricky Carroll, Garrett's Dad; Alicia Cauley; Jennifer Click; Amy Condoluci; Priscilla Cooperman; Kalita Corrigan; Cheryl Coutts; Jennifer Crouse; Carol Dean; Beth Devery, mother of Allison Devery (cancer survivor); Allison E. Ellis; Lisa N. Ellis; E. B. Engelmann; Dana Erickson; Mel Erickson; Sarah Farmer; Patty Feist; Mindi Finch; Meri-Li Forrest; Tamra Lynn Sparling Fountaine; Kerry Frank; Faith Franzen; Alana Freedman; Stacey Fundukian (mother to Rayne and Izzabella); Jenny Gardner; Merry Gibbons with daughter Gabby Ziems; Denise M. Glassmeyer; Roxie Glaze; Melanie Goldish; Susan Goldhaber; Elizabeth Guanch; Kris H.; Lisa Hall; Erin Hall; Daphne Hardcastle; Robbie Harding; Denise Glassmeyer Hendler; Kathryn G. Havemann; Connie Herron; Douglas L. Herstrom; Connie Higbee-Jones; Honna Janes-Hodder; Ruth Hoffman; Margaret Huhner; Chris Hurley; Alicia Hutchinson; Maria J.; Cheryl Putnam Jagannathan; Kelly Janzen; Theresa T. Jeniene; Karen and Brian Jordan; Fr. Joseph; Susan Kalika; Winnie Kittiko; C. J. Korenek; Cynthia Krumme; Madeline LaBonte; Marie Lappin; Joel Layfield; Missy Layfield; Bob Ledner; Pat Lee; Suzanne Lee; Kathryn C. Lim; Julie Macedo; Coramarie Marinan; Wies and Julie Matejko; Caitlin McCarthy-King; Deirdre McCarthy-King; Karen McClure; Sara McDonnall; Maria McNaught, mom to Trevor (leukemia survivor); Kimberly Mehalick; Wendy Mitchell; Amanda Moodie; Jean Morris; Leslee Morris; Laura Myer; Cathy Nell; Berendina Norton; M. Clare Paris; Jeff Pasowicz; Donna Phelps; Bev Phipps; Paula Pickering; Michelle Prymas; Mary Riecke; Jennifer M. Rohloff; Joy Rollefson (mom to Patrik); Valerie Rye; Steve and Shirlene S.; Maria and William Sansalone; Carole Schuette; Kimberly Schuetz; Donna Schumacher; Judith Mravetz Schumann; Mark W. Schumann; Sharon A. Schuster; Susan Sennett; Kurt Shedd (Dana's Dad); Lori Shipman; Mark A. Simmons, DDS; Lorrie Simonetti; Cathi Smith; Carl and Diane Snedeker; Shannon J. Snow; Marlene Sorota; Anne Spurgeon; Anabel Stehli; Becky Stephan; Kim Stimson; Dawni Summitt; Megan Thomas; Gigi N. Thorsen; Robyn Thurber; Lisa Tignor; Laura Todd-Pierce; Kathleen Tucker; Brigit Tuxen; Mike and Stacey Vasquez (parents) and Darla Cain (proud Grandma); Annie Walls; Ralene Walls; Tami Watchurst; Sheri White; Helen Wilder; Jean Wilkerson; Jan Williamson; Catherine Woodman; Amy Wright; Erika Zignego; Ellen Zimmerman; Ann; and those who wish to remain anonymous.

Despite the inspiration and contributions of so many, any errors, omissions, misstatements, or flaws in the book are entirely my own.

Chapter 1

Diagnosis

"A journey of a thousand leagues begins with a single step."
— Lao-tzu

"WE HAVE THE RESULTS of the blood work back. I'm afraid it's bad news. Your child has leukemia." For every parent who has heard those words, it is a moment frozen in time. In one shattering instant, life forever changes. Families are forced into a strange new world that feels like an emotional roller coaster ride in the dark. Every member of the family will feel strong emotions. However, with time and the knowledge that most children survive leukemia, hope will grow.

Signs and Symptoms

Parents are usually the first to notice that something is wrong with their child. Occasionally, a pediatrician sees a problem during a well-baby visit, or the disease is discovered by chance through a routine blood test. Unfortunately, because some of the signs and symptoms of leukemia mimic other conditions, diagnosis is sometimes difficult.

The onset of the disease can be slow and insidious or very rapid. Children begin to tire easily and rest often. Frequently, they have a fever that comes and goes. Interest in eating gradually diminishes, but only some children lose weight. Parents usually notice pale skin and bruising. Tiny red spots may appear on the skin. Some children develop back, leg, and joint pain, which makes it difficult for them to walk. Often lymph nodes in the neck or groin become enlarged, and the upper abdomen may protrude due to enlargement of the spleen and liver. Children become irritable, and may have nosebleeds. Parents often have an uneasy feeling that something is wrong, but they cannot pinpoint the cause for their concern.

> *Preston (10 years old) had an incredible diagnosis. We were very lucky. We were at our beach cabin for Thanksgiving. Preston was tired and listless and had a low-grade fever (99–100°) that had persisted for several days. We were bringing his younger sister into town to attend a birthday party, so we decided to bring Preston in to have him checked by the pediatrician on call. The doctor asked Preston what was wrong, and he said, "I don't know, I just feel awful." The doctor ordered blood work*

and a chest x-ray, and within 30 minutes I was told that he had a "blood cancer." I wanted to take Preston back to the cabin, but was told we needed to go immediately to the hospital, where Preston was admitted, and treatment began.

Most parents react to their concerns by taking their child to a doctor, as Preston's parents did. Usually, the doctor performs a physical exam and orders blood work, including a complete blood count (CBC). Sometimes the diagnosis is not so easy or as fast as Preston's.

I had been worried about Christine (3 years old) for two weeks. She was pale and tired. She ate nothing but toast, and had developed bruises on her shins. At preschool, she would utter a high-pitched scream whenever upset. She told me that she didn't want to go to preschool anymore, and when I asked why, she said, "It's just too much for me, Mommy."

When I took her to the doctor, he measured Christine's weight and height, pronounced them normal, and described her lack of appetite as "nothing to worry about." I told him that all she was doing was lying on the couch and asked why she would have bruises on her legs. He said bruises on shins always take a long time to heal. When I pointed out how pale she was, he stated that all children are pale in the winter. I grew more and more concerned and took her back the next week. When I told him again of Christine's difficulties with preschool, he suggested that I read a book entitled "The Difficult Child." I brought her back again and they put her on antibiotics. When her symptoms got worse, they gave her a different antibiotic.

Things continued to deteriorate and I was starting to feel frantic, so I went to talk to my neighbor who had recently retired after 40 years of nursing. She said I should take her to the doctor immediately and insist on blood work. When I took her in that afternoon, her white count was over 240,000 (normal is 10,000, the rest were cancer cells) and her hematocrit (percentage of oxygen-carrying red cells) was 12, far lower than the normal 36.

Where Should Your Child Receive Treatment?

After a tentative diagnosis of leukemia, most physicians refer the family to the closest major children's hospital for further tests and treatment. It is very important that children with leukemia be treated at a facility that uses a team approach, including pediatric oncologists, oncology nurses, pathologists, nurse practitioners, radiologists, psychologists, child life specialists, education specialists, and social workers. State-of-the-art treatment is provided at these institutions, offering your child the best chance for remission (disappearance of the disease in response to treatment) and ultimately, cure.

When we were told that Katy had leukemia, for some reason I was worried that she would miss supper during the long road trip to Children's Hospital. Why I was worried about this when she wasn't eating anyway is a mystery. The doctor told us not to stop, just to go to a drive-through restaurant. I was so upset that I only packed Katy's clothes; my husband, baby, and I had only the clothes on our backs for that first horrible week.

Usually, the child is admitted through the emergency room or the oncology clinic, where a physical exam is performed, an intravenous line (IV) is started, more blood is drawn, and a chest x-ray is obtained. Early in your child's hospitalization, the pediatric oncologist will perform a spinal tap to determine whether any leukemia cells are present in the cerebrospinal fluid and a bone marrow aspiration to identify the type of leukemia. Details of these procedures are described in Chapter 9, *Coping with Procedures*.

Physical Responses

Many parents become physically ill in the weeks after their child's diagnosis. This is not surprising, given that most parents stop eating or grab only fast food, have trouble sleeping, and are exposed to all sorts of illnesses while staying in the hospital. Every waking moment is filled with excruciating emotional stress.

The second week in the hospital, I developed a ferocious sore throat, runny nose, and bad cough. Her counts were on the way down, and they ordered me out of the hospital until I was well. It was agony.

• • • • •

That first week, every time my son threw up, so did I. I also had almost uncontrollable diarrhea. Every new stressful event in the hospital just dissolved my gut; I could feel it happening. Thankfully this faded away after a few weeks.

To help prevent illness, try to eat nutritious meals, get a break from your child's bedside to take a walk outdoors, and find time to sleep. Care needs to be taken not to overuse alcohol or drugs of any kind (prescription, over-the-counter, or illicit) to control anxiety or cope with grief. Although physical illnesses usually end or improve after a period of adjustment, emotional stress continues throughout treatment.

Emotional Responses

The shock of diagnosis results in an overwhelming number of intense emotions. Cultural background, individual coping styles, basic temperament, and family dynamics all affect a parent's emotional response to stress. There are no stages of response, and parents frequently find themselves swinging from one emotional extreme to another. Many of these emotions reappear at different times during treatment. All of the emotions described below are normal responses when your child is diagnosed. The emotional responses of children and teens are discussed in Chapter 19, *Communication and Behavior.*

> *For weeks after diagnosis, I had trouble sleeping. When I did sleep, I'd wake up abruptly thinking "Lauren might die." Then my next thought was that it was a bad dream. But, it wasn't. It took weeks for that first waking thought to disappear.*

Confusion and numbness

In their anguish, most parents remember only bits and pieces of the doctor's early explanations of their child's disease. This dreamlike state is an almost universal response to shock. The brain provides protective layers of numbness and confusion to prevent emotional overload. Pediatric oncologists understand this phenomenon and are usually quite willing to repeat information as often as necessary. Children's hospitals have nurse practitioners, physician assistants, nurses, and child life specialists who translate medical information into understandable language and answer questions from parents and children.

Don't be embarrassed to say you do not understand or that you forgot something you were told. It happens to all parents of kids with cancer. It is sometimes helpful to write down instructions and explanations, record them on a small audio recorder or smartphone, or ask a friend or family member to help keep track of all the new and complex information. These notes can be transcribed and kept with the written materials you receive from the medical providers so you can refer to them later.

> *The doctor ordered a CBC from the lab. All the while I'm still convinced my son's bleeding gums were caused by his 6-year molars. The rest happened so fast it's hard to recount. We ended up at the hospital getting a bone marrow test. My husband and I tried to tell the doctor that we would go home and let Stephen rest and that when we came back in the morning they could do another CBC. We were positive that his cell counts would go up in the morning. He said that we didn't have until morning. He said Stephen was very, very sick. After the bone marrow test, the doctor called us in a room and said that Stephen had leukemia. After that word I couldn't hear a thing. My ears were ringing, and my body was numb. There were tears in my eyes. It was actually a physical reaction. I asked him to stop explaining because I couldn't hear him. I went back to the hospital room to cry.*
>
> • • • • •
>
> *For the longest time (in fact still, three years later) I can hear the doctor's voice on the phone telling me that Brent had leukemia. I remember every tiny detail of that whole day, until we got to the hospital, and then the days blur.*

· · · · ·

I felt like I was standing on a rug that was suddenly yanked out from under me. I found myself sitting there on the floor, and I just didn't know how to get up.

Denial

Denial is when parents simply cannot believe their child has a life-threatening illness. Denial helps parents survive the first few days after diagnosis, but gradual acceptance must occur so the family can make the necessary adjustments to accommodate cancer treatment. Life has dramatically changed. When parents accept what has happened, understand their fears, and begin to hope, they are better able to advocate for their child and their family. This process takes time.

> *After our daughter's diagnosis, we had to drive two hours to the hospital. My husband and I talked about leukemia the entire trip and, I felt, started to come to grips with the illness. However, after the IV, the x-rays, and the blood transfusions, he became extremely upset that they were going to admit her. He thought that we could just go home and it would be finished. I had to say, "This will be our life for years."*

· · · · ·

> *My husband and I sat and waited in silence until the doctor came back with the test results. The next thing I knew we were in his office with a primary nurse, a social worker, and a resident listening to the sickening news that our son had leukemia. I couldn't stop crying, and just wanted to grab my 2-year-old son and run far, far away.*

Guilt

Guilt is a common and normal reaction to a diagnosis of childhood leukemia. Parents sometimes feel that they have failed to protect their child, and they may blame themselves. It is especially difficult because the cause of their child's cancer cannot be explained. There are questions: How could we have prevented this? What did we do wrong? How did we miss the signs? Why didn't we bring her to the doctor sooner? Why didn't we insist that the doctor do blood work? Why didn't we live in a safer place? Why? Why? Why? Nancy Roach describes some of these feelings in her booklet *The Last Day of April:*

> *Almost as soon as Erin's illness was diagnosed, our self-recrimination began. What had we done to cause this illness? Was I careful enough during pregnancy? We knew radiation was a possible contributor; where had we taken Erin that she might have been exposed? I wondered about the toxic glue used in my advertising work or the silk screen ink used in my artwork. Bob questioned the fumes from some wood preservatives used in a project. We analyzed everything—food, fumes, and TV.*

Fortunately, most of the guilt feelings were relieved by knowledge and by meeting other parents whose leukemic children had been exposed to an entirely different environment.

It may be difficult to accept, but parents need to understand that they did nothing to cause their child's illness. Years of research have revealed little about what causes childhood leukemia or how to prevent it.

Fear and helplessness

Fear and helplessness are two faces of the same coin. Nearly everything about this new situation is unknown, and the only thing parents really do know—that their child has a life-threatening illness—is too terrifying to contemplate. Each new revelation about the situation raises new questions and fears: Can I really flush a catheter or administer all these drugs? What if I mess something up? Will I be fired if I miss too much work? Who will take care of my other children? How do I tell my child not to be afraid when he can see I am scared to death? How will we pay for this? The demands on parents' time, talents, energy, courage, and strength are daunting.

Sometimes I would feel incredible waves of absolute terror wash over me. The kind of fear that causes your breathing to become difficult and your heart to beat faster. While I would be consciously aware of what was happening, there was nothing I could do to stop it. It's happened sometimes very late at night, when I'm lying in bed, staring off into the darkness. It's so intense that for a brief moment, I try to comfort myself by thinking that it can't be real, because it's just too horrible. During those moments, these thoughts only offer a second or two of comfort. Then I become aware of just how wide my eyes are opened in the darkness.

A child's diagnosis strips parents of control over many aspects of their lives and can change their entire world view. All the predictable and comforting routines are gone, and the family is thrust into a new world that is populated by an ever-changing cast of characters (interns, residents, fellows, pediatric oncologists, surgeons, nurses, social workers, and technicians); a new language (medical terminology); and seemingly endless hospitalizations, procedures, and drugs. This transition can be hard on all parents, particularly those who are intimidated by doctors and medical environments, and those who are used to a measure of power and authority in their home or workplace.

My husband had a difficult time after our son was diagnosed. We have a traditional marriage, and he was used to his role as provider and protector for the family. It was hard for him to deal with the fact that he couldn't fix everything.

Parents often feel utterly helpless. For example, physicians they have never met are presenting treatment options for their child. Parents are also faced with the fact that they cannot do anything that will take away their child's illness or make everything better, and parents' inability to relieve their child's suffering can lead to feelings of great helplessness. Even if parents are comfortable in a hospital environment, they may feel helpless because there is simply not enough time in the day to care for a very sick child, deal with their own changing emotions, educate themselves about the disease, notify friends and family, make job decisions, and restructure the family schedule to deal with the crisis.

> It's hard to explain how tired and terrified and empty you feel in the weeks after diagnosis. My husband and I went to Target to get our daughter some favorite foods because she had stopped eating. I needed some reading glasses and saw a display. The sign said to put your toes on the line while trying on the glasses. I was such a mess I thought it said to bend over and touch your toes. I couldn't figure out why I needed to touch my toes. Of course, I had already bent down and touched my toes. Then, we read the instructions again and burst out laughing and couldn't stop. We were laughing like hyenas! It was the first time we'd laughed since diagnosis.

Many parents explain that helplessness begins to disappear when a sense of reality returns. They begin to learn about the disease, study their options, make decisions, meet other parents of children with cancer, and grow comfortable with the hospital and staff. As their knowledge grows, so does their ability to participate constructively as members of the treatment team (for more information, see Chapter 10, *Forming a Partnership with the Medical Team*). However, don't be surprised if feelings of fear, panic, and anxiety erupt unexpectedly throughout your child's treatment.

Anger

Anger is a common response to the diagnosis of a life-threatening illness. It is nobody's fault that children are stricken with cancer. Because parents cannot direct their anger at the cancer, they may target doctors, nurses, spouses, siblings, or even their ill child. Anger directed at other people can be very destructive, so it is necessary to devise ways to express and manage the anger.

> We were sent to the emergency room after my son's diagnosis with leukemia. After the inevitable delays, an IV was started and chest x-rays taken. I struggled to remain calm to help my son, but inside I was screaming NO NO NO. A resident patted me on the shoulder and said, "We'll check him out to make sure that everything is okay." I started to sob. She looked surprised and asked what was the matter. I yelled, "He's not okay, and he won't be okay for a long time. He has cancer." I realized later that she was trying to comfort me, but I was both angry and terrified. Surprisingly, by the end of my son's hospitalization, we trusted and felt very close to that resident.

Expressing anger is normal and can be cathartic. Trying to suppress this powerful emotion is usually not helpful. Here are some suggestions from parents for managing anger.

Anger at healthcare team:

- Discuss your feelings with one of the nurses or nurse practitioners
- Share your feelings with the social worker, chaplain, or psychologist
- Talk with parents of other ill children, either locally or by joining an online support group

Anger at family:

- Exercise a little every day
- Do yoga or relaxation exercises
- Keep a journal or make an audio recording of your feelings
- Cry in the shower or pound a pillow
- Listen to music
- Talk with friends
- Join or start a support group
- Try individual or family counseling
- Live one moment at a time

Anger at God:

- Share your feelings with your spouse, partner, or close friends
- Discuss your feelings with clergy or members of your church, synagogue, or mosque
- Pray or meditate
- Give yourself time to heal

It is important to remember that angry feelings are normal and expected. Discovering healthy ways to cope with anger is vital for all parents.

> *My husband went to the gym and lifted weights during and after treatment to get his anger and worry out. I saw a therapist for a period of time, and I got on medications. I didn't want to go on meds, I didn't want to need that, but it leveled me out.*

· · · · ·

> *Here's a bit of advice: The best place to cry is in a hot shower. I would go in and cry, cry, cry, cry then come out all refreshed, clean, and warm. That really helped me.*

Sadness and grief

No one is prepared to cope with the news that their child has cancer. Intense feelings of sorrow, loss, and grief are common, even when the prognosis is good. Parents often describe feeling engulfed by sadness. They fear that they may not be able to deal with the enormity of the problems facing their family. Parents grieve the loss of normalcy and realize life will never be the same. They grieve the loss of their dreams and aspirations for their child. They may feel sorry for themselves and may feel ashamed and embarrassed by these feelings.

> *Even though my daughter's prognosis was good, I would find myself daydreaming about her funeral. Certain songs especially triggered this feeling. I invariably burst into tears because I was ashamed to be thinking/planning a funeral when I just could not imagine my life without her. When these feelings washed over me, I could actually feel a physical sensation of my heart ripping.*

> • • • • •

> *I have an overwhelming sadness and, unfortunately for me, that means feelings of helplessness. I wish I could muster up a fighting spirit, but I just can't right now.*

Parents travel a tumultuous emotional path where overwhelming emotions subside, only to resurface later. All of these are normal, common responses to a catastrophic event. For many parents, these strong emotions begin to become more manageable as hope grows.

Hope

After being overwhelmed by illness, fear, sadness, grief, guilt, and anger, most parents welcome the growth of hope. Hope is the belief in a better tomorrow. Hope sustains the will to live and gives one the strength to endure difficult times. Hope is not a way around; it is a way through. Most children survive childhood leukemia and live long and happy lives. There is reason for hope.

Many families discover a renewed sense of both the fragility and beauty of life after the diagnosis. Outpourings of love and support from family and friends provide comfort and sustenance. Many parents speak of a renewed appreciation for life and consider each day with their child as a precious gift.

> *Some people don't get it when I say that there were many good things about our journey through leukemia. I wouldn't wish it on anyone, but my daughter and I both learned that we have strengths we did not suspect; we found love and support and compassion in places we never expected it; we were honored to know people who dedicate their lives to helping children survive this disease; I found joy in the tiniest of pleasures; and I discovered that the world is unbelievably beautiful when we look at it through grateful eyes.*

A Japanese proverb says: "Daylight will peep through a very small hole."

The Immediate Future

You are not alone. The rest of this book contains stories from parents of children with cancer, as well as practical information about leukemia and its treatment. You'll learn about the choices other parents made and how they adjusted, learned, and became active participants in their child's treatment. Many have traveled this path before you, and reading about their experiences may help your family develop its own unique strategy for coping with the challenges that lie ahead.

A Mother's View

Memory is a funny thing. I'd be hard pressed to remember what I had for dinner last night, but like many people, the day of the Challenger explosion and, even further back, the day of John Kennedy's death, are etched in my mind to the smallest detail.

And like a smaller group of people, the day of my child's cancer diagnosis is a strong and vivid memory, even 7 years later. Most of the time, I don't dwell on that series of images. It was, after all, a chapter in our lives, and one that is now blessedly behind us. But early each autumn, when I get a whiff of the crisp smell of leaves in the air, it brings back that dark day when our lives changed forever.

Many of the memories are painful and, like my daughter's scars, they fade a little more each year but will never completely disappear. While dealing with the medical and physical aspects of the disease, my husband and I also made many emotional discoveries. We sometimes encountered ignorance and narrow-mindedness, which made me more sad than angry. Mistakes were made, tempers were short, and family relations were strained. But we saw the other side, too. Somehow, our sense of humor held on throughout the ordeal, and when that kicked in, we had some of the best laughs of our lives. There was compassion and understanding when we needed it most. And people were there for us like never before.

I remember two young fathers on our street, torn by the news, who wanted to help but felt helpless. My husband came home from the hospital late one night to find that our lawn had been mowed and our leaves had been raked by them. They had found a way to make a small difference that day. Another time, a neighbor came to our house bearing a bakery box full of pastries and the message that his family was praying for our daughter nightly around their supper table. The image of this man, his wife, and his eight children joining in prayer for us will never leave me. A close friend entered the hospital during that first terrible week we were there to give birth to her son. I held her baby, she held me, and we laughed and cried together.

Sometimes, when I look back at that time, I feel as though everything that is wrong with the world and everything that is right is somehow distilled in one small child's battle to live. We learned so very much about people and about life.

Surely people who haven't experienced a crisis of this magnitude would believe that we would want to put that time behind us and forget as much of it as possible. But the fact is, we grew a little through our pain, like it or not. We see through new eyes. Not all of it is good or happy, but it is profound.

I treasure good friends like never before. I view life as much more fragile and precious than I used to. I think of myself as a tougher person than I was, but I cry more easily now. And sure, I still yell at my kids and eagerly await each September when they will be out of my hair for a few hours each day. But I hold them with more tenderness when they hop off the school bus into my arms. And I like to think that some of the people around us, who saw how suddenly and drastically a family's life can change, hold their children a little dearer as well.

Do I want to forget those terrible days and nights 7 years ago? Not on your life. And I hope the smell of autumn leaves will still bring the memories back when I'm a grandmother, even if I can't remember what I had for dinner last night.

— Kathy Tucker
CURE Childhood Cancer Newsletter
Rochester, NY

Chapter 2

Overview of Childhood Leukemia

"You're braver than you believe, stronger than you seem,
and smarter than you think."

— A. A. Milne

THE WORD LEUKEMIA literally means *white blood.* Leukemia is the term used to describe cancer of the blood-forming tissues known as bone marrow. This spongy material fills the bones in the body and produces healthy blood cells. The bone marrow of children with cancer creates millions of cancerous white cells, which have lost the ability to stop multiplying. As the bone marrow becomes packed with these malignant cells, they crowd out all the healthy cells the blood needs to do its work and symptoms of leukemia begin to develop.

This chapter provides an overview of childhood leukemia. Because leukemia is a disease of the blood cells, it first looks at the function and composition of blood. It briefly describes the four types of childhood leukemia and how many children and teens are diagnosed with these diseases. It then explains the genetics of leukemia, because the results of genetic tests help determine diagnosis, treatment, and likely response to treatment. Chapter 3, *Acute Lymphoblastic Leukemia;* Chapter 4, *Acute Myeloid Leukemia;* Chapter 5, *Juvenile Myelomonocytic Leukemia;* and Chapter 6, *Chronic Myelogenous Leukemia* describe each type of leukemia in detail and the current treatments used.

Leukemia Is a Blood Disease

Blood is a vital liquid that carries oxygen, nutrients, hormones, and other necessary chemicals to the body's cells. It also removes toxins and other waste products from the cells. Blood cells carry oxygen, fight infections, and help repair injuries by slowing or stopping bleeding.

Whole blood is made up of plasma—a clear fluid—and many other components, each with a specific task. Blood contains three types of blood cells—red blood cells, white blood cells, and platelets. Red blood cells (also called erythrocytes or RBCs) contain hemoglobin, a protein that carries oxygen from the lungs to other cells in the body. RBCs carrying oxygen give blood its red color. When leukemia cells in the bone marrow interfere with production of RBCs, anemia develops. Anemia can cause tiredness, weakness, irritability, pale skin, and headaches—all due to not enough oxygen being carried to the body tissues.

Healthy white blood cells (also called leukocytes or WBCs) destroy foreign substances in the body, such as viruses, bacteria, and fungi. WBCs are produced and stored in the bone marrow and lymph nodes. They are released when needed by the body. If an infection is present, the body produces extra WBCs. There are two main types of WBCs:

- **Lymphocytes:** The three types of lymphocytes are T cells, B cells, and natural killer cells.
- **Granulocytes:** The four types of granulocytes are neutrophils, monocytes, eosinophils, and basophils.

Platelets are tiny, disc-shaped cells that help form clots to stop bleeding. Leukemia interferes with production of platelets, causing a dramatic drop in platelets in children with the disease, which can lead to excessive bleeding from the nose and gums or from cuts. Children with leukemia can develop large bruises or small red dots (petechiae) on their skin or in the mouth and throat.

> *Our daughter Emi, who has Down syndrome, was diagnosed with pneumonia at 14 months. Her blood counts showed a very low platelet count and a low white blood cell count. She was treated for the pneumonia, and when we went back for more blood work a few weeks later, her counts were even lower and the doctors thought they saw some blasts [immature white blood cells]. They sent the results to a hem-onc doctor who scheduled a bone marrow aspiration a few days later. They said they saw leukemia cells in the bone marrow, and called the next day to say it was AML. We went straight to the children's hospital and spent most of the next six months there.*

Normally, the bone marrow makes blood stem cells (immature cells) that become mature blood cells over time. A blood stem cell develops into either a myeloid stem cell or a lymphoid stem cell (see Figure 2-1). A myeloid stem cell becomes a WBC, a RBC, or a platelet. A lymphoid stem cell becomes a WBC.

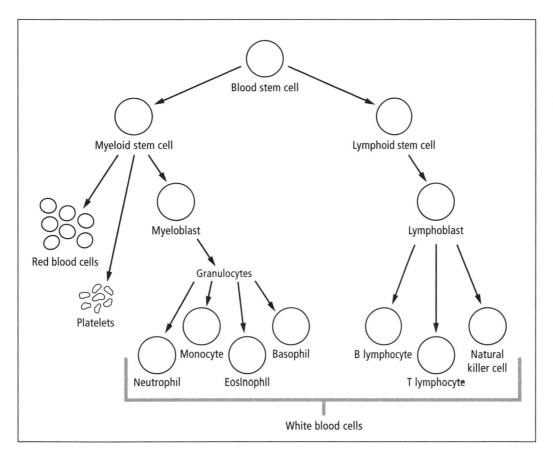

Figure 2-1: Development of mature blood cells from stem cells

The different types of leukemia are cancers of a specific WBC type. For instance, acute lymphoblastic leukemia is a cancer of the lymphocytes, and acute myeloid leukemia is cancer of the granulocytes.

Definition of a Blast

Blast is a short name for an immature WBC, such as a lymphoblast or myeloblast. Normally, less than 5% of the cells in healthy bone marrow at any one time are blasts. While in the bone marrow, normal blasts develop into mature, functioning blood cells and are then released into the bloodstream. Therefore, in healthy people, blasts are not usually found in the bloodstream. Leukemic blasts remain immature, multiply continuously, provide no defense against infection, and may be present in large numbers in the blood and bone marrow.

When Leukemia Begins

When leukemic blasts appear in the bone marrow, they multiply rapidly and do not develop into normal WBCs. They begin to crowd out the normal cells that grow from healthy blasts into mature WBCs. After accumulating in the bone marrow and lymph nodes, leukemic blasts spill over into the blood and, if left unchecked, may invade the central nervous system (CNS)—which includes the brain and spinal cord—and other organs, such as the liver and spleen.

When leukemic blasts begin to fill the bone marrow, production of healthy RBCs, platelets, and WBCs cannot be maintained. As the number of normal blood cells decreases, symptoms appear. Low RBC counts cause fatigue and pale skin. Low platelet counts may result in bruising and bleeding problems. And if mature WBCs are crowded out by blasts, the child will have little or no defense against infections.

> *Our 3-year-old daughter, Charlotte, changed from a quiet but friendly preschooler to a fearful, withdrawn one in just a few months. She didn't want to go to preschool, see her friends, or play outside. She would lie on the couch a lot. She had bruises, and we didn't know why because she hadn't been playing. She didn't look well, but the doctor couldn't find anything wrong. She became pale and didn't sleep well. Finally, the doctor took a blood sample, and when he called me on the phone to tell me she had leukemia, I dropped to my knees and couldn't get up.*

Types of Leukemia

The two broad classifications of leukemia are acute (rapid progression) and chronic (slow progression). The two forms of acute leukemia are acute lymphoblastic leukemia (ALL) and acute myeloid leukemia (AML). More than 95% of all childhood cancers are acute, with the majority being ALL.

The two types of chronic leukemia in children are chronic myelogenous leukemia (CML) and juvenile myelomonocytic leukemia (JMML), and they account for less than 5% of all children diagnosed with leukemia. The following table shows the types of childhood leukemia and the percentages of each type.

Acute		Chronic	
ALL (75%)	AML (20%)	CML (3.5%)	JMML (1.5%)

The types of childhood leukemia are explained in detail in Chapter 3, *Acute Lymphoblastic Leukemia;* Chapter 4, *Acute Myeloid Leukemia;* Chapter 5, *Juvenile Myelomonocytic Leukemia;* and Chapter 6, *Chronic Myelogenous Leukemia.*

Who Gets Leukemia?

Leukemia is the most common childhood cancer. Each year in the United States, approximately 4,100 children and teens are diagnosed with leukemia. Childhood leukemia is most commonly diagnosed in children ages 2 to 5. In the United States, leukemia is more common in white children than black children, but the incidence is highest in Hispanic children. Boys develop leukemia more often than girls. Children with certain genetic syndromes also have a higher risk of developing some types of leukemia than children who do not have these genetic syndromes.

Leukemia is not contagious; it cannot be passed from one person to another. Although the exact cause of childhood leukemia is a mystery, certain environmental or genetic factors may increase a child's risk of developing the disease. These factors are discussed in the next four chapters.

Basic Genetics

Treatment for childhood leukemia is increasingly based on genetic changes that are found in cancer cells. Therefore, having a basic knowledge of genetics will help you understand some of the terms healthcare providers may use when discussing your child's type of leukemia and proposed treatment.

Our bodies are made of cells, trillions of them. Each of these cells carries all the information the cells need to reproduce and keep our bodies functioning. Inside the nucleus of every cell are chromosomes, which contain genes that provide the instructions the body needs to live and to pass certain traits from a parent to a child. Genes are composed of DNA (deoxyribonucleic acid), which comes in strands that resemble a twisted ladder (see Figure 2-2).

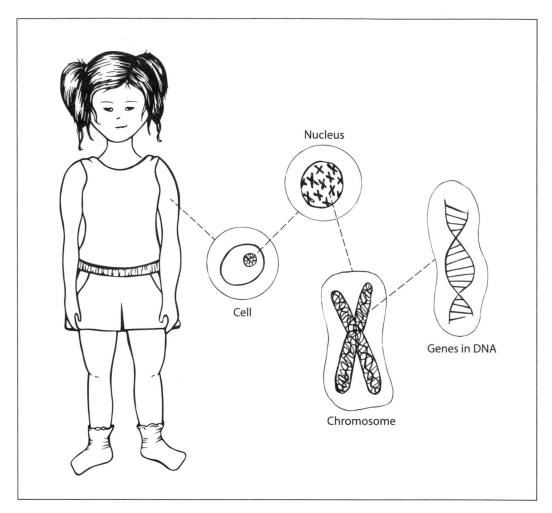

Figure 2-2: Cells, chromosomes, and DNA

Chromosomes come in pairs, and a normal human cell contains 46 chromosomes (see Figure 2-3). Of these, 44 are the same in males and females, but one pair (called sex chromosomes) is different. Females have two X chromosomes in that pair, and males have one X and one Y chromosome. In some types of childhood leukemia, the cancer cells contain too many or too few chromosomes.

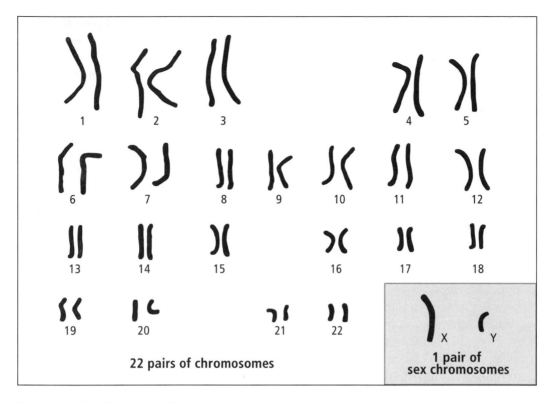

Figure 2-3: The 23 pairs of chromosomes

The cancer cells in children with leukemia often contain mutations, which are permanent changes in a gene's DNA. Genetic changes happen all the time in our cells, but the body possesses sophisticated tools for detecting and repairing the changes. A change only becomes a mutation when a repair cannot be made or is made incorrectly. These mutations come in four main varieties:

- **Duplications:** When some genes are repeated on the chromosome
- **Deletions:** When part of a chromosome is lost
- **Translocations:** When there is a break in the DNA and some genes from one chromosome attach to a different chromosome
- **Inversions:** When two breaks occur and a segment reattaches backwards, which reverses the sequence of genes

Scientists have identified many mutations in leukemia cells. Some of these mutations are associated with development of the disease. Others predict which therapies will be most effective for a particular child or how the child will react to certain drugs. For these reasons, when a child is diagnosed with leukemia, doctors immediately order numerous genetic tests on the cancer cells to gather all information possible about how the child should be treated and how she is likely to respond to treatment. This genetic knowledge has greatly improved doctors' ability to identify the best treatment for each child diagnosed with leukemia. Researchers continue to look for new genetic mutations, so you may be asked to allow an extra portion of the diagnostic marrow to be saved for research.

Best Treatments for Childhood Leukemia

At diagnosis, most parents don't know how to find the best doctors and treatments for their child. Guidelines from the American Academy of Pediatrics (AAP) describe essential services needed to treat children with cancer. The AAP says that children and teens with cancer should be treated at major children's hospitals that can deliver an accurate diagnosis and prognosis, as well as intensive medical and psychological supportive care. This includes top-notch emergency departments, pediatric intensive care units, and surgical facilities. These services are provided by multidisciplinary, family-centered teams that include:

- Pediatric oncologists
- Pediatric nurse practitioners and physician assistants
- Pediatric nurses
- Pediatric radiation oncologists
- Pediatric surgeons
- Pediatric pharmacists
- Pediatric psychologists
- Social workers
- Child life specialists
- Rehabilitation specialists
- School specialists

This type of care is available at large regional children's hospitals and from children's hospitals that are members of the Children's Oncology Group (COG). This group is made up of experts from approximately 230 hospitals that treat children with cancer. COG-affiliated children's hospitals provide state-of-the-art treatments for childhood leukemia and conduct studies to discover better therapies and supportive care for children with all types of cancer. Through this cooperative group network sponsored by the National Cancer Institute, outcomes have improved tremendously. In addition, several individual centers sometimes design their own clinical trials.

Research has shown that teenagers and young adults have better outcomes when treated on pediatric protocols at children's hospitals, rather than on adult protocols. Many children's hospitals have developed programs specifically designed to meet the medical and psychological needs of teens.

The next four chapters describe the current treatments for each type of childhood leukemia, and Chapter 8, *Choosing a Treatment*, discusses how parents make choices if more than one treatment option is available for their child.

I am at work, an ordinary day. The phone rings, "Hello?" "Can I speak to Patty?" "Speaking." "This is Anne at the University Medical Group Practice. I hate to tell you over the phone, but we think your son has leukemia."

I need to back up just a bit, to the day before. I had taken my 17-year-old son, James, to a nurse practitioner, Anne. James had been a little tired for several weeks, and he also spoke of muscle pains in varying places, such as his shoulders, back, and legs. This in itself was not unusual for him because he was in weight training. But he just didn't have his usual energy: he could not do a 25-mile bike ride anymore without getting tired. It bothered us; he was kind of acting like an old man, too tired to run up the stairs two at a time.

Anne checked him and said he looked just fine; his oxygen levels were great and his lung capacity was great. But she drew some blood for analysis—just in case—thinking mono. Thank you, Anne!

James was a junior in high school and we were turning our thoughts to colleges and dealing with him leaving home to go to college. I only took him to see Anne to set my mind at ease. After we left, I completely forgot about the visit.

The blood samples were sent off to the University Health Sciences Center and the diagnosis came back: leukemia. As Anne told me over the phone, she was in tears herself, apologizing for not telling me in person. She wanted James at the hospital ASAP. She had already booked a room for him.

Shock set in and survival instincts took over. I knew I couldn't drive safely, so a wonderful friend at work drove me the 23 miles home. There, luckily, were my son and husband, by chance home from school and work early. Back into the car for the 55-mile drive to Children's Hospital, not knowing even exactly where it was.

We were checked into Children's Hospital in Denver within 27 hours of visiting the nurse practitioner. I had an awful time opening the door that said "Oncology" and escorting my son through it. The oncology docs re-ran the tests, and two hours later, we know, yes, it is leukemia. Shock. What can you do? You deal with it, somehow. You grieve. You find out what you have to know and have to do to help him. Your life stops and starts again.

Chapter 3

Acute Lymphoblastic Leukemia

"Out of difficulties grow miracles."
— Jean de la Bruyere

TREATMENT OF CHILDHOOD ACUTE LYMPHOBLASTIC LEUKEMIA (ALL) is one of the major success stories of modern medicine. As recently as the 1960s, children with ALL usually lived only for a few months. Currently, 95% of children receiving optimal treatment attain remission, and the majority of those children are cured (defined as remaining in remission for at least five years after diagnosis).

This chapter covers risk factors for developing ALL, signs and symptoms, diagnosis, prognosis, and treatment. The treatment section is divided into five parts:

- B-cell ALL
- T-cell ALL
- Philadelphia chromosome (Ph+) ALL
- Infant ALL
- Down syndrome and ALL

The chapter ends with ways to learn about the newest treatments available for childhood ALL.

ALL Is a Blood Disease

ALL is cancer of the lymphocytes (see Figure 3-1). A normal lymphoid stem cell matures into one of three types of white blood cells (WBCs):

- B lymphocytes that make antibodies to fight infection
- T lymphocytes that help the body fight infection and disease
- Natural killer cells that kill cancer cells or viruses

In 85% of children with ALL, B lymphocytes become cancerous. In the other 15% of children with ALL, T lymphocytes become cancerous. The cancer cells multiply rapidly and have no ability to develop into mature WBCs. After accumulating in the bone marrow, cancerous lymphocytes (called leukemic blasts) spill over into the blood and enlarge the liver, spleen, and lymph nodes. If left unchecked, the cancerous cells can invade the central nervous system (CNS)—which includes the brain and spinal cord—and other organs, such as testes in boys.

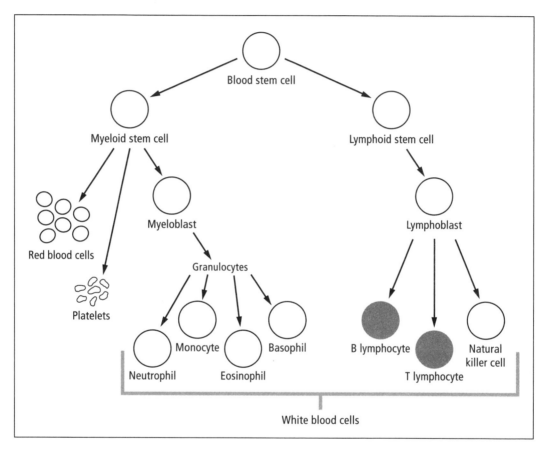

Figure 3-1: ALL is a disease of B or T lymphocytes

When leukemic blasts begin to multiply and pack the bone marrow, fewer normal red blood cells (RBCs), platelets, and WBCs are produced. As the number of normal blood cells decreases, symptoms appear. Low RBC counts cause fatigue and pale skin. Low platelet counts may result in bruising and bleeding problems. If healthy WBCs are crowded out by blasts, the child will have little or no defense against infections. To read more about blasts, blood, and genetics, see Chapter 2, *Overview of Childhood Leukemia*.

Who Gets ALL?

Approximately 3,100 children and teens are diagnosed with ALL in the United States each year. It is most commonly diagnosed in children ages 2 to 5. Hispanic children have the greatest risk of developing ALL, followed by white children, then black children. More boys than girls are diagnosed with ALL. Known risk factors include:

- Being exposed to x-rays before birth.

- Prior treatment with radiation (e.g., for an enlarged thymus).

- Being exposed to industrial chemicals such as arsenic or benzene (although few children who develop ALL were exposed to these types of chemicals).

- Having an identical twin with ALL. If one identical twin develops ALL, the risk of the other twin also developing ALL is around 25%. This is because leukemia cells are shared during fetal development (when identical twins are still inside the mother's womb). The likelihood that both identical twins develop leukemia is highest in infants. After age 7, there is no increased risk of the second twin developing the disease.

- Having a genetic condition such as Down syndrome, neurofibromatosis 1, Bloom syndrome, Fanconi anemia, ataxia-telangiectasia, Li-Fraumeni syndrome, or mutations in genes that keep DNA from repairing itself, which can cause cancers at an early age.

> *Two-year-old Levi has Down syndrome. He started being a little fussy and wasn't sleeping well. We thought that maybe he was getting an ear infection. But within a few days, his eye was swollen; he looked like "Rocky." Thankfully, Levi has the best pediatrician ever! He could not really figure out why Levi's eye would be swollen but since Levi has Down syndrome, he wanted to do a blood test just to see if everything looked okay. Levi's counts were low so they re-checked in less than a week. When those counts were still low, his pediatrician sent us to the hematology clinic at our local children's hospital where they did a bone marrow test. When his ALL was confirmed, they immediately admitted Levi to the pediatric cancer floor to begin treatment.*

Parents often search for reasons, and blame themselves, for their child's ALL. It is important to know that you did not cause and could not have prevented your child's illness.

> *My 17-year-old son and I were discussing what might have caused his ALL. I said that I had come to this conclusion: I don't have the time or mental energy to dwell on the causes. They are not important. They drain my energy and are irrelevant. Sam stated, "Right, it's kind of like a computer." I replied, "Huh?" He said, "Sometimes you know that something you do will crash the computer. But sometimes, it's something that you just can't predict, there are many factors involved and they come together to cause a crash. Sometimes you are doing the same things at another time and the computer doesn't crash. You don't try to figure out what you have done wrong. You just re-boot the computer." So I say, "Yeah, that's what we are doing:*

re-booting you." And he agrees, chuckling, "But it takes a bit longer to re-boot a person!"

Signs and Symptoms

Signs are observed by parents or doctors (e.g., pale skin), but symptoms are experienced by patients (e.g., bone pain). The most common signs and symptoms of childhood ALL are:

- Fever
- Infection
- Night sweats
- Paleness
- Weakness or feeling tired
- Easy bruising or bleeding
- Small red spots on the skin (called petechiae) caused by bleeding
- Pain in the bones (children may limp or be unable to walk)
- Pain or feeling of fullness below the ribs from an enlarged spleen and/or liver
- Swollen lymph nodes in the neck, underarm, stomach, or groin

Some children with ALL have the disease in their CNS at diagnosis. These include:

- 10 to 15% of children with T-cell ALL
- 5% of children with B-cell ALL

Few of these children have signs or symptoms of CNS disease at diagnosis. However, if they do, the most common are headaches, nausea, vomiting, and abnormal response of the pupil in the eye to light.

> *Two-year-old Austin showed no typical signs and symptoms of childhood leukemia, so it was a unique and difficult situation. Two months before he was diagnosed with ALL, he developed a lump on the top of his head that was about the size of a quarter. We had two primary care doctors look at it and we were told to just keep an eye on it. Then my father-in-law noticed that Austin had large lymph nodes on one side of his neck. They hadn't been there the day before, and so my stomach just flipped. Austin was still active, eating well, sleeping well, and no fevers. He just didn't look sick. Our pediatrician diagnosed a possible ear infection and prescribed antibiotics. Three days later, the lump on his head was red and inflamed, and the hair had dropped out of the skin over the lump. We went back to the pediatrician, and even though Austin still didn't look sick, she sent us to the emergency room. All of his initial blood results were normal and they were talking about surgically removing the*

lymph nodes. But, the WBC differential came back showing 7% blasts, so we were sent in an ambulance to the children's hospital. After they did a bone marrow biopsy and spinal tap, they told us he had ALL with CNS disease. A week after chemo started, the lump was gone.

Diagnosis

A tentative diagnosis of leukemia is made after a physical examination of the child and microscopic analysis of a blood sample. Blood tests may show too few RBCs, too few platelets, and either abnormally low or high WBC counts. Because childhood leukemia is uncommon and the signs and symptoms mimic other illnesses, diagnosis can be swift or very slow.

> *I took my 2-year old son Nico to the pediatrician because I thought he might have an ear infection. We were leaving with prescriptions for antibiotics, ear numbing drops, and a referral for an ENT when the pediatrician asked if Nico was always so pale. At that moment, I just knew. The doctor suggested that we check his hemoglobin via a finger stick, and it came back at 5.5. She assured me that the results of the finger stick were probably inaccurate, or that Nico might just be anemic from a recent virus. But to be safe she wanted to send us to the children's hospital to double-check his blood via a lab draw. As I was leaving the pediatrician's office, I asked her if the labs she had ordered would indicate if Nico had leukemia. She wanted to know how I knew. At the time I did not know how I knew, but I just knew. I cried the entire way to the hospital where Nico was diagnosed later that day.*

To confirm a diagnosis of ALL, bone marrow is sampled and tested (see Chapter 9, *Coping with Procedures*). The bone marrow is examined under a microscope by a pathologist (a physician who specializes in body tissue analysis). A leukemia diagnosis is confirmed if more than 25% of the WBCs in the marrow are cancerous blasts. A portion of the bone marrow is then sent to a specialized laboratory that analyzes many other features of the cancer cells.

> *My 2½ year old daughter Abby was diagnosed with B-cell average risk ALL in 2007. It was mid-summer when I first had the inkling that something was wrong; she'd been struggling with sniffles and seemed clumsier, some light bruising appeared, and she was just more irritable. At first I thought that she was cranky from teething and weaning from breast milk, but by fall it was clear that Abby wasn't herself. I felt panicked; I marched her to the doctor and said, "Something is wrong with my daughter and you need to find it now!" It was just 24 hours later that we learned Abby had cancer—her red blood cell level was dangerously low and her white blood cell count was low as well (5,800 with 33% blasts). Good science and intuition saved her.*

Prognosis

Prognosis is an estimate of the chance for cure. It helps determine how aggressive the treatment needs to be to have the best chance for cure with the least chance of late effects. The appropriate treatment for each child with ALL is determined by analyzing several features related to the child and to the leukemia cells.

> *I don't think hearing prognosis numbers helps. I actually asked them not to tell me those numbers because I wanted to hope. I knew my child's type of ALL was rare and many children don't survive. They told me anyway, and I found those numbers to be a huge barrier I had to scale to find my hope again. We're all different—I know parents who want the prognosis numbers. But I didn't.*

Below are some of the factors doctors consider when determining prognosis. For more detailed information about prognostic factors, you can visit the National Cancer Institute (NCI) Physician Data Query website at *www.cancer.gov/types/leukemia/hp/ child-all-treatment-pdq#section/_22.*

- **WBC count at diagnosis:** The WBC count at diagnosis helps predict response to treatment. Children with a low WBC count (<50,000) usually have a more favorable prognosis, and therefore need less intensive therapy than children with higher WBC counts.

- **Age:** Children ages 1 to 9 typically do better than infants, older children, or teens. As a result, more aggressive treatments are usually needed for infants and children older than age 9.

- **Gender:** Overall, boys have a slightly worse prognosis than girls. Possible reasons are that more boys are diagnosed with T-cell ALL, only boys have testicular relapses, and fewer boys have extra chromosomes (called hyperdiploidy) in their cancer cells.

- **Response to treatment:** One factor in a child's prognosis is how quickly the leukemia cells disappear after starting treatment. Treatment is divided into phases, the first of which is called induction. At the end of the induction phase, bone marrow is sent to a specialized laboratory to see whether any blast cells are present. This measure of residual leukemia is called minimal residual disease (MRD). If there has been a rapid reduction of blasts in the marrow, the child may need less intensive treatment.

> *Nico's white blood cell (WBC) count at diagnosis was relatively low (15,200 μL), and his cytogenetics were favorable (trisomy 4, 10). The week of diagnosis, our oncologist only discussed the low- and standard-risk treatment courses with us. We were shocked when the combination of day-8 peripheral blood and day-29 bone marrow MRD bumped our son into the high-risk category. It was like getting the diagnosis all over again. I had deluded myself into thinking that the low and standard category provided some safety net, which was really never true. The fact is some children in the low- and standard-risk protocols run into problems, while some*

children in the high- and very high-risk protocols avoid complications. I will admit that I am still jealous when I look at the standard protocol. But as someone once counseled me, "Be grateful that your child's risk category was properly identified. This enables us to adjust his treatment to give him the best chance of success."

- **CNS status at diagnosis:** If ALL is suspected, a sample of the cerebrospinal fluid (CSF) is obtained during a lumbar puncture (also called spinal tap). Children without leukemia blasts in the CSF at diagnosis have a better prognosis than those who do. The results of the first lumbar puncture at diagnosis will be described as:
  - **CNS1:** No leukemia blasts found in CSF (76% of children)
  - **CNS2:** Fewer than five leukemia blasts (per µL) found in CSF (19% of children)
  - **CNS3:** Five or more blasts (per µL) found in CSF (5% of children)
- **Number of chromosomes:** Normal cells contain 46 chromosomes (22 pairs and the sex chromosomes—XX for females or XY for males).
  - **Hyperdiploidy:** Some leukemia cells contain extra copies of entire chromosomes, giving them more than 46 (called hyperdiploidy). Approximately 20 to 25% of children with B-cell ALL have 51 to 65 chromosomes per cancer cell. Although the prognosis of children with hyperdiploidy is favorable, factors such as age, WBC count, and early response to treatment also affect prognosis. Hyperdiploidy is uncommon in children with T-cell ALL.
  - **Hypodipoidy:** Around 6% of children with B-cell ALL have fewer than 44 chromosomes in the leukemia cells. This condition is called hypodiploidy and carries a poor prognosis.
- **Extra copies of particular chromosomes:** Children with extra copies of chromosomes (e.g., chromosome 4 or 10) have an especially favorable prognosis. These extra chromosomes are called trisomies.

  When Liza was diagnosed, our oncologist told us that at the initial bone marrow aspiration he would be able to determine if she had leukemia or not, and then the other sample would go for cytogenetic testing. It took about 15 days to get the results back and Liza had hyperdiploidy, with triple trisomies 4, 10, 17.

- **Chromosome translocations (swaps between chromosomes) or rearrangements (genes swap places on the same chromosome):** Translocations and rearrangements are extremely common in B-cell ALL, and some of these are known to affect prognosis.
  - Children with the *ETV6-RUNX1* gene fusion (also known as *TEL/AML1*) need less intensive therapy unless MRD is positive at the end of induction.
  - The Philadelphia chromosome, called t(9;22) or Ph+, is found in approximately 3% of children and teens with B-cell ALL (see Figure 3-2). It is associated with a poor prognosis, especially in older children with high WBC counts who have a slow response to treatment. This translocation is found more often in teens and young

adults with ALL. Newer treatment protocols that include a tyrosine kinase inhibitor (TKI) such as imatinib have dramatically increased survival rates for children and teens with Ph+ ALL.

– Translocations and rearrangements involving the *MLL* gene are only found in 5% of children with ALL, but they are in up to 80% of infants with ALL. The most common *MLL* translocation is t(4;11). It occurs most often in infants with leukemia cells in the CNS and high WBC counts at diagnosis. It is associated with a poor outcome in infants but not in children with T-cell leukemia.

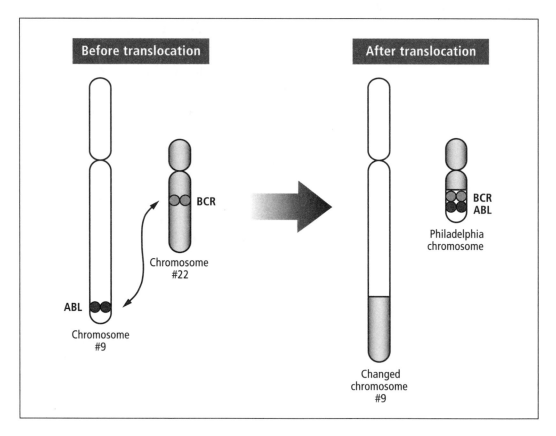

Figure 3-2: The Philadelphia chromosome

My 13-year-old son had been sick with ear and other infections for a few months. Then he started having pain in his legs and pelvis but we thought it was from growing, running track, and playing basketball. The pain got worse and he went to physical therapy for eight weeks. One night, it became unbearable and we went to the ER. When he took off his shirt, I saw that his back was covered by petechiae, which was new. They drew labs, took him off to x-ray, and the next thing I knew, a doctor and a chaplain came in and said his bone marrow was the cause of the pain and that we needed to go up to the pediatric oncology floor, where he was diagnosed with ALL. That was Tuesday. On Friday, we learned it was Ph+ ALL, which changed everything, including his chance for survival.

Different institutions and research groups use different criteria to determine prognosis and plan the best treatment. Most groups divide children with ALL into four categories—low risk, standard risk, high risk, and very high risk—based on some combination of the following:

- Age at diagnosis
- WBC count at diagnosis
- Whether the leukemia cells are B lymphocytes or T lymphocytes
- Presence of leukemia blasts in CNS at diagnosis
- Presence of leukemia blasts in the testes
- Certain changes in chromosomes or genes
- Number of chromosomes in leukemia blasts
- Response to treatment (number of leukemia blasts in the peripheral blood on day 8 and bone marrow MRD on day 29)

I focused on prognosis in an unhealthy way after my daughter was diagnosed. I kept asking the doctors why she was at a high risk for relapse. I sort of became consumed with hearing all of the prognostic percentages and where they came from. Our attending sat me down at one point and said that the prognosis was more for the doctors to determine the best treatment than it was anything to do with my individual child. When he said it was either 100% or 0% chance for us because my daughter would either live or die, something clicked and I stopped worrying about the prognosis numbers. Now that we are several years out, I so value his wisdom. I've known kids with very good prognoses who relapsed, and I know kids with really poor diagnoses who tolerated treatment well and are doing great many years later.

Treatment

Treatment for children with ALL is complicated and lasts for years. It involves chemotherapy and sometimes radiation, stem cell transplantation, or immunotherapy. Below are a few issues that apply to treatment of all types of ALL.

- **Adolescents:** Teenagers and young adults do better when they are treated on pediatric protocols at large children's hospitals, rather than on adult protocols at local or even large hospitals.
- **CNS disease:** Few children have detectable disease in their CNS at diagnosis, but most children develop disease in the brain and spinal cord if preventive chemotherapy

is not delivered to the brain. Therefore, treatment for children with ALL includes chemotherapy injected into the CSF during spinal taps (called intrathecal chemotherapy). Use of radiation to the brain to prevent CNS disease has been dramatically reduced in recent years.

- **Disease in the testes:** Around 2% of boys are found to have disease in their testes at diagnosis. Treatment may or may not include radiation to the testes.

- **Compliance affects cures:** Treatment for ALL lasts for years. Studies have shown that children who are routinely not given their oral medications on schedule have higher rates of relapse. This doesn't mean you should worry if you miss a few doses or if your child throws up a few doses. That happens to all families. The children at risk are those who routinely don't get the prescribed oral or liquid medications at home; this is particularly a problem with adolescents. Your child's treatment team should closely monitor compliance with taking medications at home and provide help to families who are having difficulties.

- **Pharmacogenetics:** Blood tests are available to assess children's genetically determined ability to metabolize some medications. These tests are discussed in Chapter 13, *Chemotherapy and Other Medications*. If children break down certain drugs slower than normal, the drug levels can build up in their bodies, resulting in increased toxicity and risk of infection. So all children who develop severe toxicities during treatment (severe infections, very low WBC counts, or high results on liver function tests) should have pharmacogenetic testing. Some institutions test children with ALL before beginning treatment.

- **Remission:** Most children with ALL are in remission (less than 5% leukemic blasts in the bone marrow) at the end of the induction phase. Children and teens not in remission by day 29 (e.g., 10% blasts in the bone marrow) are usually reclassified as very high-risk and are given intensified chemotherapy. Remission is not related to MRD. Results of MRD testing are used to determine risk level. Here are three examples:

  - A child with less than 5% blasts and less than 0.01 MRD on day 29 is in remission and would not have his risk level increased.

  - A child with less than 5% blasts and 0.2 MRD on day 29 is in remission but would require more intense treatment (risk level would increase).

  - A child with 10% blasts in the bone marrow on day 29 is not in remission and would require more intense treatment (risk level would increase).

Although the goal of treatment is to eliminate all cancer cells, there are many more cancer cells left after the induction phase of treatment. One pediatric oncologist explains as follows.

> Remission is defined as less than 5% blasts in the bone marrow. I always tell parents that friends and family may ask why chemo is still necessary if the child is in remission. I explain that MRD of zero does not mean zero cancer in the body. It means

we've reached the lowest level of detection with current technology, but we can't stop therapy. MRD is primarily used by physicians to risk-stratify patients so they get the treatment they need and no more.

The rest of this chapter contains brief descriptions of the standard ALL treatments (not clinical trial treatments) used in 2017 for children. It is divided into five sections: B-cell ALL, T-cell ALL, Ph+ ALL, infant ALL, and children with Down syndrome and ALL. Keep in mind that different institutions offer different treatments in different phases, so what follows is a general outline of the most commonly used treatments. In addition, risk level can change depending on response to treatment, so children with lower-risk disease can have phases deleted and children with higher-risk disease may be given more intensive treatment. All children with ALL receive treatment to prevent the spread of the disease to the CNS (brain and spinal cord).

Your child's pediatric oncologist will give you several documents. One is an overall plan that shows the phases of therapy. The other is called a roadmap, which clearly describes the treatment your child will receive during each specific phase. If your child is enrolled in a clinical trial, a lengthy document that covers all aspects of the protocol is also available for parents (see Chapter 8, *Choosing a Treatment*).

All treatment protocols have phases where blood counts will be very low and the risk of life-threatening infection is high. You can expect to have your child hospitalized during these phases.

B-cell ALL

Based on criteria described earlier in this chapter, children with B-cell ALL are classified as low risk, average risk, high risk, or very high risk. The Children's Oncology Group (COG) classifies the following children and teens with B-ALL as very high risk:

- All teenagers and young adults (ages 13 to 25)
- Infants younger than 1, especially those with an *MLL* gene rearrangement
- Children or teens with certain genetic abnormalities, very low number of chromosomes (<44), the Philadelphia chromosome, or the translocation called t(17;19)
- Children with high MRD levels at the end of induction (4 weeks) or a later time (e.g., 12 weeks)

> *The reports we received were: molecular diagnostics, cytogenetics, and surface markers. The reports showed that Tom had B-cell ALL with high hyperdiploidy and the presence of the triple trisomy 4, 10, 17, but without any translocations. The fact that he had the triple trisomy was supposed to carry a good prognosis. However, he was still MRD+ at the end of induction and consolidation.*

The following table shows the phases of treatment and the drugs most commonly used during each phase.

Risk level	Induction	Consolidation	Interim maintenance	Intensification	Maintenance
Low risk	dexamethasone, PEG-asparaginase, vincristine	mercaptopurine, vincristine	None	None	dexamethasone, mercaptopurine, methotrexate, vincristine
Average risk	dexamethasone, PEG-asparaginase, vincristine	mercaptopurine, vincristine	methotrexate, vincristine	cyclophosphamide, cytarabine, dexamethasone, doxorubicin, mercaptopurine, methotrexate, PEG-asparaginase, thioguanine, vincristine	dexamethasone, mercaptopurine, methotrexate, thiogruanine, vincristine
High risk	daunorubicin, dexamethasone (<10 years old), prednisone (>10 years old), PEG-asparaginase, vincristine	cyclophosphamide, cytarabine, mercaptopurine, PEG-asparaginase, vincristine	methotrexate with leucovorin rescue, vincristine	cyclophosphamide, cytarabine, dexamethasone, doxorubicin, PEG-asparaginase, thioguanine, vincristine	mercaptopurine, methotrexate, prednisone, vincristine
Very high risk	asparaginase, daunorubicin, dexamethasone (<10 years old), prednisone (>10 years old), vincristine	asparaginase, cyclophosphamide, cytarabine, etoposide, mercaptopurine, vincristine	methotrexate with leucovorin rescue, mercaptopurine, vincristine	asparaginase, cyclophosphamide, cytarabine, dexamethasone, doxorubicin, thioguanine, vincristine	mercaptopurine, methotrexate, prednisone, vincristine

Asparaginase reactions. Some children have reactions to PEG-asparaginase, and in these cases, they are usually given a related medication called Erwinia L-asparaginase for the rest of treatment. Children who have severe reactions (e.g., grade 3 or 4 pancreatitis) usually don't receive any more of this drug.

Protecting the heart. Because daunorubicin and doxorubicin can cause heart damage, some protocols include the drug dexrazoxane. This drug has been shown to protect the heart in some treatment protocols, and in some it has not been tested.

Testes. Boys who have testicular disease at diagnosis may need a testicular biopsy at the end of induction. If the biopsy shows disease, boys may receive testicular radiation during the consolidation phase.

Stem cell transplantation. Children with very high risk disease and fewer than 44 chromosomes in their cancer cells are sometimes offered a stem cell transplant after consolidation if a matched donor is available.

CNS treatment. Intrathecal chemotherapy (injected into the spinal fluid during a spinal tap) is used to prevent spread of disease to the brain for all children with B-cell ALL, with schedules depending on risk category. The chemotherapy drugs given are:

- IT methotrexate, cytarabine, and hydrocortisone (called "triples");
- IT cytarabine; or
- IT methotrexate

Cranial radiation. This is no longer used for newly diagnosed children at low, average, or high risk. Use of cranial radiation to treat children and teens with very-high-risk B-cell ALL varies among institutions and research groups. Some institutions increase systemic chemotherapy for very-high-risk children and use no cranial radiation for any children with B-cell ALL; others use cranial radiation for certain groups of children at very high risk of relapse. Children who are sometimes treated with both intrathecal medication and cranial radiation include those with:

- CNS3 disease at diagnosis (5 or more blasts in CNS fluid)
- Extremely high WBC counts at diagnosis
- Certain very-high-risk genetic characteristics of the cancer cells

> *My 2-year-old son was diagnosed with B-cell ALL with the MLL rearrangement and CNS3 disease. During induction, he developed grade 3 pancreatitis after the second dose of asparaginase and was very ill. So, he was not given any more asparaginase. Because he had disease in his CNS at diagnosis, he also had 1,200 cGy of cranial radiation. He was one of the few kids we knew who sailed through induction and felt good most of the time (except for the pancreatitis).*

T-cell ALL

T-cell ALL occurs most often in older boys and adolescents. These children often have high WBC counts (>100,000 µL) and masses in their chests (called mediastinal masses) at diagnosis. The presence of a mediastinal mass is a medical emergency, as it can press on the trachea (windpipe), causing coughing or shortness of breath. Such children will be admitted to the pediatric intensive care unit for initial evaluation and therapy. With T-cell ALL, the thymus gland in the neck may also be affected.

> *Our daughter Maya was not feeling well the week before her 5th birthday. During her birthday party, we noticed she was breathing shallowly. The next day she looked pale and her face was puffy, so my husband took her to urgent care. They took vitals and listened to her lungs and within two minutes the doctor said, "Drive straight to*

the ER or we'll call an ambulance." At the ER, they did an x-ray that showed a large mass in her chest that had collapsed one of her lungs. In the ICU, they tried to sedate her to put in a chest tube and to do a bone marrow aspiration, spinal tap, and PICC line, but she crashed. At one point, there were 20 to 30 people in the room. They did most of those tests with local anesthesia instead of sedation. At this point, Maya said, "Excuse me, I did not order this!" Diagnosis: T-cell ALL.

T-cell ALL used to carry a worse prognosis than B-cell ALL. But due to more intensive therapies, the remission rates are now almost identical. The COG standard treatment for children and teens with T-cell ALL is divided into standard risk, intermediate risk, and very high risk.

Treatment for children with standard- or intermediate-risk T-cell ALL usually includes five or six phases, as well as treatment to prevent spread of the disease to the brain. The table below shows the phases of treatment and the drugs most commonly used for children or teens at standard risk.

Induction	Consolidation	Interim maintenance	Intensification	Maintenance
daunorubicin, dexamethasone, PEG-asparaginase, vincristine	cyclophosphamide, cytarabine, mercaptopurine, PEG-asparaginase, vincristine	methotrexate, PEG-asparaginase, vincristine	cyclophosphamide, cytarabine, dexamethasone, doxorubicin, PEG-asparaginase, thioguanine, vincristine	dexamethasone, methotrexate, mercaptopurine, vincristine

Children with intermediate-risk disease may have two intensification phases, and children with very high-risk disease may have three intensification phases of treatment. Children and teens not in remission by day 29 and with MRD of more than 0.01 are usually reclassified as very high risk and are given intensified chemotherapy.

Asparaginase reactions. If children react to PEG-asparaginase, they are usually given a related medication called Erwinia L-asparaginase for the rest of treatment. Children who have severe reactions (e.g., grade 3 or 4 pancreatitis) usually do not receive any more of this drug.

Protecting the heart. Because daunorubicin and doxorubicin can cause heart damage, some protocols include the drug dexrazoxane. This drug has been shown to protect the heart in some treatment protocols, and in some it has not been tested.

Testes. Boys who have testicular disease at diagnosis may need a testicular biopsy at the end of induction. If the biopsy shows disease, boys may receive testicular radiation during the consolidation phase.

CNS treatment. Intrathecal chemotherapy (injected into the spinal fluid during a spinal tap) is used for all children with T-cell ALL. The chemotherapy drugs given to prevent spread of disease to the brain are:

- IT cytarabine
- IT methotrexate with leucovorin rescue

Cranial radiation. Some institutions use cranial radiation (1,200 or 1,800 cGy) for children who have T-cell ALL with CNS disease at diagnosis. Other do not use cranial radiation unless a child has relapsed in the CNS. Whether or not to use cranial radiation in children with T-cell ALL is the subject of ongoing clinical trials.

> *Because our 5-year-old daughter had a mass in her chest at diagnosis, she had five days of steroids before beginning treatment for the T-cell ALL. The mass dramatically shrunk during the pretreatment with steroids. We signed up for a clinical trial and were randomized to the experimental arm (included bortezomib). She had a hard time during treatment—a double lung fungal infection, pseudomonas infections on her skin that required surgical removal, multiple delays of treatment, a year of physical therapy, and more. But, she's almost finished maintenance so the end is in sight.*

Philadelphia Chromosome ALL

About 3% of children diagnosed with ALL are found to have the Philadelphia chromosome (called Ph+) in their cancer cells. It is more common in older children, teens, and young adults. In the past, this was a difficult type of leukemia to treat, but development of the targeted drug Gleevec® (imatinib) led to dramatic improvements in cure rates. Currently, treatment for children and teens with Ph+ ALL involves intensive chemotherapy and imatinib or a related medication. If imatinib stops working, a stem cell transplant from a matched donor (if available) is usually recommended. Different institutions treat this type of ALL in different ways. The table below shows the phases of treatment and drugs used by some institutions to treat children with Ph+ ALL.

Induction	Consolidation	Reinduction	Intensification	Maintenance
daunorubicin, PEG-asparaginase, dexamethasone, vincristine	cytarabine, ifosfamide, imatinib, methotrexate with leucovorin rescue, VP-16	cyclophosphamide, daunorubicin, dexamethasone, imatinib, PEG-asparaginase, vincristine	cyclophosphamide, cytarabine, etoposide, methotrexate with leucovorin rescue, PEG-asparaginase	cyclophosphamide, dexamethasone, etoposide, methotrexate with leucovorin rescue, thioguanine, vincristine

Asparaginase reactions. Some children have reactions to PEG-asparaginase, and in these cases, they are usually given a related medication called Erwinia L-asparaginase for the rest of treatment. Children who have severe reactions (e.g., grade 3 or 4 pancreatitis) usually do not receive any more of this drug.

Protecting the heart. Because daunorubicin and doxorubicin can cause heart damage, some protocols include the drug dexrazoxane. This drug has been shown to protect the heart in some treatment protocols, and in some it has not been tested.

CNS treatment. Intrathecal chemotherapy (injected into the spinal fluid during a spinal tap) is used for all children with Ph+ ALL. The chemotherapy drugs given to prevent spread of disease to the brain are:

- IT cytarabine
- IT methotrexate with leucovorin rescue

Cranial radiation. Some institutions use cranial radiation (1,200 or 1,800 cGy) for children who have CNS disease at diagnosis. Others do not use cranial radiation unless a child has relapsed in the CNS.

> *Our treatment discussion left a lot to be desired. After we found out it was Ph+ ALL, we were offered two treatment plans—one with Gleevec®, which our hospital had never used, and a clinical trial with dasatinib, also something they had no experience with. We asked for information about both options, and were told they were so new there wasn't any. When we asked how we could make a choice with no information, they said to make our best guess, and that we had 24 hours to do that. So, we started calling friends in the medical field and were connected to a person who had been involved in the initial Bristol Myers Squibb trials and he filled us in on those. We also contacted a cousin who had been on Gleevec® for years to treat his CML. We ended up enrolling in the trial, but it was mostly based on a leap of faith and anecdotal information that it did a better job of crossing the blood–brain barrier.*

A recently discovered type of ALL is called Philadelphia chromosome-like ALL. Although the leukemia cells of children with this type of ALL do not contain the BCR-ABL gene, the leukemia cells are sometimes sensitive to targeted TKI drugs, just like Ph+ ALL is. Oncologists treat children with Philadelphia chromosome-like ALL with intensive chemotherapy as well as dasatinib.

Infant ALL

About 150 infants younger than 12 months old are diagnosed with ALL every year in the United States. These infants are very challenging to treat because they often:

- Are very ill at diagnosis
- Have very high WBC counts
- Have characteristics of their cancer cells (e.g., *MLL* rearrangement) that are especially hard to treat

- Are often slow to respond to treatment
- Develop severe treatment-related toxicities (e.g., infection) at a higher rate than do older children with ALL

Many types of treatment have been tried for infants with ALL. Sometimes newly diagnosed children with very high WBC counts and CNS symptoms have an exchange transfusion in which all of their blood is replaced with donor blood. Stem cell transplant is not more effective than conventional chemotherapy for infants. Risk groups for infants with ALL often change, but the most recent are:

- **Standard risk:** No *MLL* rearrangement
- **Intermediate risk:** *MLL* rearrangement and infant is at least 90 days old
- **High risk:** *MLL* rearrangement and infant is younger than 90 days old

In general, children with no *MLL* rearrangements are treated on protocols for high-risk ALL or even more intensive treatment. Recent protocols for infants with ALL were divided into five phases—induction, post induction, reinduction, consolidation, and continuation. The drugs used were some combination of asparaginase, cyclophosphamide (with mesna), cytarabine, daunorubicin, dexamethosone, etoposide, filgrastim, mercaptopurine, methotrexate with leucovorin rescue, prednisone, and vincristine. Schedules and doses varied by risk category. Research is ongoing to identify specific genetic characteristics so targeted therapies can be developed, and clinical trials are being developed to test these drugs.

Protecting the heart. Because daunorubicin and doxorubicin can cause heart damage, some protocols include the drug dexrazoxane. This drug has been shown to protect the heart in some treatment protocols, and in some it has not been tested.

Asparaginase reactions. Some children have reactions to PEG-asparaginase, and in these cases, they are usually given a related medication called Erwinia L-asparaginase for the rest of treatment. Children who have severe reactions (e.g., grade 3 or 4 pancreatitis) usually do not receive any more of this drug.

CNS treatment. Intrathecal chemotherapy (injected into the spinal fluid during a spinal tap) is used for all infants with ALL. The chemotherapy drugs given to prevent spread of disease to the brain are methotrexate, hydrocortisone, and cytarabine (called triple intrathecals).

Down syndrome and ALL

Approximately 2 to 3% of children with ALL also have Down syndrome. It has long been known that these children are very sensitive to chemotherapy drugs and very easily develop severe infections. Efforts have been made to decrease doses to minimize toxicity while still maintaining cure rates. Currently, there is no widely accepted standard treatment for children with Down syndrome and ALL. Below is the treatment given at COG institutions in 2017 for children with standard risk B-cell ALL and Down syndrome (children with Down syndrome are rarely diagnosed with T-cell ALL). Standard risk in B-cell ALL is defined as:

- Age 1 to 9
- WBC <50,000/μL
- No *MLL* rearrangement, hypodiploidy, or Philadelphia chromosome
- Day 29 bone marrow MRD <0.01
- No CNS3 or testicular leukemia at diagnosis

> *My 11-year-old daughter, who has Down syndrome, was visiting her dad who lives eight hours from us. She had an off and on fever as well as petechiae, so he took her to his physician, who diagnosed an ear infection and put her on antibiotics. He said if it didn't improve perhaps she needed some blood work done. Then, a few days later, pus started coming out of her ear and her temperature rose to 104°. My ex took her to her former pediatrician, who took one look at the ear and petechiae, and said he was 99% sure it was leukemia. He took some blood, hugged her, and called ahead to the ER, where she was diagnosed with high-risk B-cell ALL that night.*

The table below shows the drugs most commonly used during each treatment phase for children with Down syndrome and B-cell ALL.

Induction	Consolidation	Interim maintenance	Intensification	Interim maintenance II	Maintenance
dexamethasone, PEG-asparaginase, vincristine	mercaptopurine, vincristine	methotrexate with leucovorin rescue, vincristine	cyclophosphamide, cytarabine, doxorubicin, PEG-asparaginase, thioguanine	methotrexate with leucovorin rescue, vincristine	dexamethasone, mercaptopurine, methotrexate, vincristine

Protecting the heart. Because daunorubicin and doxorubicin can cause heart damage, some protocols include the drug dexrazoxane. This drug has been shown to protect the heart in some treatment protocols, and in some it has not been tested.

Asparaginase reactions. Some children have reactions to PEG-asparaginase, and in these cases, they are usually given a related medication called Erwinia L-asparaginase for the rest of treatment. Children who have severe reactions (e.g., grade 3 or 4 pancreatitis) usually do not receive any more of this drug.

CNS treatment. Intrathecal chemotherapy (injected into the spinal fluid during a spinal tap) is used for all children with Down syndrome and ALL. The chemotherapy drugs given to prevent spread of disease to the brain are:

- Cytarabine
- Methotrexate with leucovorin rescue

Cranial radiation. This is not used to treat children with B-cell ALL and Down syndrome.

> My daughter was treated on the standard high-risk protocol for kids with Down syndrome. She was high risk because of her age. She was in the hospital for the first two weeks, then only occasionally for neutropenic fevers. They would culture her blood but nothing ever grew. She went through treatment without major toxicities or serious problems.

Information on Current Treatments

Treatments for various types of childhood leukemia evolve and improve over time. The treatments described in this chapter were the ones most commonly used when this book was written. You can learn about the newest treatments available by calling the National Cancer Institute (NCI) at (800) 422-6237 and asking for information on childhood acute lymphoblastic leukemia. This free information, also available online at *www.cancer.gov/cancertopics/pdq/pediatrictreatment*, explains the disease, state-of-the-art treatments, and any ongoing clinical trials. Two versions are available:

- One for families, which uses simple language and contains no statistics; and
- One for health professionals, which is technical, thorough, and includes citations to scientific literature.

To learn about current Phase III clinical trials for ALL in children or teens, you can visit the National Cancer Institute's website *www.cancer.gov/about-cancer/treatment/clinical-trials/advanced-search* and type "Acute Lymphoblastic Leukemia" in the "Type/condition" box. Then check the "untreated childhood acute lymphoblastic leukemia" box, choose Phase III in the "Trial Phase" box, and select the "Search" button.

When Nico was first diagnosed, I obsessively read everything that I could about leukemia. My anxiety level went through the roof. I soon discovered that most of what is on the internet is outdated. So be wary about where you are doing your research. Write down all of your concerns, and ask your oncologist to specifically address each of them. All parents fear relapse and initially focus on their child's "odds" of survival. But you will drive yourself crazy worrying about every possible thing that can go wrong at the outset. The odds are in your favor. Expect treatment to go as planned and only deal with those problems that arise. Do not look too far ahead—it is too overwhelming.

Nico's treatment course had several bumps throughout, but for us induction was still by far and away the most difficult phase. At the end of induction, while holding my screaming, hitting, kicking, biting, and bloated little boy, I told our oncologist through tears, "We already ruined him." I was wrong. My son is back and this experience has not defined him. He is still my Nico. There are bad days, but we have more good days than bad. Someone once likened this trial to fighting a forest fire. To get through it, you have to focus on extinguishing the flames just in front of you. You do not want to look at the trees in flames. You just focus on one small fire at a time. You put out the fire on the shrub at your feet and move forward. And eventually you and your child will be through the forest.

Chapter 4

Acute Myeloid Leukemia

*"We must let go of the life we have planned, so as to
accept the one that is waiting for us."*

— Joseph Campbell

LEUKEMIA IS THE TERM USED to describe cancer that begins in the bone marrow. This spongy material fills the bones in the body and produces blood cells. In a child with acute myeloid leukemia (AML), the bone marrow creates millions of cancerous white blood cells (WBCs). As the bone marrow becomes packed with these abnormal cells, they crowd out the healthy cells and symptoms of AML begin to develop.

This chapter covers risk factors for developing AML, signs and symptoms, diagnosis, prognosis, and treatment. The treatment section is divided into three parts: (1) treatment for children diagnosed with the type of AML called acute promyelocytic leukemia (APL), (2) treatment for children with Down syndrome, and (3) treatment for children with other types of AML. The chapter concludes with ways to learn about the newest treatments available for childhood AML.

AML Is a Blood Disease

AML is cancer of the blood cells called myeloblasts, which would normally develop into healthy WBCs (see Figure 4-1). A normal myeloid stem cell matures into one of three types of blood cells:

- Red blood cells (RBCs) that carry oxygen to all tissues of the body
- Platelets that form blood clots to stop bleeding
- WBCs that fight infection and disease

When cancerous myeloblasts appear in the bone marrow, they multiply rapidly and lose their ability to develop into mature WBCs. After accumulating in the bone marrow, cancerous myeloblasts spill over into the blood and, if left unchecked, may invade the central nervous system (CNS)—which includes the brain and spinal cord—and other organs, such as ovaries in girls or testes in boys.

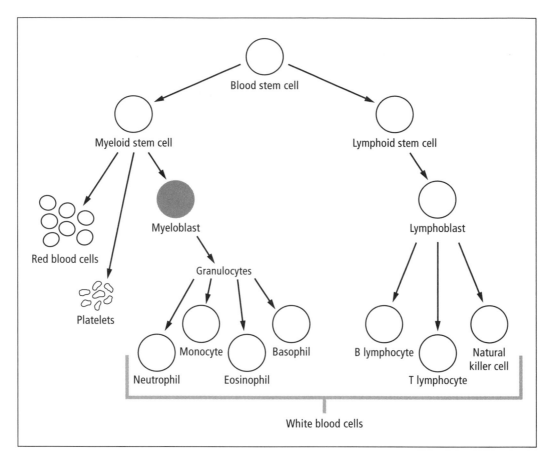

Figure 4-1: AML is cancer of the myeloblasts

When leukemic blasts begin to fill the marrow, fewer normal RBCs, platelets, and WBCs are made. As the number of normal blood cells decreases, symptoms appear. Low RBC counts cause fatigue and pale skin. Low platelet counts may result in bruising and bleeding problems. If healthy WBCs are crowded out by blasts, the child will have little or no defense against infections.

> *My 6-year-old daughter had been getting bad headaches. The school would call me to pick her up, and she would throw up all the way home. She had an appointment with the optometrist, who noticed an odd-looking vein in her eye and that she looked pale and had some bruising. He recommended taking her in for blood work. We did, and she was diagnosed with AML.*

Who Gets AML?

Approximately 730 children between the ages of 0 and 19 are diagnosed with AML in the United States each year. Boys and girls are equally affected. Risk factors include:

- Having a brother or sister (especially a twin) who has leukemia
- Being Hispanic
- Having relatives who had AML
- Having past treatment with chemotherapy or radiation
- Being exposed to high levels of certain chemicals (e.g., benzene)
- Having a genetic disorder such as Down syndrome, Fanconi anemia, Bloom syndrome, Li-Fraumeni syndrome, neurofibromatosis type 1, Diamond-Blackfan anemia, or Shwachman-Diamond syndrome. However, most children with these syndromes do not develop AML.

Environmental exposures

Several studies have found weak associations (not causes) of environmental exposures with development of childhood cancer. For example, prenatal exposure to x-rays and exposure to high levels of pesticides during pregnancy or infancy/childhood have all appeared in the news as being linked to development of AML. However, none of these has been identified as a cause. It's important for parents to remember that nothing they did or did not do caused their child's AML.

Prior treatment for cancer

Certain types of chemotherapy (e.g., etoposide, doxorubicin, daunorubicin, mitoxantrone, idarubicin, nitrogen mustard, cyclophosphamide, cisplatin, and others) used to treat other cancers can increase the risk of developing AML (called secondary AML). In these cases, AML generally develops three to ten years after exposure to these drugs. Radiation treatments for prior cancers can also increase a child or teen's risk of developing AML. However, most children diagnosed with AML have never been treated for cancer before.

Risk for twins

Identical twins. If one identical twin develops AML as an infant, the risk of the other twin also developing AML is almost 100%. This is not believed to be a genetic risk; instead, it is thought that leukemia cells are shared during fetal development (when the identical twins are inside the mother's womb). If an identical twin develops AML between ages one and seven, the other twin has twice the risk of being diagnosed with AML compared to a child in the general population.

Fraternal twins. The risk is low that both fraternal twins will develop AML, and the risk decreases with age. After age 6, there is no increased risk of the fraternal twin of a child with AML developing the disease.

Signs and Symptoms

Signs are observed by parents or doctors (e.g., pale skin) and symptoms are experienced by patients (e.g., bone pain). The most common signs and symptoms of AML are:

- Fever
- Infection
- Night sweats
- Paleness
- Weakness or feeling tired
- Shortness of breath
- Headaches
- Easy bruising or bleeding (can occur internally)
- Small red spots on the skin (called petechiae) caused by bleeding
- Pain in the bones or joints
- Pain or feeling of fullness below the ribs from an enlarged spleen
- Swollen lymph nodes
- Painful sores on skin of the arms, neck, face, and back
- Painless purple lumps (called leukemia cutis) in the neck, underarm, stomach, groin, or other parts of the body

> My 5-year-old son Aidan said his stomach hurt. It got so bad he was crying and couldn't stand. We went to the ER and he was treated for constipation. Then he had a nosebleed and started getting bruises (black, scary looking ones) all over his body. I knew something was wrong. I took him to the pediatrician who drew blood and then called two hours later to tell us to go to the children's hospital. My husband was due back from deployment overseas the next day, so my sister went with Aidan, me, and my 5-month-old daughter to the hospital. They admitted Aidan to do tests. The next morning, my sister took the baby to meet her dad for the first time, and later that day we learned Aidan had AML or APL. It was the greatest day (husband home and meeting his daughter for the first time) and the worst day (son diagnosed with cancer) of our lives.

Children with AML are sometimes diagnosed after developing a chloroma—a tumor formed from clumps of cancer cells. These pale green tumors are most often found under the skin near the eyes but may occur any place in the body.

It started six days before my daughter's fourth birthday in July. She was restless all night and in the morning said her leg hurt. We brought her to the pediatrician. He x-rayed it and said to give her Tylenol® for a week because he thought it was a soft tissue injury. After a few days the pain went away. Throughout the months of August and September, she would occasionally wake with pain in her arm or leg. In early October, she said her shoulder hurt, the doctor x-rayed it, and said it was probably growing pains. I requested blood work because I knew something was wrong. We were told, other than her sed rate being high, all else looked normal. By mid-October, she had severe leg pain again and started to limp and she didn't want to do things that she used to enjoy. I insisted on a referral, and we were sent to a pediatric rheumatologist (but we couldn't get an appointment until the next month). I started to feel like we were going to lose our little girl. The pains seemed to come more often and with a greater severity so we said we needed an earlier appointment with the rheumatologist. After the appointment and lots of tests, the rheumatologist called to say, "Her white count has dropped severely so I'm sending you to a hematologist/oncologist. I don't know what it is but there is something brewing." We were given an appointment with the hematologist/oncologist the next day. Over the next two weeks, we were in daily for blood work, x-rays, a CT scan, a bone scan, an MRI, and finally a bone marrow aspiration. The day following the bone marrow aspiration, November 12, the pediatric oncologist called to say that she had AML, and to come to the hospital immediately prepared for a long stay. The bottom fell out of our world.

Approximately 20% of children with AML have WBC counts above 100,000 µL at diagnosis. This huge number of cancerous cells in the blood can result in the following symptoms:

- Rapid and/or difficult breathing
- Fluid in the lungs
- Headache
- Sleepiness
- Confusion
- Seizures

About 10 to 13% of children with AML have the disease in their CNS at diagnosis, but few of these children have symptoms of CNS disease, such as seizures, vomiting, blurred vision, or difficulty maintaining balance.

Diagnosis

If leukemia is suspected based on symptoms and initial blood work, your child should be referred to a regional children's hospital that can provide the comprehensive services needed. At the children's hospital, bone marrow is sampled and tested (see Chapter 9,

Coping with Procedures). The bone marrow is examined under a microscope by a pathologist (a physician who specializes in body tissue analysis). A portion of the bone marrow and the chloroma biopsy, if done, undergoes other sophisticated tests to check the leukemia cells for genetic changes. The results help the doctors determine the type of AML and treatment options. A lumbar puncture (also called spinal tap) is also done to see whether leukemia cells are present in the cerebrospinal fluid.

An essential part of the diagnostic process is identifying whether the cancer is acute lymphoblastic leukemia (ALL), AML, or APL because the treatments for these diseases are very different. There also are many subtypes of AML in children, which affect both prognosis and the type of treatment needed. For example, children with Down syndrome or APL have very different treatment plans than children with other forms of AML.

To see a long list of specific genetic abnormalities found in cancer cells of children with AML, visit the National Cancer Institute's webpage about childhood AML at *https:// www.cancer.gov/types/leukemia/hp/child-aml-treatment-pdq* and then click on the section called "Classification of Pediatric Myeloid Malignancies."

> *My daughter Gabby was a 13-year-old eighth grade student when she was diagnosed with AML with the FLT 3 oncogene (putting her into the very high risk category). She had some bruising, but she is an active tomboy who frequently had bruises. In January, during flu season, she had a bellyache and vomiting. By Sunday, the belly pain was severe and we took her to the ER. The doctor said, "She either has appendicitis or leukemia." They did more tests, said she had leukemia, and asked which of the closest children's hospitals (not really close, each was almost 500 miles away) we wanted to go to. She was airlifted there and the journey began.*

APL is distinguished from other forms of AML by identifying a chromosomal translocation called t(15;17) and testing for a type of protein called *PML-RARA* fusion. Approximately 12% of children and teens with AML are diagnosed with the APL subtype. APL is most commonly diagnosed in children ages 9 to 11.

Prognosis

Prognosis is an estimate of the chance for cure. It helps determine how aggressive the treatment needs to be to have the best chance for cure with the least chance of late effects. The appropriate treatment for each child with AML is determined by analyzing several features related to the child and to the leukemia cells.

Treatment for AML has dramatically improved in the last two decades. Today, 85 to 90% of children who receive optimal treatment at a major children's hospital achieve remission. Of the children who achieve remission, 55 to 65% remain in remission for five years or more. However, there is a wide range of prognoses based on the type of AML that children have.

The WBC count at diagnosis helps predict response to treatment; a high WBC sometimes makes remission harder to achieve. Other factors that might predict more difficulty reaching remission are:

- **Secondary AML:** AML that develops after treatment for another cancer.
- **Certain leukemia cell characteristics:** Children with the following traits found in their leukemia cells have a less favorable prognosis: monosomy 7, monosomy 5/del(5q), 3q abnormalities, and *FLT3-ITD* with high-allelic ratio.
- **Race/ethnicity:** Black and Hispanic children tend to have lower survival rates than white children.
- **Weight:** Children who are very underweight or overweight at diagnosis can develop more life-threatening infections during treatment.

Factors that predict a higher likelihood of achieving remission are:

- **Age:** Children between the ages of 2 and 11 have better prognoses than do teenagers or infants.
- **Rapid response to treatment:** Minimum residual disease (MRD) is measured after the first phase of treatment (called induction). Children who have low MRD (called a rapid response to treatment) have a better prognosis.
- **APL:** Children with APL who are treated with all-trans retinoic acid (ATRA) and chemotherapy have a good prognosis, despite the fact that almost half of them have WBCs above 100,000 µL at diagnosis.
- **Down syndrome:** Most children with Down syndrome and AML are diagnosed when younger than four years old. This group of children has a very favorable prognosis.
- **Certain leukemia cell characteristics:** Children with the following traits found in their leukemia cells have a favorable prognosis: t(8;21); t(15;17); inv(16); *CEBPA* mutations, and *NPM1* mutations.

Your child's treatment team will consider a multitude of factors to determine your child's prognosis and treatment options.

Treatment

Treatment for AML can be broadly divided into three main categories: treatment for children with APL, treatment for children with Down syndrome and AML, and treatment for the other types of AML. These are discussed separately because treatment is very different for these three groups of children and teens. Children are treated in cycles of treatment (called phases) with names such as induction, intensification, consolidation, or continuation. Depending on risk level, some phases are given more than once. Most children with AML enter remission (defined as less than 5% blasts in the bone marrow). However, treatment is still needed to kill any remaining cancer cells.

Children with acute promyelocytic leukemia (APL)

Treatment for children with APL has improved considerably in the last two decades because APL cancer cells are very sensitive to the chemotherapy drugs ATRA (all-trans retinoic acid) and arsenic trioxide. Studies have shown that adding arsenic to the treatment plan allows the use of certain chemotherapy drugs to be decreased, which reduces the chance of some types of late effects. The length of treatment has also decreased from 30 months to 8 months. The current standard treatment is based on risk level:

- Standard risk (WBC count less than 10,000/μL at diagnosis)
- High risk (WBC count 10,000/μL or higher at diagnosis)

Standard risk. Current treatment for all children with standard-risk APL starts with a 28-day induction phase. During this phase, children are given ATRA and arsenic trioxide. If the WBC count goes above 10,000 then hydroxyurea and dexamethasone are added. At the end of induction, a bone marrow test is done to check for minimum residual disease (MRD). Children who have MRD of 0.01 or higher on day 29 require more intensive treatment, which may involve an additional cycle of chemotherapy (mitoxantrone, cytarabine, and ATRA).

Almost all children with APL enter remission. However, treatment is still needed to kill any remaining cancer cells. The consolidation phase of therapy for children at standard risk of relapse usually includes cycles of ATRA and arsenic trioxide (total of 28 weeks). There is no maintenance phase. In addition, a bone marrow aspiration is done during consolidation to check for a molecular remission (when disease can no longer be detected in the bone marrow).

> *When Aidan was admitted, they did a lot of tests including a bone marrow aspiration. They didn't do a spinal tap then because APL was a possible diagnosis, and kids with APL tend to bleed a lot. APL is very rare so our oncologist, who had never treated a child with APL, talked to the whole treatment team and other experts across the country to decide on a treatment. Because Aidan's WBC was low and he had no CNS disease, he was considered a low-risk patient. On Day 29, he was in remission but his MRD was positive. After induction, he had eight months of treatment that included seven cycles (two weeks on/two weeks off) of ATRA and four cycles of arsenic (four weeks on/four weeks off). Because this treatment can damage the heart, he had echoes and EKGs every month for the first year. He finished treatment two years ago, and is in remission, feeling great, and with no heart damage (although he goes for echoes and EKGs yearly).*

High risk. Current treatment for all children with high-risk APL includes a 28-day induction phase of ATRA, arsenic trioxide, IV dexamethasone, and idarubicin. Consolidation therapy for children at high risk of relapse usually includes cycles of ATRA and arsenic trioxide (total of 28 weeks). There is no maintenance phase. In addition, a bone marrow aspiration is done during consolidation to check for a molecular remission (when disease can no longer be detected in the bone marrow).

CNS treatment. Children with APL only need treatment to the brain when they have a bleed in the brain or disease in the CNS at diagnosis. Children with a bleed in their brain are given triple intrathecal therapy (methotrexate, hydrocortisone, and cytarabine) on day 29 of induction and six more doses during consolidation. Children with CNS disease receive between four and six doses of intrathecal triple therapy during induction and another six doses during consolidation. In addition, children with CNS disease are given leucovorin 24 hours after each intrathecal treatment.

Children with Down syndrome

Children with Down syndrome have a higher risk of developing AML than children without Down syndrome. But, most children with Down syndrome who develop AML have a favorable prognosis and a low relapse rate.

About 10% of infants with Down syndrome develop a disorder called transient leukemia or transient myeloproliferative disorder (TMD). This disorder usually disappears in a few months without treatment (called spontaneous remission). However, while children have this disorder, life-threatening symptoms can occur, including:

• Increased size of internal organs

• Liver damage

• Abnormal amounts of fluid in the body

• Increased bleeding due to a clotting problem

• High WBC count

Children who develop these symptoms are sometimes treated with leukopheresis (taking the WBCs out of the blood) and low-dose cytarabine. Children with Down syndrome who had TMD when they were infants have a 10 to 30% chance of developing AML in the first three years of life.

> *Our daughter has Down syndrome and we aren't sure if she had transient myeloproliferative disorder [TMD] or not. When she was 1.5 months old she became really pale and had trouble breathing. They discovered a malrotation of her intestines in addition to the heart abnormality that we already knew about. Her blood work showed low platelets (80,000) and low hemoglobin (4.4). They put in a G tube [permanent feeding tube] to replace the temporary nasogastric tube that she had been*

using because of trouble breathing and eating relating to her heart condition. They also did a bone marrow biopsy but did not find leukemia. They continued monthly blood checks after her open heart surgery at 3.5 months, and her counts were normal. One year later she was diagnosed with AML. In retrospect, they think she might have had TMD.

Children with Down syndrome are very sensitive to some chemotherapy drugs commonly used to treat AML. Recent clinical trials have reduced the intensity of treatment (e.g., reduced cytarabine dose and eliminated etoposide and dexamethasone) while maintaining survival rates. Daunorubicin dosage has also been decreased due to concerns about late effects to the heart. Thus, current standard treatment is less toxic than what was used in the past.

Our daughter was diagnosed with AML at 14 months old and she is now five years old. They did not mention a clinical trial, and she was treated with the usual AML drugs but at lower doses because she has Down syndrome. Kids with Down syndrome are very responsive to chemo drugs, and we ended up spending almost the entire six months of treatment inpatient because her absolute neutrophil count [ANC] rarely went above 500, which is expected with AML treatment. She went into remission after the first treatment cycle, but we still had to complete the entire six rounds to make sure all of the leukemia cells were completely wiped out. It was hard—she had severe sepsis after the third course, and she relied on a feeding tube the whole time. But, I was able to pump and feed her breast milk throughout treatment.

Most children younger than age four start treatment with an induction phase of cytarabine, daunorubicin, and thioguanine. Minimum residual disease (MRD) is assessed at the end of this first induction phase and the results determine treatment:

- Standard risk: MRD ≤0.05% at the end of Induction #1
- High risk: MRD >0.05% at the end of Induction #1

Up to five more treatment phases are given to children at standard risk, usually with some combination of the following drugs: cytarabine, L-asparaginase, daunorubicin, thioguanine, and etoposide. Therapy for children younger than four with high-risk disease includes those five drugs plus mitoxantrone.

Treatment was really hard for our whole family. My 1-year-old daughter was inpatient almost continuously for six months. I ran on adrenaline because I had a strong need to stay on top of everything. I needed to take care of my daughter. I needed to take care of my son. I missed time with my husband. And I didn't take care of myself. After treatment, I really crashed and experienced a lot of PTSD symptoms. I was pregnant with our third child, and I found myself really worried all of the time. It's been four years and those feelings have finally passed.

Most children with Down syndrome and AML have a very low risk of having disease in their CNS. So if no blasts are found in the CNS at diagnosis, a single dose of intrathecal cytarabine is given during a lumbar puncture.

Two groups of children are considered to have CNS disease:

- Children with cancer cells in the cerebrospinal fluid at diagnosis
- Children with chloromas in the brain at diagnosis

Children with CNS disease are given intrathecal cytarabine (during a lumbar puncture) twice weekly during induction until no cancer cells are found in the CNS fluid, and then two additional intrathecal injections of cytarabine.

Children with other types of AML

The drugs most often used to achieve remission in children with AML (who do not have Down syndrome or the APL subtype) are cytarabine, an anthracycline (e.g., daunorubicin, idarubicin), etoposide, and thioguanine. These drugs greatly depress the bone marrow, giving the child the best chance to enter remission. Side effects, however, can include severe infections and/or internal bleeding. Thus, all children with AML should be treated at a regional children's hospital that can provide state-of-the-art supportive care during treatment.

> My daughter was diagnosed with AML when she was four years old. She was on a clinical trial and was randomized to the experimental arm that used gemtuzumab—a type of targeted therapy. She had five rounds of chemotherapy (cytarabine, daunorubicin, asparaginase, etoposide) and gemtuzumab. She had a week at home between each round. In all she spent 173 days in the hospital. She breezed through the first three rounds, after the fourth round she got a very high fever (105°) and after the fifth round, she had the high fever again and her heart started to fail (she was diagnosed with a cardiomyopathy). The PICU doctor made us feel better when he told us her clinical evaluation looked much better than the tests suggested. The heart problem has resolved over time, and we don't think she has any damage from it although she goes for yearly follow-up appointments with the cardiologist.

The following information about standard treatment was accurate in 2017 when this book was being written. However, treatments evolve, so the standard or experimental treatments offered for your child may be different. Standard treatment for AML typically includes three to four cycles of treatment (called phases). The phases for AML are induction and intensification.

The number of times each phase is used depends on risk level (e.g., some children need two induction phases).The first phase (called induction #1) includes treatment with cytarabine, daunomycin, and etoposide. After this phase, several types of tests are done to determine whether children have a low or high risk of relapse. Following are the usual phases of treatment for children and teens with low-risk disease:

• Induction #1: cytarabine, daunomycin, and etoposide

• Induction #2: cytarabine, daunomycin, and etoposide

• Intensification #1: cytarabine and etoposide

• Intensification #2: cytarabine and mitoxantrone

After induction #1, children and teens with high-risk disease usually receive the following treatment:

• Induction #2: cytarabine, daunomycin, and etoposide

• Intensification #1: cytarabine and etoposide

• If a donor is available, an allogeneic stem cell transplant is done (see Chapter 16, *Stem Cell Transplantation*).

• If no donor is available, intensification #2 is completed using high-dose cytarabine.

Children with chloromas in the eyes or brain at diagnosis are treated the same as other children with AML. In almost all cases, the chloromas disappear during treatment. In cases where the chloromas do not disappear after treatment with chemotherapy, radiation may be needed.

Most children and teens with AML do not have CNS disease at diagnosis. Currently, intrathecal cytarabine is given before each induction phase to prevent disease from developing in the CNS. Children or teens who have disease in their CNS at diagnosis (5 to 15%) receive IT cytarabine twice a week until disease can no longer be found in the cerebrospinal fluid (a minimum of four intrathecal treatments, and a maximum of six treatments, may be given). Children with chloromas in the CNS at diagnosis receive six IT treatments.

> *My daughter had very high risk AML (WBC 120,000 and FLT3). At the children's hospital, they offered us the standard treatment (three intense rounds of chemo followed by a stem cell transplant) or a clinical trial, in which the tyrosine inhibitor sorafenib was added to the experimental arm. I was by myself, 500 miles away from home, and had no one else to discuss it with. I signed her up for the trial, and she was assigned to the experimental arm.*

Information on Current Treatments

Treatments for various types of childhood leukemia evolve and improve over time. The treatments described in this chapter were the ones most commonly used when this book was written. You can learn about the newest treatments available by calling the National Cancer Institute (800) 422-6237 and asking for information about childhood AML. This free information, also available online at *www.cancer.gov/cancertopics/pdq/ pediatrictreatment*, explains the disease, state-of-the-art treatments, and ongoing clinical trials. Two versions are available:

- One for families, which uses simple language and contains no statistics; and

- One for health professionals, which is technical, thorough, and includes citations to scientific literature.

To learn about current Phase III clinical trials for AML in children or teens, you can visit the National Cancer Institute's website *www.cancer.gov/about-cancer/treatment/clinical-trials/advanced-search* and type "Acute Myeloid Leukemia" in the "Type/condition" box. Then check the "untreated childhood acute myeloid leukemia" box, and choose Phase III in the "Trial Phase" box. Finally, click the purple "Search" button at the bottom of the page.

I felt strong during my daughter's six months of treatment for AML, but it hit hard after treatment ended. They told us there was a 50% relapse rate for her type of AML, so I kept doing research and obsessing about relapse. If she said her leg hurt, I'd get really scared because that was her one pre-diagnosis symptom. I think I had PTSD. I felt overwhelmed with worry and stress before each follow-up appointment. My husband was the opposite, which created a lot of stress. But, the other moms in the support group really helped me understand how common and normal those differences were. Thank goodness, those tough feelings have mostly subsided over the six years since treatment, although I still get nervous about her annual oncology checkups. No relapse and doing great!

Chapter 5

Juvenile Myelomonocytic Leukemia

"If dreams reflect the past, hope summons the future."
— Elie Wiesel

LEUKEMIA IS THE TERM USED to describe cancer of the bone marrow. In healthy people, bone marrow fills the bones in the body and produces the number of red blood cells (RBCs), white blood cells (WBCs), and platelets that the body needs. In a child with juvenile myelomonocytic leukemia (JMML), the bone marrow creates millions of abnormal WBCs. As the bone marrow becomes packed with these abnormal cells, they crowd out the healthy cells and symptoms of JMML begin to develop.

JMML is a very rare form of childhood leukemia that is most often diagnosed in the first two years of life. This chapter describes JMML and covers risk factors, signs and symptoms, diagnosis, prognosis, and treatment. It concludes with ways to learn about the newest treatments available for JMML.

JMML Is a Blood Disease

JMML is cancer of immature WBCs called monocytes, which would normally develop into healthy macrophages (see Figure 5-1). Macrophages float in the blood, killing foreign organisms, removing dead cells, and helping the body fight infection.

When cancerous monocytes appear in the bone marrow, they multiply rapidly and lose their ability to develop into mature macrophages. They begin to crowd out the healthy stem cells that would mature into WBCs, RBCs, and platelets. When this happens, infection, anemia, or bleeding may occur. After accumulating in the bone marrow, cancerous monocytes spill over into the blood and invade other organs such as the spleen, liver, and lungs.

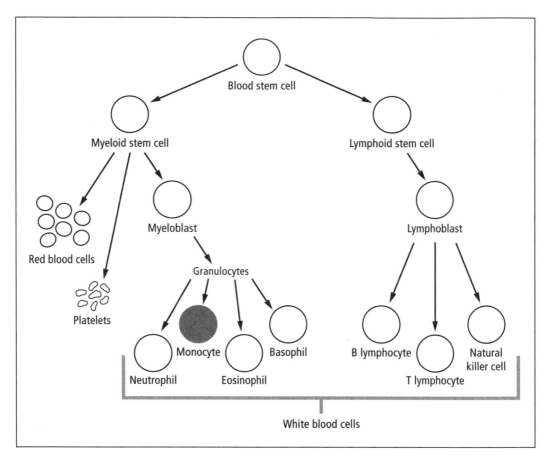

Figure 5-1: JMML is a disease of the monocytes

Because treatments for the four main types of childhood leukemia are very different, it is crucial that sophisticated laboratory studies be performed at diagnosis to identify the type of leukemia and the best treatment.

> *My daughter was diagnosed with JMML at the age of 27 months. Although it is a chronic leukemia, it is particularly fast moving. My daughter had a partial match (my husband's sister as donor) stem cell transplant four months after she was diagnosed. Today, she is eight years post-transplant, is in the fourth grade, and is the absolute joy of my life.*

Who Gets JMML?

Approximately 50 children are diagnosed with JMML in the United States every year. JMML is usually found in children younger than age two and is more common in boys than girls. It is not known why children develop this type of cancer, but a strong link exists between JMML and certain genetic syndromes, such as neurofibromatosis type 1 and Noonan syndrome. About 85 to 90% of children with JMML have a mutation in one of the following genes in their leukemia cells:

- *PTPN11* (35% of children with JMML)
- *NRAS* or *KRAS* (25% of children with JMML)
- *CBL* (10–15% of children with JMML)
- *NF1* (10–15% of children with JMML)

In addition, some children with JMML are found to have other chromosomal abnormalities. For example, about 30% of children with JMML have a deletion on chromosome 7 (called monosomy 7).

Infants with Noonan syndrome sometimes develop a JMML-like disorder during the first year of life that usually disappears before 18 months of age without treatment. It is important to identify children with Noonan syndrome who have temporary JMML from children who have the type of JMML that is caused by *PTPN11* mutations in only the leukemia cells. When *PTPN11* mutations occur only in the leukemia cells, the disease can be very aggressive and will not go away without treatment.

Signs and Symptoms

Signs and symptoms of JMML can develop over weeks or months. The table below lists the most common signs and symptoms of children diagnosed JMML.

Signs and symptoms	Percentage of children with JMML
Enlarged spleen	93%
Swollen lymph nodes in the neck, underarm, or groin	76%
Pale skin	64%
Fever	54%
Skin rash	36%

Other possible signs and symptoms are:

- Sweating
- Recurrent infections
- Smooth coffee-colored marks on the skin
- Irritability
- Bruising or bleeding
- Diarrhea (sometimes bloody)
- Shortness of breath or wheezing
- Poor weight gain and failure to thrive

These signs and symptoms can also occur from bacterial or viral infections, so your child's doctors will rule those out while they wait for genetic mutation test results in the cancer cells.

> When my son Gregory was 20 months old he had rotavirus, so I was familiar with how he looked and acted when he was severely dehydrated. When he was 3 years old and became dehydrated, lethargic, and had some behavior changes, I took him straight to the pediatrician. He did nasal swabs, didn't identify the cause, and sent us to the emergency room for fluids. He didn't perk up like most kids do after getting fluids, so they did some blood tests and told us he either had a viral infection or leukemia. We were admitted and they did numerous tests for viral infections as well as a bone marrow aspiration. We learned it was some type of leukemia. The oncologist on duty had more than 30 years of experience, but he had only seen one child with JMML. But, that's what he thought it was. They sent the bone marrow cells to another institution for a second opinion, and the consensus was JMML.

The blood of children with JMML often contains the following:

- Low numbers of mature RBCs and platelets
- Higher than normal number of WBCs (usually around 33,000/μL)
- High number of immature monocytes and other WBCs
- Immature RBCs (called nucleated RBCs)

Diagnosis

JMML is difficult to diagnose and treat. A tentative diagnosis of JMML may be made after a physical examination of the child and microscopic analysis of a blood sample. But it is extremely important that your child be seen at a major pediatric medical center that uses a certified central laboratory to identify any mutations or chromosomal abnormalities in your child's cancer cells. Because JMML is rare and the signs and symptoms mimic other illnesses, diagnosis can be swift or very slow.

My son Jacob had been sick off and on and developed bruises and red spots on his hands and feet when he was seven months old. Just before his first birthday, he developed a golf-ball sized staph-infected lymph node in his neck that was surgically removed at the local hospital. Less than a week later he developed a staph infection in his foot where the IV had been. Shortly after that, he was hospitalized with Epstein-Barr virus, and they discovered an enlarged spleen and liver. He was transferred to a regional children's hospital, where they did a bone marrow aspiration and ruled out leukemia. Within two weeks we were sent back to that hospital for another bone marrow aspiration, and 15-month-old Jacob was diagnosed with JMML with a PTPN11 mutation.

To diagnose JMML, your child's doctor will first obtain a complete medical history, do a thorough physical exam, and order a number of different tests including:

• Blood smear to check for immature monocytes, other types of immature WBCs, and nucleated RBCs

• Complete blood count (CBC), which includes:

  – The number of RBCs and platelets

  – The number and type of WBCs

  – The amount of hemoglobin (the protein that carries oxygen) in the RBCs

    The portion of the blood sample made up of RBCs (hematocrit)

• Additional blood tests (e.g., blood chemistries and evaluation of liver and kidney function)

• Bone marrow aspiration to rule out other childhood leukemias and identify mutations in cancer cells

• Tests for certain viruses and bacteria that cause symptoms similar to those of JMML

These procedures and tests are described in Chapter 9, *Coping with Procedures* and Appendix A, *Blood Tests and What They Mean.*

My infant daughter Rayne started having episodes of vomiting and gastrointestinal distress when she was three months old. At six months old, she started projectile vomiting. Her doctor thought it was an allergy to formula, but no matter what we tried, she couldn't keep anything down. We took her to the ER and they gave her a lot of fluids and took labs. Two hours later, the director of the ER came in and told us that we needed to go by ambulance to the children's hospital because her WBC count was 68,000. At that hospital, they did a bone marrow aspiration but didn't find anything wrong so they sent us home with instructions to have weekly labs. During that time, her WBC count fluctuated between 70,000 and 90,000. After six weeks, we went in for a follow-up visit at the hospital and the hematologist said, "Good news! We have a diagnosis—JMML with a CBL germline mutation."

Prognosis

Prognosis is an estimate of the chance for cure, but it is primarily used to determine treatment. Some infants with JMML can survive for years, but others need immediate treatment to survive. Your child's doctors will consider all of the information obtained during the diagnostic process to determine a prognosis and treatment options (see the table below).

Characteristic	Factors that suggest a more favorable prognosis
Sex	Male
Age at diagnosis	<3 years
Platelet count at diagnosis	>33,000/µL
Other conditions	Noonan syndrome with *PTPN11*
Hemoglobin F	<15%
Blasts in blood	<20%
Absolute neutrophil count (ANC)	>1000/µL
Mutations	Certain *RAS* or *CBL* mutations

Treatment

Most children with JMML require intensive treatment, but some do not. For example, children with Noonan syndrome and those with *CBL* syndrome sometimes develop signs and symptoms of JMML, but the illness disappears with no treatment. Doctors will adopt a "watchful waiting" strategy if they think this is the case. Sometimes treatment is needed for these children to reduce problematic symptoms, such as an enlarged spleen or low red blood cell count. However, it is difficult to determine which children need immediate treatment and which children have this slow-growing (called indolent) form of JMML.

> *When my daughter Izzabella was a year old, she fell at my mother's house, hit her head, and briefly stopped breathing. We took her to the ER where they drew some blood and did an MRI. Her platelets came back low (30,000) so her pediatrician redid the labs the next day with the same result. We were referred to a pediatric hematologist who saw her a few times. Then Izzabella started to get bruises on her legs and nosebleeds that were hard to stop. Our pediatrician sent us to the closest children's hospital, where she was diagnosed with a blood disorder called ITP [idiopathic thrombocytopenic purpura]. She had labs drawn every three months for the next year and her platelets stayed low. At that point, they did a bone marrow aspiration (negative) and sent peripheral blood for genetic testing (showed JMML with*

the CBL mutation). Because this could disappear on its own, we are in a "watchful waiting" stage, and Izzabella has blood work done every three months.

Most of the time, however, children with JMML need treatment quickly. The only treatment that can cure JMML is an allogeneic stem cell transplant (SCT). This type of transplant uses cells from:

- The bone marrow of a matched or partially matched family member
- The bone marrow of a matched unrelated donor
- An umbilical cord

An allogeneic or cord blood transplant can cure about half of the children who receive it. Usually, any child with *PTPN11, KRAS,* or *NF1*-mutated JMML needs an SCT as soon as possible after diagnosis. Infants and children with *CBL* mutations, and few of those with *NRAS* mutations, may have a type of JMML that disappears without treatment. In this situation, the decision to transplant or not needs careful consideration and discussion.

Chemotherapy

Chemotherapy is the use of drugs to kill cancer cells. Chemotherapy does not cure JMML, but it may be used to (1) treat symptoms, (2) prepare for an SCT, and (3) prevent severe graft-versus-host disease after transplant. Chemotherapy drugs that are sometimes used to treat symptoms (usually while a stem cell donor is being located) are mercaptopurine, cytarabine, and 13-cis-retinoic acid. Sometimes chemotherapy is given to reduce the amount of disease prior to transplant.

All children undergoing a SCT for JMML receive high-dose chemotherapy to make room in their bone marrow for the donated stem cells. This is called "conditioning." The chemotherapy drugs destroy cancer cells in the body and help suppress the body's immune system to prevent rejection of donated stem cells. The drugs most often used to prepare for an SCT are some combination of busulfan, fludarabine, cyclophosphamide, and/or melphalan. No standard of care currently exists for which drugs to use for conditioning. Although total body irradiation was used in the past as part of conditioning, it is rarely used today because of the late effects it causes, especially in young children.

> *My 3-year-old son needed an SCT as soon as possible. His two siblings did not match, but we were able to find three exact matches on the registry. They chose a young woman in her early 20s, and the entire process went lightning fast. He was diagnosed on February 25 and had the transplant on June 11. His conditioning included cyclophosphamide, busulfan, melphalan, and a small dose of IV methotrexate. He did not get total body radiation.*

Drugs are used after SCT to prevent severe graft-versus-host disease—usually tacrolimus or cyclosporine and methotrexate. However, methotrexate is usually not used in children who had umbilical cord transplants. In the past, steroids were given after transplant, but now the drug mycophenolate mofetil is more commonly used to keep the body's immune system from attacking and rejecting the transplanted cells. This drug belongs to a class of medications called immunosuppressants. For information about the drugs discussed in this section, see Chapter 13, *Chemotherapy and Other Medications*.

Stem cell transplant

For children with JMML, stem cells are obtained from (1) a matched or partially matched family member, (2) matched unrelated donor, or (3) cord blood. The stem cells are given to a child through their venous catheter. Children are awake during this painless process. It generally takes two to four weeks for the stem cells to multiply and make new blood cells. After SCT, the relapse rate for children with JMML is 30 to 40%. Relapse often occurs within a few months after transplant, and the risk of relapse drops considerably one year after transplant. Children who relapse after transplant will frequently receive a second transplant. For more information, see Chapter 16, *Stem Cell Transplantation*.

> *Our son with JMML needed a transplant as soon as possible. While they searched for a donor, he was treated with 6-MP. We were lucky to find an unrelated donor who was a perfect match. We went to a major transplant center where he received nine days of conditioning with mephalan, cyclophosphamide, and busulfan. The transplant was in November 2015 and he relapsed in March 2016. We were lucky that our donor was willing to donate a second time. After a year away from home, we were able to return home. We found out just a month ago that he is in remission. His central line is finally out and he is doing all of the things little boys are supposed to do.*

Information on Current Treatments

Treatments for various types of childhood leukemia evolve and improve over time. The treatments for JMML described in this chapter were the ones most commonly used when this book was written. You can learn about the newest treatments available by calling the National Cancer Institute (NCI) at (800) 422-6237 and asking for information about JMML. This free information explains the disease, state-of-the-art treatments, and any ongoing clinical trials. Two versions are available:

- One for families, which uses simple language and contains no statistics; and
- One for health professionals, which is technical, thorough, and includes citations to scientific literature.

For accurate and up-to-date online information about JMML, visit the NCI website at *www.cancer.gov/types/myeloproliferative/patient/mds-mpd-treatment-pdq.*

It has been eight years since my son's successful stem cell transplant for JMML. He had his share of side effects and a few long-term effects, but he is doing fine now. It was a hard journey, but when I look back, it made all of us who we are today. The science behind my son's treatment changed my career—I'm now training to become a nurse. My two other children really suffered because I was focused on their little brother and basically disappeared for three years. We are just starting to unpack all of those emotions now with the help of good therapists. We all need a few more tools in our toolboxes. All of my kids are amazing! A friend of the family coined a phrase that I think captures how we feel: "We are the most fortunate of the least fortunate."

Chapter 6

Chronic Myelogenous Leukemia

*"I can be changed by what happens to me,
but I refuse to be reduced by it."*

— Maya Angelou

LEUKEMIA IS THE TERM USED to describe cancer of the bone marrow. This spongy material fills the bones in the body and produces blood cells. In a child with chronic myelogenous leukemia (CML), the bone marrow creates millions of cancerous white blood cells (WBCs). As the bone marrow becomes packed with these abnormal cells, they crowd out the healthy cells and symptoms of CML begin to develop.

CML is rare in children, accounting for less than 3% of all childhood leukemias. It is most often diagnosed in adolescents and is rarely found in children younger than age 6. This chapter describes CML and covers risk factors, signs and symptoms, diagnosis, prognosis, and treatment.

CML Is a Blood Disease

CML is cancer of WBCs that begins in the bone marrow (see Figure 6-1). When cancerous cells appear in the bone marrow, they multiply rapidly and begin to crowd out the normal cells, particularly red blood cells (RBCs). When this happens, anemia may occur. After accumulating in the bone marrow, cancerous WBCs spill over into the blood and invade other organs, such as the spleen.

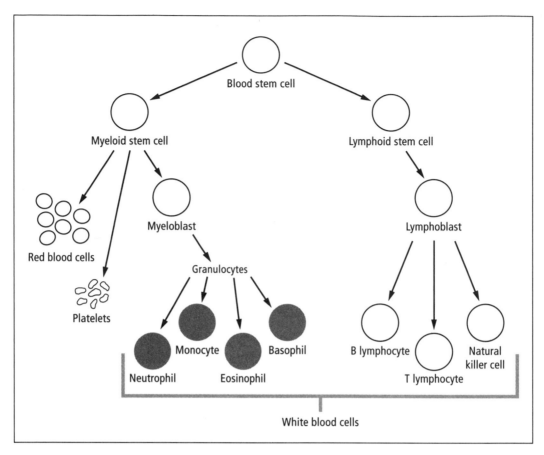

Figure 6-1: CML is a disease of myeloid cells

Who Gets CML?

Approximately 120 adolescents and children are diagnosed with CML in the United States every year. It is usually diagnosed in older children and adolescents and is found in equal numbers in males and females. This disease affects children of different races equally, unlike some of the other childhood leukemias (e.g., ALL is more common in Hispanic children).

> My 7-year-old daughter, Madison, was diagnosed with CML in 2010. Her pediatrician deserves a big pat on the back because he saved her life. She had always been thin, but her abdomen started to protrude. I took her in and her pediatrician said it might be constipation, but he would feel better if she had some blood work done. Her white blood cell count was over 500,000. He called and said, "You need to go to the hospital right now; she has leukemia." Looking back, I think she might have had low energy and maybe was pale, but our pediatrician did the right thing on the first visit and if I thanked him a hundred times, it would not be enough!

Doctors do not know why children develop this type of cancer, although adults who have been exposed to high levels of radiation (e.g., persons who have been treated with radiation for other illnesses) have an increased risk of developing CML years after the radiation exposure. However, few children or teens diagnosed with CML have been exposed to that amount of radiation.

Signs and Symptoms

CML develops over months or years, and there are usually no signs or symptoms in the early stages. It is sometimes discovered when a child or teen is having a routine blood test. If the disease is not found from a routine blood test, a child may develop some of the following signs and symptoms:

- Abdominal pain or feelings of fullness due to an enlarged spleen
- Swollen lymph nodes in the neck, underarm, stomach, or groin
- Pale skin
- Poor appetite
- Weight loss
- Fatigue or weakness
- Bruises
- Headaches
- Fevers
- Night sweats
- Bone and joint pain

Because CML is rare in children and these symptoms are common to many childhood illnesses, it's often hard to diagnose early. When a complete blood count (CBC) test is done, the following results are usually found in children with CML:

- High WBC count of mostly neutrophils and other types of WBCs
- High platelet count
- Low RBC count

When a child's WBC is extremely high at diagnosis, other signs and symptoms may be present, including:

- Rapid breathing
- Visual changes
- Hearing loss

- Hemorrhage of the retina
- Priapism (long-lasting and painful erection in males)

Diagnosis

If CML is suspected, it is extremely important that your child be evaluated and treated at a major pediatric medical center that uses a certified central laboratory to identify any mutations or chromosomal abnormalities in the cancer cells. Accurate identification of changes in the cancer cells determines the diagnosis and best treatment.

To diagnose CML, your child's pediatric oncologist will first obtain a complete medical history, do a thorough physical exam, and order many tests, including:

- A complete blood count, including:
  - The number and type of WBCs
  - The number of RBCs and platelets
  - The portion of the blood sample made up of RBCs (hematocrit)
- Additional blood tests (e.g., blood chemistries and evaluation of liver and kidney function)
- Bone marrow aspiration or biopsy to evaluate the cancer cells and confirm the diagnosis
- Genetic studies on the cancer cells

These procedures and tests are described in Chapter 9, *Coping with Procedures* and Appendix A, *Blood Tests and What They Mean*.

> *My daughter, Dana, was 9 years old when she had a stomachache that began in the middle of a soccer tournament. We took her to the doctor who examined her and ordered some routine blood work. They called us that day to say her white blood cell count was 65,000 and that she needed to come in right away for more tests. After the results came back, the doctor said that Dana probably had leukemia. Dana later told me, "Dad, that's the first time I've ever seen you cry." They started her on Gleevec®, we got another opinion from an expert across the country, then we just tried to make life as normal as possible. Fast forward 11 years, and Dana is in college, playing on the college soccer team, volunteers at the college radio station as a DJ, and is still taking Gleevec® every evening.*

In more than 90% of children with CML, analysis of cancer cells shows a genetic abnormality called the Philadelphia chromosome (see Figure 6-2). This chromosome contains a translocation (or swap) of genetic material involving chromosomes 9 and 22, called t(9;22). This rearrangement creates a new gene (called BCR-ABL) that codes for a protein that causes the cancerous cells to rapidly reproduce. These chromosome changes are not inherited from a parent—they happen during a person's lifetime.

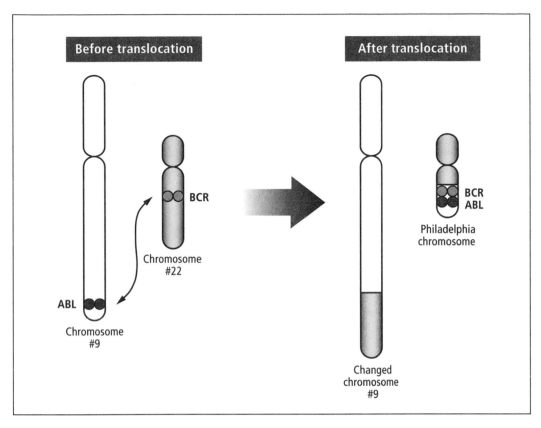

Figure 6-2: The Philadelphia chromosome

CML has three phases: 1) chronic phase, 2) accelerated phase, and 3) blast phase. The following table shows how your child's doctor will determine the phase of the disease.

Chronic Phase Must meet all of the following:	Accelerated Phase Must meet one or more of the following:	Blast Phase Must meet one or more of the following:
Documented t(9;22) or BCR-ABL fusion gene	Peripheral blood or bone marrow has 15% to 19% blasts	Blasts in peripheral blood or bone marrow >20%
Blasts in bone marrow <15%	Persistent low platelet count (<100,000) that is unrelated to therapy	Blast accumulation in organs other than the spleen
Does not meet any criteria for accelerated or blast phase	Increasing spleen size and WBC count despite treatment	Clusters of blasts found in bone marrow biopsy

Approximately 95% of children with CML are diagnosed in the chronic phase. If untreated, the chronic phase usually lasts about three to five years. With current treatments, the majority of children remain in remission for many years.

> My son was 3 years old when he was diagnosed with CML. We noticed that his abdomen was distended—sometimes it was hard and sometimes it was soft. First we were told it was constipation. Then we went to another doctor for an unrelated medical issue. He was concerned and ordered an ultrasound, which showed a very enlarged spleen and kidneys. They called and asked us to come back in for blood work the next day. So we went back in for that. That same night, after our son was asleep, they called and said to go to the children's hospital immediately because his white blood cell count was over 300,000.

Prognosis

Prognosis is an estimate of the chance for cure, but it is primarily used to determine treatment. The prognosis of a child with CML greatly depends on:

- Phase of disease at diagnosis
- Genetic abnormalities of the cancer cells
- The cancer's response to treatment with imatinib (Gleevec®) or another drug in the same family

A small percentage of children diagnosed during the chronic phase are found to have genetic abnormalities in addition to the Ph+ translocation. Many of these changes have no impact on prognosis, although children with an abnormality of chromosome 17 may have a slightly worse prognosis.

Tyrosine Kinase Inhibitors

The Philadelphia chromosome makes a protein called BCR-ABL that activates enzymes called tyrosine kinases, causing cells to divide uncontrollably. Drugs that specifically target this protein (e.g., imatinib) are called tyrosine kinase inhibitors (TKIs). Other drugs in the TKI family are:

- Dasatinib (Sprycel®)
- Nilotinib (Tasigna®)
- Bosutinib (Bosulif®)
- Ponatinib (Iclusig®)

TKIs are currently the first choice to treat CML. If your child is prescribed one of these drugs, make sure you understand that TKIs can interact with other drugs, over-the-counter medications, vitamins, herbal supplements, and even certain foods, such as grapefruit and pomegranate. They also can harm the fetus of a pregnant teen. Because drugs in the TKI family target a specific protein, they do not damage healthy cells like chemotherapy drugs do. Treatment with these drugs is called targeted therapy.

Treatment

Some children diagnosed with CML have extremely high WBC counts at diagnosis. Large numbers of WBCs can cause the blood to become thick and viscous, sometimes leading to problems such as tumor lysis syndrome (when large amounts of cancerous cells are rapidly killed by therapy, which can lead to kidney failure) or blockages in blood vessels in the brain. Therefore, children with extremely high WBC counts at diagnosis (>200,000) may be treated with the following:

- The chemotherapy drugs hydroxyurea or allopurinol.
- A process called leukapheresis, in which blood is taken from body, put through a machine to remove the WBCs, and then transfused back into the child's body.

> When we took Madison to the hospital after we learned she had a WBC count of over 500,000, they did a bone marrow aspiration that confirmed it was CML. The first thing they did was leukapheresis, which is a way to take blood out of the body, remove white cells, and put the blood back in the body. This is to reduce the number of white blood cells before giving treatment and to protect organs from side effects. She had both a femoral line in her groin and a line in her arm, so they took blood out of one, ran it through the machine to take out the white cells, then put the blood back in through the other line.

In the past, children and teens with CML were first treated with hydroxyurea, followed by interferon-alpha (sometimes with cytosine arabinoside added) and then an allogeneic stem cell transplant if a matched donor was available. But, the development of imatinib (Gleevec®) has revolutionized treatment for CML. Use of this drug has resulted in 80 to 90% of children diagnosed in the chronic phase entering and remaining in remission for many years.

> When my 7-year-old daughter was diagnosed with CML, they did leukapheresis, gave her two units of red blood cells, then started her on Gleevec® (300 mg) immediately. Within two weeks, her WBC count was cut in half. At 11 years old, they increased her dose to 450 mg a day. She had many of the usual side effects—her growth was slowed (went from 90th percentile in weight and height to the 25th) and she had some joint pain. Within four months of diagnosis, she was in a major molecular response.

Imatinib and other TKIs work differently than chemotherapy, because they specifically target the BCR-ABL protein and do not damage healthy cells. These drugs are usually very good at controlling CML for long periods of time and with far less severe side effects than chemotherapy drugs. However, they do not cure CML when used alone, and they must be taken every day. More information is available in Chapter 13, *Chemotherapy and Other Medications*. To monitor the effectiveness of the medication, a very sensitive test called PCR (polymerase chain reaction) is done periodically to measure the amount of BCR-ABL present. It is done on blood or bone marrow samples and can detect very small amounts of BCR-ABL.

> *Our son was one of the first kids put on Gleevec® at our children's hospital. It began to work right away, cutting his WBC count in half within a couple of weeks. He had several difficult side effects, such as foot and leg pain, a rash on his face, as well as nausea from the pills. We didn't feel heard about these side effects; his doctors thought the symptoms were unrelated because most adult patients do really well with these "easy" pills. We are members of a pediatric CML online support group, and we learned that these effects are quite common. For some kids, these side effects subside after a few months. But, seven years into treatment, our son still has considerable fatigue, nausea, and if he's been on his feet all day, the area behind his knees becomes painful.*

Currently, imatinib is the primary treatment used for children diagnosed with CML in the chronic phase. Doctors do not yet know when to stop treatment of children with imatinib; currently children remain on the drug indefinitely. If the drug stops working (or never worked well), the dose is increased or one of the second-line drugs from the same family (dasatinib, nilotinib, bosutinib, or ponatinib) is used. However, the long-term effects of these second-line targeted drugs are not known.

Treatment options for children or teens in the accelerated phase or in blast crisis are designed to eliminate as much disease as possible before doing a stem cell transplant (SCT). Treatments may include a targeted drug such as imatinib for accelerated phase, or a high-dose combination chemotherapy plus a targeted drug for blast crisis. For these children, treatment with chemotherapy and TKIs is most often followed by an SCT.

In the past, surgical removal of the spleen was part of CML treatment. This is no longer done because it significantly increases the risk of survivors developing life-threatening infections later in life. Radiation of the spleen is sometimes used if treatment with imatinib does not reduce the size of a very enlarged spleen.

At the present time, a SCT is the only known cure for children and teens with CML. But transplants can have severe and even life-threatening complications, and the short- and long-term toxicities are well known. Because targeted treatments (e.g., imatinib, dasatinib) can keep the disease at bay for years, the best use and timing of SCT for children with CML in the chronic phase is not known. SCT is generally reserved for children who do not respond well to targeted treatments, are unable to tolerate these drugs, or relapse on targeted therapy.

> Families of kids with CML live with a cloud of uncertainty over our heads. It isn't known how long Gleevec® and related medications work for kids. At the beginning, Tommy had bone marrow aspirations every three months, and his PCR results stayed low, but never reached zero. One year it went up quite a bit, and our team suggested that he take his Make-a-Wish® trip because he might need a stem cell transplant. But, luckily, they decided to watch and wait and the PCR result went back down and stayed there. His numbers fluctuate a bit but overall have remained stable. His sister is a perfect match should we ever have to go that route.

If targeted drugs are no longer working, high-dose chemotherapy with a SCT is sometimes suggested, especially if a matched donor is available. The types of transplant used to treat children with CML are:

- Syngeneic (from an identical twin)
- Allogeneic (from an HLA-identical sibling or a matched unrelated donor)
- Umbilical cord blood

Children and teens who receive imatinib before transplant have higher cure rates. Although the effect has not yet been studied, most transplant doctors give children imatinib for a year after transplant. More information about SCTs is available in Chapter 16, *Stem Cell Transplantation*.

> My daughter has never complained about her cancer and treatment. She never asked, "Why me?" I have tried hard not to let this define who she is. She is smart, demure, and quiet, and she lives her life like every other child. I didn't put her in a bubble and it was a good decision. It has changed who I am, however. I know who the people around me really are. People I was close to disappeared, but people I didn't know well stepped up and filled the gap. My children had a good life before the diagnosis of CML, but they have a great life now. We try hard to live life as normally as possible. When we have to go to the hospital for tests, we make a weekend of it. We go to a nice hotel, a Broadway show, and a fancy dinner. Girls' night out!

Information on Current Treatments

Treatments for various types of childhood leukemia evolve and improve over time. The treatments for CML described in this chapter were the ones most commonly used when this book was written. You can learn about the newest treatments available by calling the National Cancer Institute (NCI) at (800) 422-6237 and asking for information on childhood CML. This free information explains the disease, state-of-the-art treatments, and any ongoing clinical trials. Two versions are available:

- One for families, which uses simple language and contains no statistics; and
- One for health professionals, which is technical, thorough, and includes citations to scientific literature.

For accurate and up-to-date online information about CML, visit the NCI website at *www.cancer.gov/types/leukemia/patient/cml-treatment-pdq.*

My daughter has taken Gleevec® for 11 years. The first couple of years she had the normal side effects—nausea, rashes, headaches. Those gradually faded away so now, 11 years later, she only has a little rash and occasionally feels more tired than usual. But, her body seems to have adjusted so it has become much easier for her. That said, she only missed two days of school because of the CML and few people know she has cancer. She doesn't want to be treated differently than any other young woman. She's living a great life and has touched many people's lives. Because of the "magic bullet" Gleevec®, she was able to play varsity soccer throughout high school and now in college. One of our favorite 4-letter words is HOPE.

Chapter 7

Telling Your Child and Others

"To name things is to tame them."
— Tim O'Brien
Tomcat in Love

YOU HAVE JUST LEARNED your child has leukemia. There is so much to take in, so much to do, and all you really want to do is wake up and end this nightmare. But you are the only one who knows this news. What will you tell your sick child? And what can you say to your other children, or your parents? Should you tell your friends and neighbors? What can you possibly say?

Telling Your Child

Children and teens need age-appropriate information soon after diagnosis to create a supportive climate and help them begin to understand what is happening and feel comfortable asking questions. In the past, shielding children from the painful reality of cancer was the norm. Most experts now agree that children feel less anxiety and cope with treatments better if they are given age-appropriate explanations. Your child needs to know what is happening now and be prepared for what is to come. Because you are coping with a bewildering array of emotions yourself, sharing information and providing reassurance and hope may be difficult. Remember that sharing strengthens the family, allowing all members to face the crisis together.

When to tell your child

You should tell your child as soon as possible after diagnosis. Sick children know they are sick, and all children know when their parents are upset, frightened, and withholding information. In the absence of the truth, children imagine—and believe—scenarios far more frightening than the reality. It's nearly impossible for children to make sense of their new world without an explanation: they're in a strange place, none of their normal activities continue, strangers are performing scary and painful procedures on them, their parents are upset, and they see sick children everywhere they look. They may not talk about their fears, but they know something is very wrong.

> We felt we had to tell our 4-year-old daughter the truth from the very beginning. She needed to know that she could trust us. Talking about it helped her understand why the treatments were necessary. We told her that her hair would fall out, but that it would grow back. We told her when something would hurt and when it wouldn't. We told her we were all in this together and that we would discuss everything every step of the way.

The most loving thing a parent can do is to tell the truth before the child is overwhelmed by fear of what she has imagined. Staying silent has another side effect: it undermines the credibility of the parent with the child. This will be a long and frightening journey, and your child must believe you are in this together and that she can always count on you to support her and tell her the truth.

> We feel that you have to be very honest or the child will not be able to trust you. Meagan (5 years old) has always known that she has cancer and thinks of her treatments and medications as the warriors to help the good cells fight the bad cells.

Who should tell your child

You can decide who should first talk to your child about the cancer, based on his age, level of understanding, and whether you think your child would rather hear this news from you or the doctor. This conversation usually takes place in the hospital at a quiet time soon after diagnosis. Generally, you'll have time to talk with the medical team about the best way to explain the diagnosis to your child.

Some parents tell their child in private. Others prefer to have the treatment team (oncologist, nurse, social worker) present when explaining the diagnosis; this may help show that everyone is united in their efforts to help your child get well. Most children's hospitals have child life specialists who can help explain the diagnosis and treatment to young children in an age-appropriate way. Often, they use age-appropriate materials (e.g., books, pictures, dolls) to help with the conversation. Staff members can answer the child's questions and provide comfort for the entire family.

Children sometimes feel guilty and responsible for their illness. They may harbor fears that the cancer is a punishment for something they did wrong. Parents, social workers, psychologists, and child life specialists can help explore these concerns and provide reassurance.

> My 6-year-old son Brian was sitting next to me when the doctor called to tell me that he had cancer. I whispered into the phone, "What should I tell him?" The doctor said to tell him that he was sick and needed to go to a special children's hospital for help. As we were getting ready to go to the hospital, Brian asked if he was going to

die, and what were they going to do to him. We didn't know how to answer all the questions, but told him that we would find out at the hospital. My husband told him that he was a strong boy and we would all fight this thing together. I was at a loss for words. At the hospital, they were wonderful. What impressed me the most was that they always talked to Brian first, and answered all his questions before talking to us. When Zack (Brian's 8-year-old brother) came to the hospital two days later, the doctors took him in the hall and talked to him for a long time, explaining and answering his questions. I was glad that we were all so honest, because Brian later confided to me that he had first thought he got cancer because he hadn't been drinking enough milk.

Adolescents have a powerful need for control and autonomy that should be respected. At a time when most teens are becoming independent, teens with cancer are suddenly dependent on medical personnel to save their lives and on parents for emotional support. Teenagers sometimes feel more comfortable discussing the diagnosis with their physician in private. In some families, a diagnosis of cancer can force unwelcome dependence and add new stress to the already turbulent teen years. Other families report that the illness helped forge closer bonds between teenagers and their parents.

Children and teens react to a cancer diagnosis with a wide range of emotions, as do their parents. They may lapse into denial, feel tremendous anger or rage, or be extremely optimistic. As treatment progresses, both children and parents experience a variety of unexpected emotions.

We've really marveled as we watched Joseph go through the stages of coping with all of this just as an adult might. First of all, after he was diagnosed in April, he was terrified. Then for three months, he was alternately angry and depressed. When we talked to him seriously during that time about the need to work with the doctors and nurses against the cancer no matter how scary the things were that they asked him to do, he looked us right in the eye and screamed, "I'm on the cancer's side!" Over the course of a few weeks, he seemed to calm down and made the decision to fight it, cooperate with all the caregivers as well as he possibly could, and live as normal a life as he could. It's hard to believe that someone could do that at 4 years old, but he did it. By his 5th birthday in late July, he'd made the transition to where he is now: hopeful and committed to "killing the cancer."

What to tell your child

Children need to be told that they have leukemia and what that means, using words and concepts that are appropriate for their age and level of emotional development. The sooner they are comfortable with the word leukemia, and with the name of their disease, the less mysterious it will seem and the more powerful they will feel as they deal with it. Very young children might be satisfied to hear, "Leukemia is a disease that makes part of your blood sick, and we need to go to the hospital for medicine to make it better." Older children may benefit from reading books alone or with a parent, reading information on reliable internet sites, or asking members of the treatment team questions to get the information that matters most to them.

Older children and teens may have some knowledge of cancer, which might mean they will need a more detailed explanation of their cancer and how it is treated. They may also have a lot of worries, fears, and misconceptions. Providing them with encouragement and reasons to feel optimistic and empowered is as important as making sure they have accurate information.

> When my daughter went into the hospital to get the mediastinal mass diagnosis, I told her doctor if she got a bad report that I wanted him to tell her father and me and not give her any such news. Her doctor, who I had never met before this encounter, informed me that she was 15 years old and would be the one dealing with cancer and it was very necessary that she be told everything and that nothing be kept from her. I thought that was so mean of him, but I liked him and had never shown any disrespect for a doctor before, so I decided since he had dealt with kids with cancer before and I hadn't that he must know something I didn't know. He did! There have been so many times I have been so thankful that he had the wisdom to tell me that right off the bat.

It is important to share the name of the disease and an age-appropriate description of it with your child. Here are some other key concepts to talk about:

- No one knows what causes cancer, and it is not the child's fault she got sick.
- Some things about cancer are scary—for the child and the parents—and it is okay to feel afraid, confused, angry, or sad.
- It may be necessary to spend a lot of time in the hospital.
- There might be some unpleasant side effects, such as hair loss and nausea, but most of them are temporary.
- The parents, the child, and the healthcare team all have jobs to do to help the child get well, and everyone will work together to make that happen.
- Questions or worries are normal, and your child should feel free to ask a parent or someone on the healthcare team any questions she wants to ask.
- There are many things you as parents cannot control, but you will never lie to him and will always try to make sure there are no surprises.
- School-age children might not be able to go to school for a few months, but there are ways they can keep in touch with their classmates while they are out of school.
- Cancer is not contagious; friends and family cannot catch it, and your child did not catch it from anyone.
- Cancer is caused by cells that grow the wrong way, and it is no one's fault.

My 4-year-old daughter told me very sadly one day, "I wish that I hadn't fallen down and broken inside. That's how the cancer started." We had explained many times that nothing she did, or we did, caused the cancer, but she persisted in thinking that falling down did it. She also worried that if she went to her friend Krista's house to play that Krista would catch cancer.

· · · · ·

My daughter Kathleen Rea knew she had cancer when she was three. She knew that her motor oil wasn't running her engine right—but she called it cancer. Young children need to be reassured that they did nothing to cause the disease. It is important that they understand the disease is not contagious and they cannot give it to their siblings or friends. They need to have procedures described realistically, so that they can trust their parents and medical team.

Children will have many questions throughout their treatment. Parents must assure their child that this is normal and that they will always answer the child's questions honestly. Gentle and honest communication is essential for the child to feel loved, supported, and encouraged.

When I told Christine (3 years old) that she had a disease in her blood, I told her I would always be with her, and that I would make sure that there were never any surprises. (This is difficult sometimes in the hospital setting, but it can be done.) She is very artistic and wanted me to draw a picture of the cells that were a problem. We drew lots of pictures of white cells being carried off by chemo drugs to be "fixed." Although many of the other parents successfully used images of good cells killing off bad cells, I thought that would upset my extremely gentle daughter. So we imagined, drew pictures, and talked about chemo turning problem cells into helpful cells.

When your child asks a question, take a moment to be sure you heard and understood it correctly, and then formulate a thoughtful answer your child will understand. Parents are under tremendous stress and have many things on their minds. In this distracted state, it is easy to toss off a superficial answer or answer a question the child did not ask; but doing so can increase the child's confusion and undermine trust in the parent as a source of information. Barbara Sourkes, PhD, explains the importance of understanding the child's question before responding:

Coping with the trauma of illness can be facilitated by a cognitive understanding of the disease and its treatment. For this reason, the presentation of accurate information in developmentally meaningful terms is crucial. A general guideline is to follow the child's lead: he or she questions facts or implications only when ready, and that readiness must be respected. It is the adult's responsibility to clarify the precise intent of any question and then to proceed with a step-by-step response, thereby granting the child options at each juncture. He or she may choose to continue listening, to ask for clarification, or to terminate the discussion. Offering less information with the explicit invitation to ask for more affords a safety gauge of control for the child. When these guidelines are not followed, serious miscommunications may ensue. For example, an adult who hears "What is going to happen to me?" and does not clarify the intent of the query may launch into a long statement of plans or elaborate reassurances. The child may respond with irritation, "I only wanted to know what tests I am going to have tomorrow."

Telling the Siblings

The diagnosis of cancer is traumatic for siblings. Family life is disrupted, their time with parents decreases, and the ill child receives a lot of attention. Older children and teens who understand the seriousness of a cancer diagnosis will be worried and fearful, but may hesitate to burden their parents with their concerns. Brothers and sisters need as much knowledge about what is going on as their sick sibling does. Information provided should be age appropriate, and all questions should be answered honestly.

Healthcare providers (e.g., physicians, physician assistants, nurse practitioners, child life specialists, and social workers) can help parents educate the siblings. Brothers and sisters can be extremely cooperative if they understand the changes that will occur in the family, and their role in helping the family cope. Maintaining open communication and respecting their feelings helps siblings feel loved and secure.

> *We always, always explained everything that was happening to Brian's older brother (8 years old). He never asked questions, but always listened intently. He would say, "Okay. I understand. Everything's all right." We tried to get him to talk about it, but through all these years, he just never has. So we just kept explaining things at a level that he could understand, and he has done very well through the whole ordeal. The times that he seemed sad, we would take him out of school and let him stay at the Ronald McDonald House with his brother and one parent (we alternated parents—one at the Ronald McDonald House and one at home) for a few days, and that seemed to help him.*

· · · · ·

We have tried to spend one-on-one time with each of the other kids. These are some other things that have been good for us:

- *The kids have been going to the hospital with Ethan one at a time, and getting a sense that this is no picnic, what he is going through.*

- *If one of us is out of town and Ethan is in the hospital, I have hired a babysitter to be with him in the evening and have done something special with the other kids for one of the nights. This works great if you live close enough to the hospital where your child is being treated.*

- *My husband and I have each taken the older kids on the traditional summer trips. This has been hard on Ethan, but none of this is perfect.*

- *My husband and I have each taken one school subject for the kids and have really spent time with them on it. I did reading with Tucker (I read everything he does and we talk about it), French with Abe, and Spanish with Jake. My husband has different topics, and we do something every day. We were too dysfunctional to be able to do more than one subject, so we decided to focus, and it has been a lot of fun for us.*

We talk about lots of things as a family and help the kids as needed, but these are "special" things. This has been a long year for us, but I think these things helped.

Even with good communication and support, parents may see siblings struggling with tough emotions that may lead to behavioral changes, such as regression, school problems, and trouble sleeping. Chapter 17, *Siblings*, explores sibling issues in detail and includes many suggestions from both parents and siblings who have gone through this experience.

Notifying the Family

Notifying relatives is one of the first painful jobs for parents of a child newly diagnosed with leukemia. Depending on the family dynamic, the family may be a refuge or a source of additional stress.

I called my mom and asked her to tell everyone on my side of the family. My husband called his sister and asked her to tell everyone. We asked that they not call us for a few days because we needed a little time to feel less fragile and didn't want to cry in front of Christine too much.

· · · · ·

I called my sister and asked her to take care of telling everyone. She called my other sister, and together they told my frail mother.

· · · · ·

I waited three days after the diagnosis to call anyone. The doctors had trouble determining whether it was ALL or AML, and I wanted to be able to give the prognosis on the first call.

Family members often react in surprising ways, with unexpected help coming from some people and a disappointing lack of support from others. Parents must be prepared for these unexpected responses and try not to take them personally. Usually, the other person is struggling to process this difficult news in his or her own way and may be trying to spare the parent from more stress by not asking too many questions.

My dad had always been my rock, but when I told him about my son's illness, he basically didn't say anything and he never came to the hospital. I was furious with him. It took me a long time to realize that he needed me to be strong for him, too. He was just devastated by the thought that his only grandchild might be taken from him and that there was nothing he could do to stop it.

Notifying Friends and Neighbors

The easiest way to notify friends and neighbors is to delegate one person to do the job. Most parents are at their child's bedside and want to avoid more emotional upheaval, especially in front of their child. Parents need to recognize that friends' emotions will mirror their own: shock, fear, worry, helplessness. Because most friends want to help but don't know what to do or say, they will welcome any suggestions you can give about what might be helpful (e.g., whether you want phone calls or cards). The more clarity you can provide, the less stress you will experience and the better your friends can support you. If you want visitors, for example, let people know when visiting hours are and whether there are any restrictions set by the hospital (or by you or your child) about who can come and how long they can stay.

There were many days I wanted to hide in bed and pull the covers over my head. I know everyone meant well and genuinely cared, but the constant stream of people through the house and phone ringing added to the stress we were already under. We already had a home care nurse coming five days a week, a physical therapist coming three days a week, in addition to constant phone calls to follow up on blood work and tests, appointments to schedule, and family members to keep track of. Bubba, our dog, loved all the commotion, but the rest of us tired quickly.

Not everyone you know will want or need the same level of detailed information. You may wish to encourage hospital or home visits from your closest friends, but ask others to wait for phone or email updates. However, think twice before leaving anyone off the notification list. Many parents report that people they barely knew ended up being some of their most helpful and supportive resources.

It can be helpful to choose a trusted friend or family member to provide information via email, text messages, or social media so you're not exhausted with repeated phone calls and messages and can focus on your child. You may want to create a dedicated Facebook page that you and your "social director" control, where either of you can post updates and photos. This makes sharing information simple and quick. Consider making it a private page that can only be read and commented on by people you allow, giving you more control over your family's privacy. There are also online services such as *www.CaringBridge.com, www.CarePages.com,* and *www.LotsaHelpingHands.com* that you can use to update friends, family, and supporters, and enlist help with meals, sibling child care, fundraisers, and other tasks. More information is available in Chapter 18, *Family and Friends*.

Notifying Your Child's School

You should notify the principal as soon as possible about your child's diagnosis. It is a good idea to do this in writing; an example of a notification letter is contained in Chapter 20, *School*. You can also express your hope that you, the school, and the hospital will work together to ensure that your child's education has as few interruptions as possible. You may wish to ask the principal to share your letter with the teacher (or multiple teachers) or you can send a separate note. If you want to ask the teacher(s) and students to stay in touch with your child, inform them that she may sometimes feel too tired to answer right away. Personal visits may not be feasible or welcome, at least at first, but cards, letters, pictures, classroom videos, or other updates will make your child feel less isolated and will remind him that there are people who care for him at school. The wishes of teens about notification of school and friends should be respected. Much more information is available in Chapter 20, *School*.

When I was diagnosed with leukemia, I felt like I was trapped in a room with no windows or doors, and the walls were closing in on me. I thought that I would never be able to smell my grandmother's hand cream, or feel the way my dad's face felt in the morning before he shaves, or the way my mom's silk blouse feels when I hug her. I thought that I would never have the sensation of turning one year older again. I thought that I would never again be able to feel how I feel after it rains, when it smells so fresh and clean like the whole world just took a bath. I thought that I would never be able to taste my first glass of champagne on New Year's and feel all bubbly and warm like I was flying in a hot-air balloon. And all of a sudden my dream popped, and I realized that this wasn't a dream, it was reality.

Right now, there are thousands of kids like me across the country who are feeling the same way I felt eight years ago, and I would just like to wish them good luck. Because it's a long, hard journey full of needles, blood tests, and chemotherapy, but when you finally get to the end, you feel like you've been freed after years and years of darkness, and I'll tell you one thing—that is the greatest feeling you could have.

Chapter 8

Choosing a Treatment

*"The challenge remains clear: to strive for the cure
and health of all children through the development of more
effective yet less damaging treatment for our young patients."*

— Daniel M. Green, MD, and Giulio J. D'Angio, MD

THE FIRST FEW WEEKS AFTER DIAGNOSIS are utterly overwhelming. In the midst of confusion, fear, and fatigue, you might need to make an important and sometimes difficult decision: whether to choose the best-known treatment (standard treatment) or enroll your child in an experimental treatment (clinical trial). This chapter explains helpful things to know before deciding on a treatment for your child, including the difference between standard treatment and clinical trials. It also covers questions to ask, informed consent, and stories from parents about the decisions they made.

Treatment Basics

To receive the best available treatment, it is essential that a child with leukemia be treated at a pediatric medical center by board-certified pediatric oncologists with extensive experience treating your child's type of leukemia. For most children, treatment begins within days (sometimes hours) of diagnosis and requires aggressive supportive care. The goal of treatment is to achieve complete remission by killing all cancer cells as quickly as possible.

Treatment of childhood leukemia includes one or more of the following:

- Chemotherapy and other medications (see Chapter 13)
- Radiation therapy (see Chapter 15)
- Stem cell transplantation (see Chapter 16)

Treatment for children with leukemia begins with a course of chemotherapy, usually involving several different drugs in carefully controlled combinations. For most children, the only treatment is chemotherapy that lasts for many months or years. For certain leukemias, a stem cell transplant is done after one or more courses of chemotherapy. Doctors try to avoid radiation therapy because of the potential for permanent damage. Radiation is normally used only when leukemia cells are found in the cerebrospinal fluid or testes at diagnosis, if the child is at very high risk of central nervous system relapse, or prior to a stem cell transplant (SCT).

Standard Treatment

The standard treatment (also sometimes called the standard of care) for each type of leukemia is the treatment that has worked best for the most children up to that point in time. The current standard treatments are the result of decades of clinical research studies. As researchers analyze the results from ongoing or completed clinical trials, they accumulate knowledge and make changes in standard treatments. In the 1980s, for example, most children with acute lymphoblastic leukemia (ALL) received cranial radiation as standard treatment. Carefully controlled clinical trials later showed that most children with ALL do not require cranial radiation, and even those who do can be given a lower dose than was used in the 1980s. As a result, the standard treatment for children with ALL was changed.

To learn about the standard treatment for your child's type of leukemia, contact the National Cancer Institute at (800) 422-6237 or go to the pediatric section of its website at *www.cancer.gov/cancertopics/pdq/pediatrictreatment*. The NCI provides accurate information about childhood leukemias, state-of-the-art treatments, and ongoing clinical trials. Two versions are available online:

- One for families, which uses simple language and contains no statistics; and

- One for professionals, which is technical, thorough, and includes citations to scientific literature.

The standard treatments for each type of leukemia are covered in the following chapters:

- Chapter 3, *Acute Lymphoblastic Leukemia*
- Chapter 4, *Acute Myeloid Leukemia*
- Chapter 5, *Juvenile Myelomonocytic Leukemia*
- Chapter 6, *Chronic Myelogenous Leukemia*

The Protocol

If your child receives the standard treatment, you will be given a written copy of the treatment plan, called a protocol. Just like a recipe for baking a cake, a protocol has a list of ingredients, the amounts to use, and the order to use them in for the best chance for success. The protocol lists the treatments, drugs, dosages, and tests for each segment of treatment and for follow-up care.

The portion of the protocol devoted to the schedule for treatments and tests may be quite long. The family may also be given an abbreviated version (one to two pages) for quick reference on a daily basis. This shortened part of the protocol is often called the "roadmap." Parents and teenage patients should review these documents carefully with the treatment team to ensure they understand them.

> *It took me a long time to get over my hang-up that things needed to go exactly as per protocol. Any deviations on dose or days were a major stress for me. It took talking to many parents, as well as doctors and nurses, to realize and feel comfortable with the fact that no one ever goes along perfectly and that the protocol is meant as the broad guideline. There will always be times when your child will be off drugs or on half dose because of illness or low counts or whatever. It took a long time to realize that this is not going to ruin the effectiveness, that the child gets what she can handle without causing undue harm.*

Clinical Trials

If a clinical trial is open for your child's particular type and risk level of leukemia, within days of diagnosis you will be asked to consider enrolling your child in it. You then must choose between standard treatment and the clinical trial.

Clinical trials are carefully controlled research experiments that use human volunteers to develop better ways to prevent or cure diseases. Pediatric clinical trials attempt to improve existing treatments. A clinical trial can involve a totally new approach that seems promising, or it may fine-tune existing treatments by reducing their toxicity or developing new ways to assess responses to treatment. Many children are needed in each clinical trial for the results to be statistically meaningful.

Sometimes, parents choose to enroll their child in a clinical trial because they want to contribute to better treatments in the future. Other parents may be wary of participating in an experimental program and may opt for standard treatment. There is no right choice. Obtain all the information you can, weigh the pros and cons, and make a decision based on your values and comfort level.

> *The study that our institution was participating in at the time of my daughter's diagnosis was attempting to lessen the treatment to reduce toxicity yet still cure the disease. My family began a massive research effort on the issue, and we had several family friends who were physicians discuss the case with the heads of pediatric oncology at their institutions. The consensus was that since my daughter was at the high end of the high-risk description, it was advisable to choose the standard treatment, which was more aggressive than one of the parts of the proposed clinical trial.*

Your treatment team may also tell you about studies that are sponsored by pharmaceutical companies, especially those designed to help with the side effects of treatment. Such supportive care trials evaluate antibiotics, antinausea drugs, and new agents to raise blood counts, minimize pain, or control other symptoms. The oversight and control of these trials is entirely different than the oncology treatment studies discussed in this chapter. Ask your doctor or nurse to discuss these studies with you if your child is invited to participate in one.

Types of clinical trials

The three main types of clinical trials for children with leukemia are described below.

Phase I. If laboratory evidence suggests a drug might work in humans, it is first tested in a Phase I study. These studies:

- Examine how the body processes (metabolizes) the drug
- Establish the highest dose that can safely be given (the maximum tolerated dose, or MTD)
- Evaluate side effects

In pediatric Phase I trials, the dose of a new drug is gradually increased in small groups of children until it becomes too toxic; essentially, one small group of children gets a low dose, the next small group gets a slightly higher dose, and so on, until an unacceptable number of children experience unacceptable side effects.

Phase I studies are experiments, and their purpose is not to cure the participants. The true beneficiaries of Phase I studies are future patients. In most cases, parents are not asked to enroll their child in a Phase I study unless all other treatment options have failed. Parents often enroll their children in these trials in the hope that a new and untried drug will be effective against their child's disease, but they need to recognize that the chances of that are low.

Phase II. Phase II trials test new drugs to see whether they are effective for specific diseases. This is the stage at which many drugs fail—meaning they are not as effective as originally predicted or they have unexpected or serious side effects.

Phase III. These clinical trials determine whether a new treatment is better or worse than the standard therapy. Some Phase III trials are designed solely to improve survival; others are done to try to maintain survival rates while lowering the toxicity of treatment. In pediatric Phase III studies, some children will receive the standard therapy, while others receive the experimental treatment. Some children will derive direct benefit if a new treatment is superior to the standard therapy; other children might be on an experimental therapy that is later learned to not be as effective as the standard therapy.

To ensure the results are accurate, Phase III studies require hundreds to thousands of participants and take several years to complete.

The National Cancer Institute (NCI) offers several resources to help parents understand the clinical trial process. You can call the NCI at (800) 422-6237 or visit its clinical trials website at *www.cancer.gov/clinical_trials*.

The information in the rest of this chapter pertains to Phase III trials that are reviewed and funded by the NCI. Enrolling in Phase I and Phase II trials is very different, as is enrolling in trials sponsored by pharmaceutical companies.

Design of clinical trials

In 2000, four pediatric cancer research groups merged to form a single pediatric cancer research organization called the Children's Oncology Group (COG), which is supported by the NCI. Approximately 230 institutions that treat children with cancer are members of COG (*www.childrensoncologygroup.org*). Researchers from these institutions contribute to the design of new clinical trials for children with cancer. In addition, the NCI and some large children's hospitals design their own clinical trials for children. When designing pediatric clinical trials, the first priority is to protect the children from harm. Researchers are ethically bound to offer treatments they think will be at least as safe and effective as the standard treatment.

Study arms

Phase III clinical trials sort participants into different groups that receive different treatments (called arms). Every Phase III trial has one arm that is the current standard treatment, called the standard arm. Each of the other arms contains one or more experimental components, such as the following:

- New drugs
- Old drugs used in a new way (e.g., different dose or new combinations of old drugs)
- Duration of treatment that is shorter or longer than standard treatment
- The addition, deletion, or change in dose or timing of certain treatments (e.g., radiation therapy)
- The use of new supportive care interventions (e.g., preventative antibiotics or new drugs to control nausea)

Once the trial is complete, the effectiveness of each experimental arm is compared to the standard arm.

Randomization

Phase III trials require a process called randomization, meaning that after parents agree to enroll their child in a clinical trial, a computer randomly assigns the child to one arm of the study. The parents (and the doctors) will not know which treatment their child will receive until the computer assigns one. The purpose of computer assignment is to ensure that children are evenly assigned to each arm without bias from doctors or families. One group of children (the control group) always receives the standard treatment to provide a basis for comparison to the experimental arms. At the time the clinical trial is designed, there is no conclusive evidence to indicate which arm will be superior. As a result, it is impossible to predict whether your child will benefit from participating in the study.

> We had a hard time deciding whether to go with the standard treatment or to participate in the study. The "B" arm of the study seemed, on intuition, to be too harsh for her because she was so weak at the time. We finally did opt for the study, hoping we wouldn't be randomized to "B." We chose the study basically so that the computer could choose and we wouldn't ever have to think "we should have gone with the study." As it turned out, we were randomized to the standard arm, so we got what we wanted while still participating in the study.

> • • • • •

> We decided not to participate in a study for several reasons. One arm would require extra spinal taps, and our son was just so little that we couldn't bear the thought of any more treatments than were required in the standard arm. Another arm contained a second induction, and since we were on Medicaid, we just didn't feel it was right for the taxpayers to pay for anything extra. We felt we were only entitled to basic healthcare.

Researchers closely monitor each ongoing clinical trial and modify it if one arm is identified as superior during the course of the trial or if an arm has unacceptable side effects.

Supervision of clinical trials

The ethical and legal codes governing medical practice also apply to clinical trials. In addition, most research is federally funded or regulated and has rules that protect patients. For example, all COG trials are federally funded and have review boards that meet at prearranged dates for the duration of each trial to ensure the risks of the trial are acceptable relative to the benefits.

The treating institution is required to report all adverse side effects to COG, which reports them to the U.S. Food and Drug Administration. If concerns are raised, the study may be put on hold while an independent Data Safety and Monitoring Board and the study committee review the situation. If one arm of the trial is causing unacceptable side effects, that arm is stopped, and the children enrolled are given the better treatment.

All institutions that conduct clinical trials have an Institutional Review Board (IRB)—made up of scientists, doctors, nurses, and citizens from the community—that reviews and approves all research taking place there. The purpose of the IRB is to protect patients. Funding agencies (e.g., National Cancer Institute) also review and approve trials before children are enrolled.

Questions to ask about clinical trials

To fully understand the clinical trial proposed for your child, here are some important questions to ask the oncologist:

- What is the purpose of the study?
- Who is sponsoring the study? Who monitors patient safety?
- What tests and treatments will be done during the study? How do these differ from standard treatment?
- What are the possible benefits?
- What are the possible disadvantages?
- What are the possible side effects of the study compared to those of standard treatment?
- What are the possible long-term impacts of the study compared with the standard treatment?
- Will the study require more hospitalizations than standard treatment?
- Does the study include long-term follow-up?
- Will you compare the study versus standard treatment in terms of possible outcomes, side effects, time involved, costs, and quality of life?
- Will our insurance cover the costs of the clinical trial?

After discussing the clinical trial with the team, you will need a copy of the information to review later. Many parents record the conversations or bring a friend to take notes; others write down all the doctor's answers for later reference.

> *A clinical trial involving very high-dose chemotherapy followed by stem cell transplant was proposed for our 2-year-old daughter. We asked numerous questions, and I wrote down all the answers in my notebook. The two primary questions were: How many kids die during and after this treatment? Are her chances of long-term survival worth the pain we were going to put her through? We struggled with the concept of hurting her if it wasn't going to do any good. We also asked about the specific drugs, their side effects, and what to expect from each treatment. It was a very difficult process and decision.*

Things to consider about clinical trials

Deciding whether to enroll your child in a clinical trial is often difficult. The following lists describe why some families choose to enroll and why others choose not to enroll. These lists may help clarify your feelings about this important decision.

Why some families choose to enroll:

- Children receive either state-of-the-art investigational therapy or the standard therapy.
- Clinical trials can provide the chance to benefit from a new therapy before it is widely available.
- Children enrolled in clinical trials may be monitored more frequently throughout treatment.
- Review boards of scientists oversee clinical trials.
- Participating in a clinical trial often makes parents feel they did everything medically possible for their child.
- Information gained from clinical trials will benefit children with cancer in the future.

Reasons why families choose not to enroll:

- The experimental arm may not provide treatment that is as effective as the standard therapy, or it may cause additional side effects or risks.
- Some families do not like the feeling of not having control over choosing the child's treatment.
- Some clinical trials require more hospitalizations, treatments, clinic visits, or tests that may be more painful than the standard treatment.
- Some families feel additional stress about which arm is the best treatment for their child.
- Insurance may not cover investigational studies. Parents need to carefully explore this issue prior to signing the consent form.

Making a Decision

As soon as possible after diagnosis, parents and older children sit down with the medical team to discuss treatment options. If your child is being treated at a COG hospital, the first discussion is usually about standard treatment and a clinical trial (if a trial is open and your child qualifies). Parents are sometimes very conflicted about choosing a treatment.

The choice to opt for standard treatment or a clinical trial is a strictly personal one, but parents should only make it after they are certain they understand the implications of each path. The treatment team is legally and ethically bound to inform parents of the full range of appropriate treatment options available to their child, and to help them understand what each option entails before asking them for written consent to begin a particular treatment plan. Members of the treatment team may not coerce or deceive the parents into choosing a treatment. Once the parents have consented to standard treatment or a clinical trial, the doctor must abide by their decision.

Informed consent process

Before a child is enrolled in a clinical trial, the parents need to sign an informed consent form. True informed consent is a process, not merely an explanation and signing of documents. Informed consent requires that:

- All treatments available to the child have been explained—not just the treatment available at your hospital or through your doctor, but all the treatments that could be beneficial, wherever they are given.
- All treatment options are thoroughly discussed, with all the possible benefits and risks clearly explained.
- The parents and, to the extent possible, the child, have discussed these options and chosen the treatment they want.
- Aspects of the study that are considered experimental and those that are standard are clearly described.

An informed medical decision is one that weighs the relative merits of a therapy after full disclosure of benefits, risks, and alternatives. During the discussions between the medical team and family, all questions should be answered in language that is clearly understood by the parents and child or teen, and there should be no pressure on parents to enroll their child in a study. The objective of the informed consent process is that all family members understand their options, are comfortable with their choice, and can comply with it. Studies show that the more questions parents ask during the informed consent process, the better they understand what they are agreeing to.

> We had many discussions with the staff prior to signing the informed consent to participate in the clinical trial. We asked innumerable questions, all of which were answered in a frank and honest manner. We felt that participating gave our child the best chance for a cure, and we felt good about increasing the knowledge that would help other children later.

Informed consent is a process that occurs over several meetings. During the meetings, the pediatric oncologist and sometimes other members of the treatment team provide information and the parents ask questions (and get answers). However, the informed consent process does not always work as it should for a variety of reasons, including the parents' state of mind, the communication style of the doctor, and the system in place to discuss treatment options. Most often, this situation is the result of miscommunication arising from some combination of the following:

- No formal meeting times were set in advance to discuss treatment options, so parents didn't understand the importance of the discussion they were having with the doctor and the treatment team.
- Parents, who are tired, confused, and mentally numb, appear to understand things they are barely hearing.
- The doctor does not recognize that the parents aren't following what he is saying and that they need more guidance and time to absorb the choices.
- The doctor is unconsciously promoting the choice she believes is the best one and she interprets the lack of questions as agreement.
- There is no one in the room except the doctor and the parents; therefore, there is no one to help with communication.

Parents may want to invite a trusted friend or their child's pediatrician to attend the informed consent meetings to ensure they understand their options. These people can be physically present, on the telephone, or can use software such as Skype®.

> When my son was diagnosed, we were told we had two options: a clinical trial or standard treatment. We decided to get a second opinion before making our decision. Our pediatrician, my husband, and I met in the pediatrician's office for a telephone conference with a pediatric oncologist from a major treatment center. We each presented our concerns. Our pediatrician thought of some issues neither my husband nor I had considered. I think we all came away better informed of our options.

Some families seek a second opinion to help sort out their options. It is most useful to get a second opinion from a center that treats significant numbers of children with your child's diagnosis. Most pediatric oncologists are willing to arrange the second opinion for you.

> My son Justin was diagnosed with standard risk B-cell ALL when he was 8 years old. We were at a small hospital with one oncologist who had just completed her residency. We were offered standard treatment or ALL0331, a COG phase III trial that had one standard arm and three experimental arms. We consulted with ped-onc staff at a large and respected children's hospital in another state, and they said those were the same options they offered their families in similar circumstances, so we signed up. We were randomized to one of the experimental arms—same induction but an intensification with an additional medication.

Studies have shown that when treatment team members who are not doctors are present during the informed consent meetings, parents have a better understanding of their choices. You may want to ask for a nurse or a social worker to be present during the meetings.

Two days after my child was diagnosed, the oncologist told me it was time to begin treatment. I do remember him talking a lot, but I swear it actually sounded like "Wah, wah, wah, protocol, wah, wah, wah, very successful, wah, wah, wah, sign here." And I did. It was several days before it sank in that I had authorized an experimental treatment protocol and not the standard treatment. The irony is that I worked in clinical research. I knew how this was supposed to go. But I was alone and tired and frightened and went along like a sheep. In the end it was my responsibility to hold it together and ask what needed to be asked. But it just wasn't in me at the time. Later, I told the doctor this and he was astonished to learn that I hadn't heard a word he said.

Assent

Assent means that children and adolescents are involved in decisions about their treatment. Children younger than age 18 do not have the legal right to refuse standard treatment for their cancer. They do, however, have the right to participate in decisions about experimental treatments. All clinical trials are considered experimental treatments. Regardless of whether children will receive the standard treatment or an experimental treatment, they have the right to have the disease, treatment, and procedures explained to them at an age-appropriate level.

Doctors and parents are required to allow children to make their wishes known about their treatment. According to the American Academy of Pediatrics (AAP), assent means that the child:

- Is aware of the nature of his or her disease
- Understands what to expect from tests and treatments
- Has had his or her understanding assessed
- Has had an opportunity to accept or reject the proposed treatment

Parents can read or download a copy of the AAP policy statement ("Informed Consent, Parental Permission, and Assent in Pediatric Practice") from the AAP website. In part, the policy states, "In situations in which the patient will have to receive medical care despite his or her objection, the patient should be told that fact and should not be deceived." This policy applies to standard treatment.

Clinical trials, however, are research, and IRBs decide whether the child's assent is needed. If parents and the child or teen disagree about treatment, discussions are usually held with a mediator (for example, a social worker or pediatric psychologist) to try to reach an agreement. If parents and their child or teen still disagree, an advocate for the child is appointed and a decision about treatment is made by the hospital ethics committee.

In short, parents can legally make decisions about standard care, but both parents and children have decision-making rights about whether or not to participate in clinical trials.

Saying no to a clinical trial

Parents, children, and teens have the legal right to decide whether or not to participate in a clinical trial. If the family chooses for the child not to participate in the proposed clinical trial, or if their insurance refuses to pay for the treatments given in the clinical trial, the child or teen is given the best-known treatment (standard treatment) for his type of leukemia.

> We just were not comfortable with the concept of a clinical trial. It seemed like gambling to us. We also felt totally overwhelmed about making decisions on important subjects that we didn't understand. Even though we asked many, many questions, we just couldn't come to grips with the whole idea in the two days after our daughter was diagnosed. So, we declined the trial and had the best known treatment. We are happy with our decision.

Saying yes to a clinical trial

If you decide to enroll your child in a clinical trial, the form you sign will have language similar to the following: "The study described above has been explained to me, and I voluntarily agree to have my child participate in this study. I have had all of my questions answered, and understand that all future questions that I have about this research will be answered by the investigators listed above." It is a good idea to keep a copy of the signed form.

> Sean missed the deadline for enrolling in a clinical trial when he was diagnosed. However, when his cancer returned, we did enroll him on a trial. The particular trial he was in was a randomized computer trial that decided if he was getting one or two extra chemotherapy agents. We felt if we enrolled him in the trial, maybe the results would help other children.

Removing your child from a clinical trial

Parents have the legal right to withdraw their child from a clinical trial at any time, for any reason. But before doing so, it's a good idea to discuss questions or concerns with your child's oncologist. The decision to withdraw from a trial should not be held against the parent, and the child will still receive the best available care for his type of leukemia. On the consent form signed by parents, there will be language similar to this: "You are free not to have your child participate in this research or to withdraw your child at any time without penalty or jeopardizing future care."

> Jesse was enrolled in a clinical trial to assess long-term consequences of radiation. The testing was free, and we were glad to participate. Unfortunately, the billing

department of the hospital continually billed us in error. We tried to correct the problem, but it became such a hassle that we withdrew from the study.

The Entire Clinical Trial Document

If your child is enrolled in a clinical trial, the roadmap described earlier is actually a very small portion of a lengthy document describing all aspects of the study. The entire document usually exceeds 100 pages and covers the following topics: study hypothesis, experimental design, scientific background and rationale with relevant references from the scientific literature, patient eligibility and randomization, therapy for each arm of the study, required observations, pathology guidelines, radiation therapy guidelines (if applicable), supportive care guidelines, specific information about each drug, relapse therapy guidelines, statistical considerations, study committee members, record-keeping requirements, reporting of adverse drug reactions, and a consent form.

The clinical trial that my child was enrolled in had three arms—A, B, and C. He was in the A portion, so we only referred to the A section of the protocol, which clearly outlined each procedure and drug to be given for the duration of the trial. It also listed the follow-up care required by that particular clinical trial.

The full protocol is intended for use by specialists in oncology. It is highly technical and may be confusing or overwhelming for some parents.

However, some parents are medical professionals or people who want to better understand their child's illness and treatment. These parents may want to have a copy of the full study document for several reasons. First, it provides a description of some previous clinical trials and explains the reasons the investigators designed this particular study. Second, it provides detailed descriptions of drug reactions, which may comfort parents who worry that their child is the only one exhibiting extreme responses to some drugs. Third, motivated parents who have only one protocol to keep track of sometimes prevent errors in treatment. Finally, for parents who are adrift in the world of cancer treatment, it can give them a bit of control over their child's life.

Since knowledge is comfort for me, I really wanted to have the entire clinical trial document, despite its technical language. Whereas the brief protocol that I had listed day, drug, and dose, the expanded version listed the potential side effects for each drug, and what actions should be taken should any occur. I needed all of that information.

Other parents may find that reading hundreds of pages of technical information is overwhelming or not helpful. As with almost every topic discussed in this book, families need to make choices based on what works best for their unique situation.

If your child is enrolled in a clinical trial and you would like a copy of the entire document, ask your child's oncologist for a copy. If the oncologist will not provide it, call COG (626-447-0064) and ask for a copy. Informed consent documents for COG trials specifically state that families will receive a copy of the full protocol upon request. After reading the document, it may be helpful to schedule an appointment with your child's oncologist, nurse practitioner, or research nurse to discuss any questions or concerns.

The full clinical trial document is not for general distribution because it is unethical to use these protocols outside a controlled research setting. Parents who obtain a copy should not share it with others.

Protocol Changes

Many parents express anguish when their child's doses or schedules for chemotherapy change during treatment. It is very common for doses to be lowered or treatment to be delayed while a child recovers from low blood counts, infection, or toxic reactions to the treatment. In fact, almost every child has dose reductions or delays in treatment. The protocol is a guideline that will be modified, depending on your child's response to treatment.

> When we were struggling with the decision of whether to join the study, I asked the oncologist how would we ever know if we made the right decision. He said something very wise, "You will never know and you should never second guess yourself, no matter how the study turns out. Statistics are about large groups of kids, not your child. Your child might respond no matter which arm she is on or she might show no benefit from a treatment arm where most other kids do well. Statistics for you will be either 100 percent or 0 because your child will either live or die. I can't tell you which will be the better treatment—that is why we are conducting the study. But no matter what, we will be doing absolutely the best we can.

Chapter 9

Coping with Procedures

"Mommy, I didn't cry but my eyes got bright."
— 4-year-old with leukemia

THE PURPOSE OF THIS CHAPTER is to prepare children and parents for several common procedures by providing detailed descriptions of each. Because many procedures are repeated frequently during treatment for childhood cancer, it is important to establish a routine that is comfortable for you and your child. The procedure itself may cause discomfort, but a well-prepared, calm child fares far better than a frightened one. This chapter covers planning for procedures, pain management, and descriptions of the most common procedures used to treat childhood leukemia.

Planning for Procedures

Procedures are needed to make diagnoses, check for the possible spread of disease, administer treatments, and monitor response to treatment. Some procedures are pain-free but others can cause both physical and psychological distress. All procedures are easier to tolerate when parents and the child are prepared and know what to expect.

> My daughter (3 years old) took an old stuffed animal to the clinic with her. Having the nurse and doctor perform the procedure first on "bear" helped her immensely.

The best way to prepare a child is for parents to prepare themselves, intellectually and emotionally, to provide the support and comfort their child needs during procedures. Although having the procedure is non-negotiable, options are usually available to lessen the pain and stress. Parents need to know what these choices are to be effective advocates for their child.

Most children's hospitals have a child life program. These programs try to minimize psychological trauma and maintain, as much as possible, normal living patterns for hospitalized children. The American Academy of Pediatrics considers child life programs the standard of care for hospitalized children. As soon as possible after admission, find out whether your hospital has a child life program or an equivalent support team.

Matthew was in sixth grade when he was diagnosed, and he was worried about the surgery to implant the port. The child life specialist came in and really helped. She showed him what a port looked like; then they explored the pre-op area, the actual surgery room, and post-op. She showed him on a cloth doll exactly where the incision would be and how the scar would look. Then she introduced him to "Fred," the IV pump. She said that Fred would be going places with him, and that Fred would keep him from getting so many pokes. She told Matthew that he could bring something from home to hang on Fred. Of course, he brought in a really ugly stuffed animal. Throughout treatment, she really helped his fears and my feelings about losing control over my child's daily life.

Child life specialists or other team members may provide support before and during procedures. They establish relationships with children based on warmth, respect, and empathy. They also communicate with the other members of the treatment team about the psychosocial needs of children and their families.

You can do quite a bit to prepare your child for procedures. Discuss with the child life professional or social worker when and how to prepare for upcoming procedures. Although it may not always be possible, try to schedule procedures so the same person does the same procedure each time. Call ahead to check for unexpected changes to prevent any surprises for your child. Repetition can provide comfort and reassurance to children. Ritual can also be important. A child may prefer a precise sequence of steps or the use of certain cue words to signal the start of a procedure. If staff members know the child and comply with her wishes, the child is usually calmer and more cooperative.

I started giving my 4-year-old daughter two days' notice before procedures. But she began to wake up every day worried that "something bad was going to happen soon." So we talked it over and decided to look at the calendar together every Sunday to review what would happen that week. She was a much happier child after that.

Parents should have a choice whether or not to be present during a medical procedure. If your child does better when you aren't in the room, ask the child life specialist or another member of the treatment team to be present solely to comfort your child. Teens often want to handle the procedure on their own and it is normally best to respect their wishes.

During procedures, a parent's role is to be supportive and loving. In most cases, the best place to position yourself is at your child's head, at eye level. Speak calmly and positively to your child. You can tell stories, sing songs, or read a favorite book. It helps to praise your child for good behavior, but don't reprimand or demean your child if problems occur. Giving children some control over what happens helps tremendously, but only give choices when they truly exist.

Oncology clinics usually have a special box full of toys or a selection of rewards for children who have had a procedure. It sometimes helps for the child to have a treat to look forward to afterward. Some parents bring a special gift to sneak into the box for their child to find.

We decided from the very beginning that, even though it's no fun to have procedures, we were going to make something positive out of it. So we made it a party. We'd bring pizza, popcorn, or ice cream to the hospital. We helped Kristin think of the nurses as her friends. We'd celebrate after a procedure by going out to eat at one of the neat little restaurants near the hospital.

Pain Management

The goal of pediatric pain management should be to minimize discomfort while performing the procedure. The two methods used to achieve this goal are psychological (using the mind) and pharmacological (using drugs).

Psychological methods

It is essential to prepare for every procedure, because unexpected stress is more difficult to cope with than anticipated stress. If parents and children understand what is going to happen, where it will happen, who will be there, and what it will feel like, they will be less anxious and better able to cope. Here are some ways to prepare your child:

- Verbally explain each step in the procedure
- Meet the person who will perform the procedure, if possible
- Tour the room where the procedure will take place
- Let small children use dolls to play-act the procedure
- Let older children observe a demonstration on a doll
- Let adolescents watch a video that demonstrates the procedure
- Encourage discussion and answer all questions

For my child, playing about procedures helped release many feelings. Parents can buy medical kits at the store or stock their own from clinic castoffs and the pharmacy. We had IV bottles made from empty shampoo containers, complete with tubing and plastic needles. Several dolls had accessed ports, and many stuffed animals in our house fell apart after being speared by the pen during countless spinal taps. Christine's younger sister even ran around sometimes with her own pretend port taped onto her chest. Some suggestions for a child's medical kit are: gauze pads, tape, tubing, stethoscope, reflex hammer, pretend needles, syringes, medical chart, and toy box. Of course, lots of dolls or stuffed animal patients are required.

Children and teens can learn mindfulness-based, stress-reduction techniques, using thoughtful awareness to help manage anxiety. A psychologist or other specialist who is experienced in mindfulness meditation can teach specific techniques that help children cope with difficult situations. This can be very helpful for your child during and after cancer treatment. You can ask the psychologist at your treatment center to provide a referral to an experienced practitioner (e.g., psychologist or counselor who has training in mindfulness work), preferably one who is covered by your medical insurance.

Guided imagery is another technique children can learn to help manage pain. It is an active process that helps children feel as if they are actually entering an imagined place. Focusing on pleasant images allows the child to shift attention from the procedure. Ask whether the hospital has someone to teach your child this very effective technique.

A 17-year-old wrote the following description of using imagery during procedures. It is reprinted with permission from the *Free to Be Yourself* newsletter of Cancer Services of Allen County, Indiana.

My Special Place

Many people had a special place when they were young—a special place that they still remember. This place could be an area that has a special meaning for them, or a place where they used to go when they wanted to be alone. My special place location is over the rainbow.

I discovered this place when I was 12 years old, during a relaxation session. These sessions were designed to reduce pain and stress brought on by chemotherapy. This was a place that I could visualize in my mind so that I could go there any time that I wanted to—not only for pain, but when I was happy, mad, or sad.

It is surrounded by sand and tall, fanning palm trees. The blue sky is always clear, and the bright sun shines every day. It is usually quiet because I am alone, but often I can hear the sounds of birds flying by.

Every time I come to this place, I like to lie down in the sand. As I lie there, I can feel the gritty sand beneath me. Once in a while I get up and go looking for seashells. I usually find some different shapes and sizes. The ones I like the best are the ones that you can hear the sound of the ocean in. After a while I get up and start to walk around. As I walk, I can feel the breeze going right through me, and I can smell the salt water. It reminds me of being at a beach in Florida. Whenever I start to feel sad or alone or if I am in pain, I usually go jump in the water because it is a soothing place for me. I like to float around in the water because it gives me a refreshing feeling that nobody can hurt me here. I could stay in this place all day because I do not worry about anything while I am here.

To me this place is like a home away from home. It is like heaven because you can do anything you want to do here. Even though this place may seem imaginary or like a fantasy world to some people, it is not to me. I think it is real because it is a place where I can go and be myself.

Distraction can be used successfully with all age groups, but it should never be used as a substitute for preparation. Babies can be distracted by colorful, moving objects. Parents can help distract preschoolers by showing them picture books or videos, telling stories, singing songs, or blowing bubbles. Many youngsters are comforted and distracted from pain by hugging a favorite stuffed animal. School-aged children can watch videos or TV, or listen to music. Some institutions use interactive video games on tablets to help distract older children or teens.

Relaxation, biofeedback, massage, acupuncture, Reiki (Japanese energy healing), and accupressure are all also used successfully to manage pain. Ask the hospital's child life specialist, psychologist, or nurse to discuss and practice different methods of pain management with you and your child.

Pharmacological methods

Most pediatric oncology clinics sedate or anesthetize children for procedures that are painful or that require them to lie completely still. If your clinic does not offer this option, strongly advocate for it. Sedation and anesthesia have the advantage of calming children, reducing pain, and, in many cases, removing all memory of the procedure.

My job as an oral surgery assistant requires me to be very familiar with different types of sedation. From the first day of Stephan's diagnosis, I quietly insisted on Versed® for bone marrows and spinal taps. We have been in treatment for two years, and they still fight me every time, saying that it's just not necessary. When I make the appointment I tell them we want Stephan sedated, and then I call and remind them so that all will go smoothly.

Three types of drugs are used for pain management during procedures:

• Sedatives, which depress the central nervous system and result in relaxation. The child or teen may fall asleep, but will remain conscious.

• General anesthetics, which induce a loss of consciousness to prevent the child or teen from experiencing pain or remembering a procedure.

• Local anesthetics, which temporarily interrupt nerve transmission at a specific site on the body to lessen pain.

Sedatives and general anesthetics. These anesthetics are given intravenously in the operating room (OR) or the clinic sedation room. Certain drugs must be administered by an anesthesiologist (a doctor specializing in anesthesia) in a hospital setting. Drugs commonly used during procedures for children with cancer include:

- **Valium® (diazepam) or Versed® (midazolam), plus morphine or fentanyl:** Valium® and Versed® are sedatives that are used with pain relievers such as morphine or fentanyl. These drugs can be given in the clinic, but the possibility of slowed breathing requires expert monitoring and the availability of emergency equipment. The combination of a sedative and a pain reliever will result in your child being awake but sedated. Your child may move or cry, but he will not remember the procedure.

> My son was treated from ages 14 to 17. During his spinal taps he would get Versed® once he was positioned on the table. I would always sit at his head and keep his shoulders forward while his head rested on my arm. (Kind of a hug.) As the Versed® took effect, he would look up at me with huge eyes and give me a grin a mile wide, then he would say something off the wall. He had to spend an hour flat after the spinal tap. He'd be groggy the whole time, constantly asking me what time it was and how soon we could leave. He'd forget he asked and ask me again 5 minutes later. This continued for the whole hour. Later, we'd laugh about it. He never remembered anything from the spinal taps.

- **Propofol:** Propofol is a general anesthetic that will cause your child to lose consciousness. It must be administered in a hospital by an anesthesiologist. It is given intravenously and has the benefit of acting almost immediately with little recovery time. Propofol prevents memory of the procedure but it does not relieve pain, so it is often used with a local anesthetic (discussed later).

> Patrick (12 years old) hates the lack of control involved when having a procedure and getting propofol. He attempts to regain some control by verbally explaining to the doctors just exactly how he wants it done each time. He has his own little routine—tells them jokes, sings "I Want to Be Sedated" (you know, the Ramones' song), etc. Patrick's biggest problem is the taste from the propofol. We have tried so many different things when he wakes up to mask the taste—Skittles®, gum, Gatorade®. We now have a supply of Atomic Fireballs®. I give him one as soon as they bring him out, and he says that really helps cover the taste.

An anesthesiologist, who is also the father of a young child with ALL, said this:

> Let's face it, kids don't care about lab work or protocols, they just want to know if they are going to be hurt again. I think that one of our most important jobs is to advocate, strongly if necessary, for adequate pain control. If the dose doesn't work and the doctor just shrugs her shoulders, say you want a different dosage or drug used. If you encounter resistance, ask that an anesthesiologist be consulted. Remember that good pain control and/or amnesia will make a big difference in your child's state of mind during and after treatment.

Because treatment for leukemia may take months or years, some children build up a tolerance for sedatives and pain relievers. Over time, doses may need to be increased or drugs may need to be changed. If your child remembers the procedure, advocate for a change in the drugs or dosage. It is reasonable to request the services of an anesthesiologist to ensure the best outcome for your child. Over three years of treatment, this family needed to work with the team to find methods that were tolerable for their child at different ages:

> Sedation is tricky with kids. What worked great for my son at one point in treatment did not work at others. We changed clinics during treatment. At our first hospital, we started out with an anesthesiologist who typically used either gas (a mask) plus propofol, or Versed® plus propofol. My son was just miserable after gas—crying and crying and crying for about an hour. But he was even worse after the IV Versed®/ propofol combo. He would try to throw himself out of the bed, scream, bite, and basically just act psychotic for about an hour (he was two years old during this period). Next, they tried ketamine and Versed®. My son was out of it, but never totally asleep (sort of a trance) and within about 10 minutes, he seemed to recover and acted normally. Then we moved, and the new clinic's standard sedation was Versed® and propofol, which I warned them not to use but they did anyway. That was when my son was diagnosed with "emergence delirium." We had a lot of back and forth with anesthesia and they tried different combos. We decided to try oral Versed®, which made him act really drunk. It was uncomfortable to see a drunk 3 year old, but it was better than emergence delirium, and they were able to do the lumbar puncture even though he was awake. The oral Versed® worked for about nine months, and then it just didn't sedate him enough anymore. After a lot of discussion, we tried propofol alone and that was okay—not great, but mostly not terrible.

Your child will not be allowed to eat or drink for several hours before sedation or anesthesia. After a procedure, your child may eat or drink when she is alert and able to swallow.

Local anesthetics. There are several types of local anesthetics used to prevent discomfort or pain during procedures.

- **EMLA® or LMX®:** These are anesthetic creams, which contain a combination of lidocaine and prilocaine or lidocaine alone. The cream is placed on the skin one to two hours before a painful procedure. It is held in place on the skin by an occlusive dressing or adhesive cling wrap.

- **Synera®:** This anesthetic patch contains lidocaine and tetracaine and is placed on the skin 20 to 30 minutes before a needle poke or other painful procedure for children age 3 or older.

- **Ethyl chloride spray:** This anesthetic spray can be used right before a procedure to anesthetize the surface of the skin.

- **Injectable medications:** Some medications, such as xylocaine or lidocaine, are injected into tissues to prevent pain during procedures such as lumbar punctures.

For more information about these local anesthetics, see the section called the section called "Topical anesthetics to prevent pain" in Chapter 13, *Chemotherapy and Other Medications*.

> *Danica was age 5 at diagnosis and she learned quickly how to be comfortable with getting her port accessed. She would pop into the chair, pull up her shirt, and be ready to go. The first time her port was accessed, it was still bruised from the insertion of the port, and they didn't tell me to put the EMLA® patch on it an hour before. That really hurt. After we learned about EMLA®, she did fine and would even remind me to put it on her.*

There is also a non-drug option called Buzzy® that parents can purchase without a prescription. It is popular for children who either don't like or have an allergy to topical anesthetics. Buzzy® uses cold and vibration to block the pain of needle pokes.

Procedures

Knowing what to expect will help lay the foundation for months or years of tolerable procedures. Because hospitals and practitioners have their own guidelines and preferences, the descriptions of procedures in the rest of this chapter may not exactly mirror your experience, but the fundamentals are the same everywhere. Reading the rest of this chapter may lessen your fears and help you to calm and prepare your child. The procedures are listed in alphabetical order.

Questions to ask before procedures

You need information prior to procedures to prepare yourself and your child. Consider asking your doctor these questions:

- Why is this procedure needed and how will it affect my child's treatment?
- What information will the procedure provide?
- Who will perform the procedure?
- Will it be an inpatient or outpatient procedure?
- Would you explain the procedure in detail?
- Is there any literature available that describes it?
- Is there a child life specialist on staff who will help prepare my child for the procedure? If not, are there nurses, social workers, or psychologists who can talk to me about how to prepare my child?
- Is the procedure painful?

- How long will it take?
- What type of anesthetic or sedation is used?
- What are the risks, if any?
- What are the possible side effects?
- When will we get the results?

Accessing implanted catheters

The procedure that occurs most often during treatment is accessing your child's implanted central venous catheter. This procedure is described in detail in Chapter 12, *Central Venous Catheters*.

> *My daughter had a terrible time having her port accessed. She would scream and cry (probably terrifying the other kids waiting outside the room for their turn!) and I became an expert at holding her down. I'd lie down next to her, holding down her hands, pressing my knee on her legs to keep her from kicking, and with my head on her forehead. It was horrible. I don't think it was particularly painful, just a terrible invasion for her, and she knew she'd feel badly after her treatment. We ended up meeting with the neuropsychologist on staff at the hem-onc office. The doctor was wonderful and warm, she talked to my daughter about why having her port accessed bothered her so much, and we talked about ways that she might cope. The doc made some good suggestions: listening to music, looking at a book, dreaming herself somewhere else. The neuropsychologist then accompanied her into the procedure room. My daughter was calm and completely still through the whole procedure, and never made a fuss again about having her port accessed. I'm very grateful.*

Blood draws

Frequent blood samples are a part of life during treatment for leukemia. Three common laboratory tests performed on blood are a complete blood count (CBC), blood chemistries, and blood cultures. A CBC measures the types and numbers of cells in the blood. Blood chemistries measure substances in the blood plasma to determine whether organs (e.g., liver, kidneys) are functioning properly. Blood cultures help evaluate whether a child is developing a bacterial or fungal infection. For a list of normal blood cell counts, see Appendix A, *Blood Tests and What They Mean*.

A finger poke provides enough blood for a CBC, but blood chemistries or cultures require one or more vials of blood. Children with catheters usually have blood drawn from the catheter rather than the arm or finger. If the child does not have a catheter, blood is usually drawn from the large vein on the inside of the elbow. The procedures for a blood draw are similar to those for placing an IV, which are described later in this chapter.

Bone growth test

A bone growth test is an x-ray of your child's non-dominant hand and wrist; for example, if your child is right-handed, the left hand and wrist will be x-rayed. It is performed to determine whether your child's growth is appropriate for her age. Your child's x-ray film will be compared with a series of photographs of wrist films of children of all ages so the radiologist can define your child's "bone age" compared to her chronological age. The results help determine whether endocrine testing is needed. This test takes only a few moments to perform and is not painful.

> My daughter wasn't growing much while she was taking Gleevec® from age 7 to 13. We went for an endocrine consult and they ordered a bone growth test. The test showed she was a couple of years behind in closure of the growth plates, which was great news because it meant she had more time to grow. When she was switched to Sprycel®, she started to grow again.

Bone marrow aspiration

Protocols for children with leukemia require bone marrow aspirations, a process by which bone marrow is removed with a large-bore needle. The purpose of the first, or diagnostic, bone marrow aspiration is to see what percentage of the cells in the marrow are abnormal blasts. Then these cells are analyzed to determine which type of leukemia is present. For children or teens with acute lymphoblastic leukemia, the next bone marrow aspiration usually is done on day 29 of treatment to see how many blasts are still present. This information, along with other test results such as the amount of minimal residual disease (MRD), is used by oncologists to decide how intensive treatment should be.

> Our son never got sick, didn't lose his hair, and gained weight during the nine months of treatment for APL. He was able to keep going to preschool because his counts never dropped. He does have PTSD from the many bone marrow aspirations he's had. He gets very upset on the way to the sedation room and wakes up vomiting and very emotional. He is pretty much wiped out for the whole day. So, now they premedicate him with Ativan® and they changed from ketamine to other sedatives, and things have improved.

Doctors usually take a sample of the marrow from the iliac crest of the hip (the top of the hip bone). This bone is right under the skin and contains a large amount of marrow. The child lies face down on a table, sometimes on a pillow to elevate the hip. The doctor puts on sterile gloves, finds the site, and then wipes it several times with an antiseptic to eliminate any germs. The nurse places sterile paper around the site, then an anesthetic (usually xylocaine) may be injected into the skin and a small area of bone. The doctor then pushes a hollow needle (with a plug inside) through the skin into the bone, withdraws the plug, and attaches a syringe. She then aspirates (sucks out) the liquid marrow through the syringe. Finally, she removes the needle and bandages the area.

> *Melissa (age 5) has had several bone marrow aspirations since her diagnosis. We always use propofol (which I refer to as the "milk of human kindness," because of its milky appearance) before the procedure. After the aspiration is over, Melissa wakes up from a very deep sleep and has felt no pain whatsoever. She's usually hungry and ready to go ASAP. Propofol has worked exceptionally well for her.*

Without sedation, bone marrow aspiration is very painful, so most doctors anesthetize children for this procedure. Do not hesitate to advocate for this at your hospital. Here are some descriptions from children and teens who have experienced it:

> *It was the worst thing of all. It felt really, really bad.*

· · · · ·

> *It hurts a lot. It feels like they are pulling something out and then it aches. It feels like they are trying to suck thick Jell-O® from inside the bone. Brief but incredible pain.*

Echocardiogram

Some drugs used to fight cancer can damage heart muscle, decreasing its ability to contract effectively. Many protocols require a baseline echocardiogram to measure the heart's ability to pump before any chemotherapy drugs are given. Echocardiograms are then given periodically during and after treatment to check for heart muscle damage.

An echocardiogram uses ultrasound waves to measure the amount of blood that leaves the heart each time it contracts. The percentage of blood ejected during a contraction compared to blood in the heart when it is relaxed is called the ejection fraction.

The echocardiogram is performed by a technician, nurse, or doctor. The child or teen lies on a table and has conductive jelly applied to the chest. Then the technician puts a transducer (which emits the ultrasound waves) on the jelly and moves the device around on the chest to obtain different views of the heart. The technician might apply some pressure on the transducer, which could cause very mild discomfort. The test results are displayed on a videotape and photographed for later interpretation.

> *Meagan used to watch a video during the echocardiogram. Sometimes she would eat a lollipop or a Popsicle®. She found it to be boring, not painful.*

Finger pokes

Finger pokes are different from blood draws because only a quick puncture of the skin is needed to obtain a few drops of blood. The technician will hold the finger and quickly prick it with a small sharp instrument. Blood will be collected in narrow tubes or a small container. Most often the technician needs to squeeze the fingertip to get enough blood. If a Buzzy® or numbing cream is not used, the squeezing part is uncomfortable and the finger may ache for a while.

One way to lessen the discomfort of a finger poke is to put a blob of EMLA® on the tip of the middle finger, cover the fingertip with plastic cling wrap, and then use tape or a bandage to hold it in place. Another method is to buy long, thin balloons with a diameter a bit wider than your child's finger. Cut off the open end, leaving only enough balloon to cover the finger up to the first knuckle. Fill the tip of the balloon with EMLA® and slide it on the fingertip. EMLA® needs to be applied an hour before a finger poke to be effective. When it's time for the poke, remove the plastic wrap or balloon, wipe off the EMLA®, and ask for a warm pack. Wrapping this heated pack around the finger for a few minutes opens the capillaries to allow the blood to flow out more readily. Now your child is ready for a pain-free finger poke.

> Even though we use EMLA®, Katy (5 years old) still becomes angry when she has to have a finger poke. I asked her why it was upsetting if there was no pain, and she replied, "It doesn't hurt my body anymore, but it still hurts my feelings."

Some children are more anxious about the anticipation of a poke than the actual poke itself, so using EMLA® may cause them to worry more. As you try various methods, you and your child will learn what works best. Children who choose their own routines for pain control may feel more comfortable and secure.

Gastrostomy

A gastrostomy is the creation of an external opening in the abdominal wall through which a feeding tube (usually called a G-tube) is placed in the child's stomach. A G-tube is used for children who can't eat normally because of chronic swallowing problems or long-term pain in the mouth or throat, or for children who have lost their appetite for a long time because of disease or treatment. The stomach end of the feeding tube has a small balloon on it that prevents it from being accidentally pulled out.

> My daughter was diagnosed when she was three months old. During her second round of chemo, I told them that the sound of her crying had changed, and she was coughing a lot while nursing. It turns out her vocal cords were paralyzed from the vincristine. She was in a lot of pain and needed to be on a continuous drip for that. I couldn't nurse her anymore so they put a G-tube in because they were afraid she might aspirate and get pneumonia. She needed a way to get nutrition, but it was very hard not to be able to nurse her.

A skilled gastroenterologist or surgeon can perform the procedure in about 10 minutes. Most children have general anesthesia for the procedure and remain in the hospital for one to two days after the operation to receive pain medication and make sure they can tolerate tube feedings. After two to three months, the tube may be replaced with an unobtrusive skin-level device called a button. After a short recovery, children may play, bathe, and swim normally.

The G-tube is used for liquid feedings and medications for as long as the child needs it. If a child no longer requires the tube, it is removed and a bandage is placed over the site. The wound closes in a day or two.

Spinal tap (lumbar puncture or LP)

The body has a structure, called the blood–brain barrier, to protect the brain from toxins that may be circulating in the blood. Due to this barrier, systemic chemotherapy usually cannot destroy any blasts in the central nervous system (brain and spinal cord). Chemotherapy drugs must be directly injected into the cerebrospinal fluid (CSF) to kill any blasts present and prevent a possible central nervous system relapse; this is called intrathecal administration. The drugs most commonly used are methotrexate, ARA-C (cytarabine), and hydrocortisone. The number of spinal taps required and when they are done varies, depending on the child's risk level, the clinical study, and whether radiation is used (most often there are fewer spinal taps if cranial radiation is used).

Most hospitals sedate children for spinal taps. To perform a spinal tap, the doctor or nurse practitioner positions the child on his side with his head tucked close to the chest and knees drawn up. A nurse usually helps hold the child in this position. The doctor, wearing sterile gloves, finds the designated spot in the lower back, swabs it with antiseptic several times, and injects one or two shots of an anesthetic (usually xylocaine) into the skin and deeper tissues. It is necessary to wait a few moments to ensure the area is fully anesthetized.

> In the beginning of treatment, they used Versed® when doing spinal taps on my 11-year-old daughter who has Down syndrome. She hated it and would growl at her beloved doctor and scream to "Stop it!" So, we started doing spinal taps in the OR under general anesthesia, and it was much better.

The doctor will push a spinal needle between two vertebrae and into the space where CSF is found. The CSF will begin to drip out of the hollow needle into a container. After collecting a small amount of CSF, the doctor removes the needle, bandages the spot, and sends the CSF to the laboratory to see whether any cancer cells are present.

Some facilities will suggest your child lie flat for at least 30 minutes after a spinal tap to reduce pressure changes in the CSF. If your child develops a persistent severe headache following the procedure that lessens while he lies flat but throbs when he sits up, notify the doctor or nurse. The nurse will likely have your child lie flat and will offer him a high-caffeine beverage (such as Mountain Dew®) to drink. If the headache persists, an anesthesiologist sometimes does a procedure called a "blood patch," during which your child lies in the same position as for the spinal tap. The anesthesiologist will draw a small amount of blood from your child's arm or central line. She will then inject the blood at the site of the prior spinal tap, where CSF may be slowly leaking into the tissues. If this is the cause of the headache, the relief is immediate. You can stay with your child during the procedure.

Starting an intravenous (IV) line

Most children with cancer have a permanent venous catheter implanted in their chest within a week of diagnosis to avoid the pain of multiple IV sticks (see Chapter 12, *Central Venous Catheters*). However, there may be instances when your child will also need an IV line started.

Children's hospitals either use nurses or technicians with specialized training to start IVs and draw blood. The IV technician will generally use a vein in the lower arm or hand. First, a constricting band is put above the site to make the veins larger and easier to see and feel. The technician feels for the vein, cleans the area, and inserts the needle. She will then withdraw the needle, leaving only a thin plastic tube in the vein. The technician will make sure the tube is in the proper place, then will cover the site with a clear dressing and secure it with tape.

Here are a few ways to make this procedure a bit easier:

- **Stay calm:** The body reacts to fear by constricting the blood vessels near the skin's surface. Small children are usually more calm with a parent present, but teenagers may prefer privacy. Listening to music, visualizing a tranquil scene (such as floating in a pool or watching snow fall in the mountains), or using the same technician each time can help.

- **Keep warm:** Cold temperatures cause the surface blood vessels to constrict. Wrapping the child in a blanket and putting a warm pack or heating pad on his arm can enlarge the veins.

- **Drink lots of fluids:** Dehydration decreases fluid in the veins, making them harder to find.

- **Let gravity help:** If your child is lying in bed, she can hang her arm down over the side to increase the amount of blood in the vessels in her arm and hand.

- **Let your child have control, as appropriate:** If your child has a preference, let him pick the arm to be stuck. If he is a veteran of many IVs, let him point out the best vein.

- **Stop if problems develop:** The art of treating children requires spending lots of time on preparation and not much time on procedures. If a conflict arises, take a time-out and regroup. Children can be remarkably cooperative if they feel you are respecting their needs and if they are given some control over the situation.

> *You'll think I'm crazy, but I'll tell you this story anyway. After getting stuck constantly for a year, my daughter (5 years old) lost it one day when she needed an IV. She started screaming and crying, just flew into a rage. I told the tech, "Let's let her calm down. Why don't you stick me for a change?" She was a sport and started a line in my arm. I told my daughter that I had forgotten how much it hurt and I could understand why she was upset. I told her to let us know when she was ready. She just walked over and held out her arm.*

· · · · ·

> *I request a portable ultrasound each time for Lillia, as her veins are very deep and hard to get to. It used to take 30 minutes of poking, multiple collapsed veins, and techs finally giving up or Lillia saying "no more." With the ultrasound, the whole thing takes just a few moments and they never miss getting the best vein. It is heaven sent!*

Traditionally, infants and young children have been restrained on their backs to insert IVs. This technique lessens the risk of misplacing the IV, but it can cause a lot of fear and distress. Many treatment centers now allow parents to hold children upright in their laps to reduce stress. Child life specialists can teach parents ways to hold a young child to help him feel secure while undergoing procedures.

Subcutaneous injections

Some children require medications given by subcutaneous (under the skin) injection during their treatment. For example, growth hormone is given by subcutaneous injection. If you will be giving shots at home, make sure a nurse has trained you to do it and ask her to write down any tips she has for making the shot as easy for your child as possible.

> *We found that giving 4-year-old Joseph as much power in the process as possible really helped. The shots themselves are non-negotiable, but there are many parts of the process where the child can have some control (where to put the EMLA® cream, where to be sitting for the cream and/or the shot, who holds him, what toy to hold during the procedure, etc.). We also made sure to have a consistent little treat available afterwards, although this became unnecessary after a while. Even at 4, Joseph loved money, so for a long time he kept a pint jar, which would travel to the hospital and back home again, and he'd get to drop in a nickel for each pill successfully swallowed (a huge chore for him) and a quarter for each shot. Of course, adults would*

look very surprised when we told them we gave Joseph "quarter shots." Something tells me the bar scene will be very confusing to him when gets to college.

To minimize pain caused by subcutaneous injections, apply numbing cream one to two hours before the shot, and then cover it with a Tegaderm® patch or plastic cling wrap held in place with paper tape. Parents can also numb the site prior to the injection by using a Buzzy® device for 30 to 60 seconds or by rubbing ice over the skin.

We always used EMLA® cream before our son needed a subcutaneous injection. I think part of the benefit to him was pharmacological, and part of it was psychological. He just seemed to be more at ease with the injections when he knew the EMLA® was applied an hour before the needle was given.

Taking oral medications

As the parent of a child with a leukemia, one of your most important jobs is to give each dose of all oral medications to your child on time, every day. To do this, it is essential to get off to a good start and establish cooperation early in the process. Children with leukemia need to be able to swallow pills, and they will need to learn how to do it in a short span of time. Some pills must be swallowed whole, but others can be chewed without affecting efficacy. However, some medications (e.g., prednisone, dexamethasone) should not be chewed because they have a bitter aftertaste and may cause your child to develop an aversion to all oral medications.

To teach Brent (6 years old) to swallow pills, when we were eating corn for dinner I encouraged him to swallow one kernel whole. Luckily, it went right down and he got over his fear of pills.

Children and teens can learn how to swallow pills by practicing with candy. One method, developed by the Child Study Center at New York University Langone Medical Center, starts with a child swallowing a tiny candy such as Nerds®. When the child is able to easily do this five times, he practices swallowing a slightly larger candy. The size of the candies is gradually increased (e.g., mini M&Ms®, Tic Tacs®, and then full-sized M&Ms®). This method allows your child or teen to practice swallowing in a relaxed setting at home with as much repetition as needed. With lots of encouragement from parents, the stress is minimal. If this method does not work for your child, a more gradual way to learn to swallow pills is described online at *http://research4kids.ucalgary. ca/pill-study*.

I wanted Katy (3 years old) to feel like we were a team right from the first night. So I made a big deal out of tasting each of her medications and pronouncing it good. Thank goodness I tasted the prednisone first. It was nauseating—bitter, metallic, with a lingering aftertaste. I asked the nurse for some small gel caps, and packed them with the pills which I had broken in half. I gave Katy her choice of drinks to take her pills with and taught her to swallow gel caps with a large sip of liquid. Since I gave her more than 3,000 pills and 1,100 teaspoons of liquid medication during treatment, I'm very glad we got off to such a good start.

Empty gel caps come in many sizes, and you can purchase them at a pharmacy or ask a nurse for them if your child is in the hospital. Many parents put pills inside gel caps to mask the taste and make them more slippery and easier to swallow. Number 4s are small enough for a 3- or 4-year-old child to swallow. Children develop different taste preferences and aversions to medications, and gel caps are useful for those that bother them.

After much trial and error with medications, Meagan's method became chewing up pills with chocolate chips. She's kept this up for the long haul.

• • • • •

I always give choices such as, "Do you want the white pill or the six yellow pills first?" It gives him a little control in his chaotic world.

For younger children who aren't able to swallow pills, many parents crush the pills into a small amount of pudding, applesauce, jam, ice cream, frozen juice concentrate, or another favorite food. However, your child may develop a lifelong aversion to these foods after treatment is over. Before mixing pills with food, check with the doctor or pharmacist, because some foods can negate the effects of some medications.

Jeremy was 4 when he was diagnosed, and we used to crush up the pills and mix them with ice cream. This worked well for us.

• • • • •

Our son was 2 ½ years old when diagnosed. We put the med in an oral syringe and put very hot water in a tiny glass. Then we would draw a wee bit of the hot water into the oral syringe and then we would cap it. Then you gently shake the syringe and turn it back and forth while the med completely dissolves. Then we would take off the cap and fill it the rest of the way with nice cold Kool-Aid®. Alexander would get to choose the flavor of Kool-Aid® each day and we would just mix up a couple different batches of flavors and keep them in the fridge. He felt like he was in control because he chose the flavor, and it covered up the lousy taste of the medication. We asked our oncologist about this at the very beginning, and he said it was a great way to do it because neither the water nor the Kool-Aid® had any unwanted effects on the medication. Anyway, we never once had any problem with this method.

• • • • •

The method we used for getting my son to take his foul-tasting chemo/meds was the mixing agent Syrpalta®. This is a grape-flavored syrup available from the pharmacy. It doesn't react with most meds and the flavor can hide almost anything. We used quite a bit of the stuff. First, we crushed his pills with a pill crusher/cutter, then we mixed them in a cup before putting them in a syringe to squirt in his mouth. (Keep in mind he was only about 15 months old when he got sick.) We had to make sure he got every drop though, since some of the pills were really small and a little bit of syrup could hide a significant portion of the dose. You should make sure that any med you do this with is safe to crush or mix with Syrpalta® (or chocolate, or anything else for that matter). Meds with time-release or slow-release agents should never be crushed.

Pharmacists can flavor oral medications with a product called FlavorX®, allowing your child to choose from a variety of flavors such as banana, strawberry, mango, watermelon, and chocolate. The pharmacist can advise you about which flavors will work best to cover up the taste of each medication. You can find a local pharmacy that offers FlavorX® by visiting the website *www.flavorx.com.*

Most children on maintenance take SMZ-TMP (sulfamethoxazole and trimethoprim), Bactrim®, or Septra® two to three times a week to prevent a specific type of pneumonia that can develop in children with suppressed immune systems. These drugs come in either liquid or pill form and are produced by a variety of manufacturers. Ask your pharmacist for a kid taste test. Letting your child choose a medicine that appeals to him encourages compliance.

Because children associate taking medicine with being sick, it is helpful to explain why they must continue taking pills for years after they feel well. Some parents say, "We need these pills to gobble up the last few bad cells" or "The medicine keeps your blood strong." Others explain that the leukemia can return, and the medicine prevents it from growing again.

We had a lot of issues with dexamethasone. Our pharmacy provided a liquid version, but one of our nurses warned us that this form tasted worse than the crushed tablets of dex. My 2-year-old son fought hard. I tried everything—hiding dex in a melted Starburst®, applesauce, ice cream, chocolate syrup. I read that chocolate is supposed to mask bitterness better than anything else. But ultimately, I found that I had to keep the volume of medication as tiny as possible to get my son to swallow it. So I never mixed it so that it was more than 3 mls. Then I found the thinnest syringe I could get my hands on. I would slide the syringe down the side of his mouth (avoiding his tongue) and he could get all the liquid down in one quick swallow. I also used bribery at first (I think stickers), but eventually it became no big deal. So the concoction that worked best for us was super concentrated tropical punch Kool-Aid® mixed with extra powdered sugar! I crushed the dex, added just 2 cc's of this disgustingly sweet liquid, and then let it dissolve in the syringe. It was gross, but it worked for us.

Taking a temperature

Fever is the enemy during treatment because it can signal infection, and children on chemotherapy cannot fight infection effectively if their white blood cell counts are depressed. Parents take hundreds of temperatures, especially when their child is not feeling well.

Temperatures can be taken under the tongue, under the arm, on the forehead, or in the ear using a special type of thermometer. Rectal temperatures are not recommended due to the risk of tears and infection. Here are a few tips that might help:

- **Use a digital thermometer under the tongue or arm:** Some have an alarm that beeps when it's time to remove the thermometer (usually only one minute).

  We bought a digital thermometer that we only use under his arm. It has worked well for us because he likes the beep.

- **Use a tympanic (ear) thermometer:** Be sure you read the directions so you use it properly. This thermometer gives a read out in only a few seconds.

  When my in-laws asked at diagnosis if there was anything that we needed, I asked them to try to buy a tympanic thermometer. The device cost over 100 dollars then, but it worked beautifully. It takes only one second to obtain a temperature. I can even use it when she is asleep without waking her. They are now sold at pharmacies and drug stores, and cost much less.

- **Use a pacifier thermometer for infants and toddlers:** The thermometer is in the nipple of the pacifier and the toddler's mouth must be closed on the nipple for three minutes to get an accurate reading.

Before you leave the hospital, you should know when to call the clinic because of fever. Usually, parents are told not to give any medication for fever and to call if their child's temperature goes above 101° F (38.5° C) or below 96.8° F (36° C). It is particularly important for parents of children with implanted catheters to know when to call the clinic, as an untreated infection can be life-threatening. It is also helpful to have a copy of your child's most recent blood cell counts when you call to notify the doctor about fever.

Teens and medication

Teenagers usually have completely different issues around taking pills than do young children. Most problems with teens revolve around autonomy, control, and feelings of invulnerability. It is normal for teenagers to be noncompliant, and they cannot be forced to take pills if they choose not to cooperate. Trying to coerce teens fuels conflict and frustrates everyone. If you need help, ask the psychosocial team at the hospital to work out a plan for treatment adherence. Everyone will need to be flexible to reach a favorable outcome.

I think the main problem with teens is making sure that they take the meds. Joel (15 years old) has been very responsible about taking his nightly pills. I've tried to make it easy for him by having an index card for the week, and he marks off the med as he takes it. I also put a list of the meds on a dry erase board on the fridge as a reminder. As he takes the med, he erases it. That way it's easy for him (and me) to see at a glance if he's taken his stuff. The index card alone wasn't working because sometimes he couldn't find a pen or forgot to mark it off.

• • • • •

One of the biggest concerns with teens and maintenance is noncompliance. I think it's a delicate balancing act to allow the teen to be responsible for taking his own meds and yet have some supervision of the process. Our meds are kept in a small plastic basket on the kitchen counter. All meds are taken there. I'd never want him to keep his meds in his room where I would have no idea if he had taken them or not. On Friday nights when he is to take his weekly methotrexate—a 16-pill dose—I will count it out and put it in a medicine cup on the counter. I am not always an awake and alert person when he comes home at midnight on Friday night. When I get up Saturday morning, I know immediately if he's taken his meds. If he had shown any resistance to taking the meds, or any sign of telling me that he had taken them when he had not, I'd be doing this differently. But he's aware of the importance of each dose and the importance of his participation in the team beating the leukemia. My only other advice is to be sure and ask the doctors what to do about a missed dose for each med. In 3-plus years of treatment, you are going to have a missed dose, and it helps to know how to handle it.

Transfusions (blood)

Leukemia treatment can cause severe anemia, which is a low number of oxygen-carrying red blood cells (RBCs). This is because the normal lifespan of a RBC is three to four months, and as old cells die, the chemo-stressed marrow cannot replace them. Many children require transfusions of RBCs when they are first admitted to the hospital and periodically throughout treatment.

Whenever my son needed a transfusion, I brought along bags of coloring books, food, and toys. The number of video players at the clinic was limited, so I tried to make arrangements for one ahead of time. When anemic (hematocrit below 20%), he didn't have much energy, but by the end of the transfusion, his cheeks were rosy and he had tremendous vitality. It was hard to keep him still. After one unit (bag) of red cells, his hematocrit usually jumped up to around 30.

One bag (called a "unit") of RBCs takes two to four hours to administer and is given through an IV or catheter. Mild allergic reactions are common. If your child is prone to allergies or experiences an allergic reaction, you may need to premedicate her with an antihistamine such as Benadryl® (diphenhydramine) before transfusions. Acute allergic reactions are rare, but they do happen. If your child develops chills and/or fever or any difficulty breathing during a transfusion, notify the nurse immediately so the transfusion can be stopped.

RBC transfusions carry some risks of infection. Excellent tests are used to detect the most serious viruses in donated blood. The risk of exposure to the HIV virus from a blood transfusion is now less than 1 in 2 million. The risk of acquiring hepatitis B is 1 in 800,000, and hepatitis C is 1 in 1.6 million. Exposure to cytomegalovirus is also a small possibility. These very small risks are the reason transfusions are given only when absolutely necessary.

> My daughter received several transfusions at the clinic in Children's Hospital with no problems. After we traveled back to our home, she needed her first transfusion at the local hospital. Our pediatrician said to expect to be in the hospital at least eight hours. I asked why it would take so long when it only took four hours at Children's. He said he had worked out a formula and determined that she needed two units of packed cells. I mentioned that she only was given one unit each time at Children's. He called the oncologist, who said it was better to give only one unit. We went to the hospital, where a unit of red cells was given. Then a nurse came in with another unit. I questioned why he was doing that and he said, "Doctor's orders." I asked him to verify that order, as we had already discussed it with the doctor. He went into another room to call the doctor, and came back and said the pediatrician thought my daughter needed 30 cc more packed cells. I called Children's and they said she didn't need more, so I refused to let them administer any more blood. It just wasn't worth the risk of hepatitis to get 30 cc of blood. Even though I was pleasant, the nurse was angry at me for questioning the pediatrician.

Transfusions (platelets)

Platelets are an important component of blood. They help form clots and stop bleeding by repairing breaks in the walls of blood vessels. A normal platelet count for a healthy child is 160,000 to 450,000/mm^3. Chemotherapy can severely depress the platelet count. If a child's platelet count is very low, it may be necessary to transfuse platelets so uncontrollable bleeding doesn't occur. Many centers require a transfusion when a child's platelet count goes below 10,000 to 20,000/mm^3, and sometimes more transfusions are required every two or three days until the marrow recovers. Most platelet transfusions take less than an hour.

As with other blood products, an allergic reaction is possible and platelets are capable of transmitting infections such as hepatitis, cytomegalovirus, and HIV. Even though the chance of contracting these viruses is extremely low, platelets are transfused only when necessary.

> Three-year-old Matthew had countless platelet transfusions, and only once did he have a reaction. It was an awful thing to watch, but the nurse who was monitoring him was very calm and professional, which helped both of us. Matthew was always premedicated for his platelet transfusions with Benadryl®, which made him very drowsy. Most often he would sleep through the entire transfusion.

Urine specimens

Children taking chemotherapy often need to provide urine specimens. One way to help obtain a sample is to encourage your child to drink lots of liquids the hour before. Explain to the child why the test is needed. Ask the nurse to show how the dip sticks work. They change color, so they are quite popular with preschoolers. You can use a shallow plastic bucket (called a hat) under the toilet seat to catch urine.

> Turn on the water while the child sits on the toilet. I don't know why the sound of running water works, but it does.

As all parents learn, eating and elimination are functions that the child controls. If she just can't or won't urinate in the hat, go out, buy her the largest drink you can find, and wait.

It may be necessary to obtain a sterile specimen of urine, or "clean catch," if infection is suspected. You or your child will need to cleanse the perineal area with soap or an antiseptic wipe, and she will need to urinate into a small sterile container.

If your child is not yet toilet trained, if a clean catch is impossible, or if your child is unable to urinate, it may be necessary to insert a urinary catheter. This procedure can be quite stressful, because it involves placing a sterile, flexible tube up the urethra and into the bladder. It is definitely appropriate to ask that your child be given a mild sedative or muscle relaxant before the procedure if he is anxious, and to request that the most skilled person available perform the procedure. In skilled nursing hands, the procedure takes less than five minutes to perform.

X-rays

X-rays, a type of electromagnetic radiation, provide the doctor with a quick and simple way to view organs and structures inside your child's body. X-rays are performed for many reasons during a child's treatment. Some of the most common reasons for taking x-rays are because they are:

• Needed before operations

- Needed after your child's central venous catheter is placed to confirm it is in the proper location
- Used to determine whether your feverish child has pneumonia

For chest x-rays, your child may be asked to breathe in, hold his breath, and remain perfectly still for a few seconds. The technologist leaves the room during the time the x-rays are taken. If you are planning to stay with your child, you need to wear a lead apron to protect yourself from radiation. Your child may also have to wear a lead apron or lead shield to protect specific areas of his body. Pregnant women should not be in the room when x-rays are taken.

Meagan is scheduled to go off therapy this May. She's doing well and is very happy. A father at our support group was advising a new set of parents to remember to view life from the child's perspective. He said that, especially with the little ones, parents sometimes agonized more than the child. He told us that at the end of the first year of treatment, he and his wife were reflecting on how much misery their child had endured, and then she piped up and said, "This has been a great year for me!" Meagan is the same. When I have bad days and get preoccupied with the uncertain future, I see Meagan skipping along and saying as she frequently does, "I'm such a happy girl!"

Chapter 10

Forming a Partnership with the Medical Team

"The good physician treats the disease; the great physician treats the patient who has the disease."

— William Osler, MD

IT IS EXTREMELY IMPORTANT that parents and the medical team establish and maintain a relationship based on excellent medical care, good communication, and caring. Trust is essential in this partnership. Doctors rely on parents to make and keep appointments, give the right medicines at the correct times, prepare their child for procedures, and monitor their child for signs of illness or side effects. Parents rely on doctors for medical knowledge, expertise in performing procedures, good judgment, compassion, and clear communication. It is a delicate balance that spans years of trauma and emotional upheaval. Cooperation and respect between the healthcare team and parents supports children and helps them cope. This chapter explores ways to create and maintain that environment.

Choosing a Hospital

At diagnosis, if your family is not initially referred to a specific children's hospital, or if there is more than one excellent children's hospital in your area, you may be able to choose where you would like your child to be treated. Parents can obtain a free referral to an accredited center from the National Cancer Institute (800) 422-6237 or from the:

Children's Oncology Group (COG)
(626) 447-0064
https://childrensoncologygroup.org/index.php/locations

> *We decided to have treatment at our local children's hospital (member of COG) instead of going far away to a big city hospital. My daughter was 4 when she was diagnosed with AML, her sister was 2½, and her brother was 9 months. I was nursing my son, so we moved the whole family into the hospital. The nurses were great— they moved a second bed into the room for us to use in addition to the pull-out couch. It was a mixed pediatrics floor, not just oncology, so we were put in a laminar air*

flow room to reduce the risk of infection. We had special hallway slippers to use when we left the room, and we washed our hands every time we had been out of the room. I stayed in the room with all three kids, and my husband came after work and slept with us there at night. I wanted to make it as normal as possible, so I brought in wheeled shelves with books and toys and a little wood table and chairs. The child life specialists brought in a play mat, and we covered the walls with the girls' drawings and pictures. We were in the hospital almost continuously from November to June, and we celebrated a third birthday and a first birthday there.

In recent years, the way health care has been planned and delivered to children has changed. It is now based on the concept of family-centered care. The core concepts of family-centered care are respect, dignity, information sharing, participation, and collaboration, which foster healthy relationships among healthcare providers, parents, and children. At most children's hospitals, a family-centered team is assigned to each family with a newly diagnosed child. This team—composed of physicians, physician assistants, nurses, child life specialists, psychologists, social workers, physical and occupational therapists, and others—strives to ensure that the emotional, social, and developmental needs of every family member are addressed, in addition to the medical care of the child. Members of your child's team will be there to answer questions and provide emotional support while recognizing that you are the expert about your child.

The day my 3-month-old daughter was diagnosed, we met the team—oncologist, nurse, nurse practitioner, child life specialist, and social worker. They are the ones who take care of us during our frequent hospitalizations; they provide consistency and much, much more. The nurses just get it. They understand why sometimes I burst into tears when they say, "How are you doing?" They have been our family in the darkest of hours. They are the only thing I am going to miss when this is all over.

The Doctors

At large children's hospitals, there are doctors at all levels of training—from first-year medical students to experienced professors of medicine. It's often hard to sort them all out in the chaotic early days after diagnosis. This section describes each type of doctor you might meet at a large children's hospital.

A **medical student** is a college graduate who is attending medical school. Medical students often wear white coats, but they do not have MD (i.e., Doctor of Medicine) after their name on their name tags. They are not doctors.

An **intern** (also called a first-year resident) is a graduate of medical school who is in the first year of postgraduate training. Interns are doctors who are just beginning their clinical training.

A **resident** is a graduate of medical school in the second or third year of postgraduate training. Most residents at pediatric hospitals will be pediatricians when they complete their residencies. Residents are temporary: they rotate into different services (e.g., cardiology, neurology, oncology) every four weeks.

A **fellow** is a doctor who has completed residency training and is now focusing on a particular specialty. Most fellows you encounter will be specializing in pediatric oncology.

Attending doctors (or simply, attendings) are highly trained doctors hired by the hospital to provide and oversee medical care and to train interns, residents, and fellows. They have completed a residency and a fellowship program. Many of them also teach at a medical school.

Consulting doctors are doctors from other services who are brought in to provide advice or treatment to a child in the oncology unit. The attending may ask for consults with other specialists, who may appear in your child's hospital room unexpectedly. If questions arise about who these doctors are and what role they play, you should ask any member of your family-centered team.

> *I've been very lucky that our doctors have been very open with us. When Samantha was first diagnosed, our doctor spent two hours explaining and answering our questions, and it has never stopped. Even if we haven't asked, but the doctors notice concern in our faces, they sit and take the time to find out our worries. They've all been great—the nurses, hospital, and support staff.*

Each child in a teaching hospital is assigned an attending, who is responsible for that child's care. This doctor should be board certified or have equivalent medical credentials. This means the doctor has taken rigorous written and oral tests given by a board of examiners in his or her specialty and meets a high standard of competence. You can call the American Board of Medical Specialties at (866) ASK-ABMS (275-2267) or visit *www.certificationmatters.org/is-your-doctor-board-certified.aspx* to find out whether your child's attending is board certified.

If your family is insured by a health maintenance organization (HMO), or an insurance company that maintains a list of preferred hospitals, you probably will be sent to an affiliated hospital, which will have one or more pediatric oncologists on staff. If this hospital is not a regional pediatric hospital, you can go elsewhere to get state-of-the-art care (see the "Choosing a hospital" section earlier in this chapter). However, make sure your insurance will cover care at the institution you choose.

The Nurses

An essential part of the hospital hierarchy is the nursing staff. The following explanations will help you understand which type of nurse is caring for your child.

An **LPN** is a licensed practical nurse. LPNs complete certificate training and must pass a licensing exam. In some hospitals, LPNs are allowed to perform most nursing functions, except those involving administration of medications. Many pediatric oncology services limit the involvement of LPNs to personal care, such as patient hygiene and monitoring fluid input and output.

An **RN** is a registered nurse who obtained an associate's degree or higher in nursing and then passed a licensing examination. RNs who have a bachelor's degree in nursing are also referred to as BSNs. RNs supervise all other nursing and patient care staff (such as nurses aides or nursing assistants), give medicines, take vital signs (e.g., heart rate, breathing rate, blood pressure), monitor IV machines, and change bandages. Many RNs in the pediatric oncology service have received specialized training in pediatric oncology nursing and have taken an examination to receive the credential of Certified Pediatric Hematology/Oncology Nurse (CPHON).

A **nurse practitioner** or **clinical nurse specialist** is a registered nurse who has completed an educational program (a master's or doctoral degree) that teaches advanced skills. For example, in some hospitals and clinics, nurse practitioners perform procedures such as spinal taps. Nurse practitioners or clinical nurse specialists are often the liaison between the medical teams and patients and their families.

The **head** or **charge nurse** is an RN who supervises all the nurses on the hospital floor for one shift. If you have any problems with a nurse in the hospital, your first step in resolving the issue should be to talk to the nurse involved. If this does not fix the problem, the next step is a discussion with the charge nurse.

The **clinical nurse manager** is the administrator for an entire unit, such as a surgical or medical floor or outpatient clinic. The clinical nurse manager is in charge of all nurses on that unit.

> At our hospital, each of our nurses is different, but each is wonderful. They simply love the kids. They throw parties, set up dream trips, act as counselors, best friends, and stern parents. They hug moms and dads. They cry. I have come to respect them so much because they have such a hard job to do, and they do it so well.

Finding an Oncologist

Parents do not have the luxury of time in choosing a pediatric oncologist. At diagnosis, the family is usually sent to the nearest children's hospital where the child is assigned a pediatric oncologist (attending) or fellow who is in charge of all treatment. Often the assigned oncologist is a good match, and the family finds the doctor to be competent, caring, and easy to communicate with.

> Justin's oncologist had remarkable interpersonal skills. At our first meeting he said, "Justin has leukemia. There are two kinds of leukemia, and both of them are treatable." So right away he emphasized the positive. He then wrote on his notepad what all of Justin's blood counts were; he told us what normal counts were and explained clearly what we needed to do next. He was very reassuring. It has been years since that day, and he has always been very caring. He still frequently calls us on the phone.

If you don't develop a good rapport with the oncologist assigned to your child, you can ask to be assigned to a different oncologist you may have met on rounds or during clinic visits. Most parent requests are accommodated, as hospitals realize the importance of good communication between family members and doctors. Your child will, however, still be seen by several different doctors throughout treatment, because most institutions have rotating doctors on call.

Types of Relationships

Three types of relationships tend to develop between doctors and parents.

Paternal. In a paternal relationship, the parent is submissive, and the doctor assumes a parental role. This dynamic may seem desirable to parents who are uncomfortable or inexperienced in dealing with medical issues, but it places all the responsibility for decisions and monitoring on the doctor. Although you may feel overwhelmed and nervous at the beginning, it is important to remember that you are the expert when it comes to your child, and you know best how to gauge his reactions to drugs and treatments.

> I once asked a fellow about my daughter's blood work. She literally patted me on the head and said it was her job to worry about that, not mine. I said in a nice voice that I thought it was a reasonable question and that I would appreciate an answer.

Some parents are intimidated by doctors and fear that if they question the doctors their child will suffer. This behavior prevents the child from having an adult who speaks up when something seems wrong.

Adversarial. Some parents adopt an "us against them" attitude, which is counterproductive. They seem to feel the disease and treatment are the fault of the medical staff, and they blame staff for any setbacks that occur. This attitude undermines the child's confidence in her doctor.

> I knew one family that just hated the children's hospital. They called it the "house of horrors" or the "torture chamber" in front of their children. Small wonder that their children were terrified.

If you or someone in your family has had negative interactions with medical professionals in the past, it can be difficult to get past those feelings and work comfortably with doctors and nurses. The pediatric oncology world is often more collaborative and open to family input than other arenas of medical care. It's helpful to find out which people are responsible for various parts of your child's tests and treatments, and to try to get to know each of them. That way you can feel more comfortable asking them questions and will have a better sense of when care is being handled well. Also, if something goes wrong, you will have good relationships with the people you need to call on to correct it.

Collegial. This is a true partnership in which parents and doctors are all on the same footing and respect each other's domains and expertise. The doctor recognizes that the parents are the experts on their child and are essential in ensuring that the protocol is followed. The parents respect the doctor's expertise and feel comfortable discussing various treatment options or concerns that arise. Honest communication is necessary for this partnership to work, and the effort is well worth it. The child has confidence in his doctor, the parents have lessened their stress by creating a supportive relationship with the doctor, and the doctor feels comfortable that the family will comply with the treatment plan, giving the child the best chance for a cure.

> We had a wonderful relationship with our daughter's oncologist. He perfectly blended the science and the art of medicine. His manner with our daughter was warm, he was extremely well-qualified professionally, and he was very easy to talk to. I could bring in articles to discuss with him, and he welcomed the discussion. Although he was busy, he never rushed us. I laughed when I saw that he had written in the chart, "Mother asks innumerable appropriate questions."

Another mother relates a different experience:

> We tried very hard to form a partnership with the medical team but failed. The staff seemed very guarded and distant, almost wary of a parent wanting to participate in the decisions made for the child. I learned to use the medical library and took research reports in to them to get some help for side effects and get some drug dosages reduced. Things improved, but I was never considered a partner in the healthcare team; I was viewed as a problem.

Communication

Clear and frequent communication is the foundation of a positive doctor/parent relationship. Doctors need to be able to explain clearly and listen well, and parents need to feel comfortable asking questions and expressing concerns before they grow into grievances. Nurses and doctors cannot read parents' minds, nor can parents prepare their child for a procedure unless it has been explained well. A pediatric oncologist shares her perspective:

> All parents are different and have different coping styles. Some deal best with a lot of information (lab results, meds, study options) up front, while others are overwhelmed and want the information a little bit at a time. There is no way for the doctor to know the parents' coping styles at the beginning. (Even the parents may not yet know!) So if they let the doctor know how much information they want or don't want, it is very helpful.

The following are parent suggestions about how to establish and maintain good communication with your child's medical team.

* Tell the staff how much you want to know.

> I told them the first day to treat me like a medical student. I asked them to share all information, current studies, lab results, everything, with me. I told them that I hoped they wouldn't be offended by lots of questions, because knowledge was comfort to me.

· · · · ·

> If the doctors at Children's told me to do something, I didn't question it because I trusted them.

* Inform the staff of your child's temperament, likes, and dislikes. You know your child better than anyone, so don't hesitate to tell the clinic staff about what works best.

> Whenever my daughter was hospitalized, I made a point of kindly reminding doctors and nurses that she was extremely sensitive, and would benefit from quiet voices and soothing explanations of anything that was about to occur, such as taking temperatures, vital signs, or adjustments to her IV.

* Encourage a close relationship between doctor, nurse, and child. Insist that all medical personnel respect your child's dignity. Do not let anyone talk in front of your child as if she is not there. A child with cancer shared her feelings in *Advice to Doctors and Other Big People*:

> The best part about the doctor is when he gives me bubble gum. The worst part is when he's in the room with me and my mom and he only talks to my mom. I've told him I don't like that, but he doesn't listen.

- Most children's hospitals assign each child a family-centered team, including a primary nurse. Try to form a close relationship with your child's nurse. Nurses usually possess vast knowledge and experience about both medical and practical aspects of cancer treatment. Often, the nurse can fix misunderstandings between doctors and parents.

- Children and teenagers should be included as part of the team. They should hear the explanations of treatments and procedures and be given age-appropriate choices.

> Leeann's doctor has been great. She knows how to talk to kids without talking down to them. She would take the time during her hospital rounds to help Leeann with her homework and laugh at all of our stupid jokes. A good sense of humor was a must for all of us.

- Coordinate communication. If your hometown pediatrician will handle blood work or other routine testing, find ways to facilitate communication between the oncologist and pediatrician.

> During maintenance, we had a problem with the pediatrician's office not calling me with the results of my daughter's blood work in time for me to call the hospital ped onc clinic. This would result in worry for me and a delay in changes to her chemotherapy doses. I told the pediatrician's nurse that I knew how busy they were and I hated having to keep calling to get the results. I asked her if it was possible for them to give the lab authorization to call me with the results. They thought it was a great idea, and it worked for years. The lab would fax the doctor the results, but call me. Then I would call the hospital clinic and get the dose changes. The clinic would then fax that information to the pediatrician's office. It was a win/win situation: the pediatrician's office received no interruptions, they got copies of everything in writing, and I got quick responses from the clinic on how to adjust her meds to her wildly swinging blood counts.

- Go to all appointments with a written list of questions. This prevents you from forgetting something important and avoids the need for numerous follow-up phone calls.

- Ask for definitions of unfamiliar terms. Repeat back the information to ensure you understood it correctly. Writing down answers or recording meetings are both common practices.

- Ask about access to medical records. Some parents want to read their child's medical chart to get more details about their child's condition and to help in formulating questions for the medical team. Sometimes the doctor or nurse will let the parents read the chart in the child's hospital room or in the waiting room at the clinic, but some hospitals have policies that prohibit this. As access to online medical records becomes more common, you may be able to log in to the chart from home to read the physicians' notes, and keep track of blood counts and other test results. Most states and provinces have laws that allow patient access to all records. Keep in mind that hospitals may restrict parental access to the full medical record if the child is a teen; this is done to protect your child's confidential medical discussions with his physician. Your teen can choose (or not) to sign a form allowing you complete access to the records.

• If you have questions or concerns, discuss them with the nurses or residents. If they are unable to provide a satisfactory answer, ask the fellow or attending doctor assigned to your child.

> We found that sitting down and talking things over with the nurses helped immensely. They were very familiar with each drug and its side effects. They told us many stories about children who had been through the same thing and were doing well years later. They always seemed to have time to give encouragement, a smile, or a hug.

• Remember you have the right to make requests about who does certain procedures. The medical team includes many specialists: doctors, nurses, child life specialists, social workers, physical therapists, nutritionists, x-ray technicians, radiation therapists, and more. At training hospitals, many of these people will be in the early stages of their training. If a procedure is not going well, you have the right to tell the person to stop and to request that a more skilled person do the job.

> At our children's hospital, family practice residents rotate through, and are often assigned to do the spinal taps. My son was on a high-dose methotrexate protocol, which required a rescue drug to be administered at a certain time. Once, the resident tried for an hour to do the tap, and just couldn't do it. My son was very late getting the rescue drug, and I was worried. Later, I requested a conference with the oncologist and asked him to perform the spinal taps in the future to prevent the residents from practicing on my child. He agreed, but I didn't intervene that first time and I felt very guilty.

• Know your rights—and the hospital's. Legally, your child cannot be treated without your permission. If the doctor suggests a procedure you do not feel comfortable with, keep asking questions until you feel fully informed. You have the legal right to refuse the procedure if you do not think it is necessary.

> One day in the hospital, a group of fellows came in and announced that they were going to do a lung biopsy on Jesse. I told them that I hadn't heard anything about it from her attending, and I just didn't think it was the right thing to do. They said, "We have to do it," and I repeated that I just didn't think it needed to be done until we talked to the attending. They seemed angry, but I stood my ground. When the attending came later, he said that they were not supposed to do a biopsy because the surgeon said it was too risky of an area in the lung to get to.

- However, if the hospital staff feels you are endangering the health of your child by withholding permission for treatment, they can take you to court. Everyone must remember that the most important person in this circumstance is the child.

- Use "I" statements. For example, "I feel upset when you won't answer my questions," rather than, "You never listen to me."

- If it helps you feel more comfortable, keep track of your child's treatments to check for mistakes.

> *A nurse thought my daughter had a double-lumen catheter and put two incompatible drugs through her single lumen line. It immediately turned to concrete. Arielle had to have the line removed. When they took it out, we saw the drugs had precipitated and formed what looked like little tablets. If this had become dislodged into her bloodstream (a very real possibility) it could have been fatal. Scary! I check everything now.*

- Be specific and diplomatic when describing problems.

> *Noah was 5 months old and receiving radiation treatment. I felt very strongly that an infant should be able to wake up to his mother (and that not having the mother present was emotionally damaging to the baby). I was upset that the anesthesia team was not honoring this concern, and I was simply told, "He won't remember." I made the point that "He may not remember here," pointing to my head, but that "He does remember here," pointing to my heart. I arranged to be called to the treatment room shortly before he awakened from anesthesia.*

- If you have something to discuss with the doctor that will take some time, request a care conference. These are routinely scheduled between parents and doctors and should be planned to allow enough time for a thorough discussion. Grabbing the attention of a busy doctor in the hallway is not fair to her and may not result in a satisfactory answer for you.

> *One technique I use to keep from forgetting what I want to say at the doctor's appointment is to type out an agenda for the appointment. I also make a copy for the doctor. This helps me stay calm and focused on the agenda, and it gives me and my doctor a written record of what our concerns were, and what was discussed during the appointment.*

- Do not be afraid to speak up when you are right or to apologize if you are wrong.

> *When my daughter was in the hospital one time, the nurse came in with two syringes. I asked what they were, and she said immunizations. I said that it must be a mistake because my daughter was immunosuppressed from treatment, and the nurse said that the orders were in the chart. So I checked my daughter's chart, and the orders were there, but they had another child's name on them.*

- Show appreciation.

  I sent thank-you notes to three residents after my daughter's first hospitalization. The notes were short but sweet. I wanted them to know how much we appreciated their many kindnesses.

  • • • • •

  I always try to thank the nurse or doctor when they apologize for being late and give the reason. I don't mind waiting if it is for a good cause, and I feel they show respect when they apologize.

  • • • • •

  Erica's doctor would sometimes call up just to say, "How's my little chickadee?" He really cared. It touched me that he took the time to call, and I often told him that I appreciated it.

The Tumor Board

Many hospitals have a committee to review surgery, pathology, and radiology findings and discuss potential treatment plans for individual children or teens with cancer. This committee is called the tumor board. Members consist of representatives from the child's multidisciplinary team, a pathologist, a radiologist, and other senior specialists who deal with childhood cancer. Often, the consensus opinion from the tumor board is the treatment offered to the family. Many centers present individual cases to the tumor board at various times during treatment, such as when the effects of treatment need to be assessed.

Getting a Second Opinion

There are times during your child's treatment when getting a second opinion may be advisable. Parents are sometimes reluctant to request a second opinion because they are afraid of offending their child's doctor or creating hard feelings. The majority of doctors will not resent a parent for seeking a second opinion. If your child's doctor does resist, ask why. Second opinions are a common and accepted practice, and they are sometimes required by insurance companies.

There are two ways to get a second opinion: see a pediatric oncologist at a different center of excellence or ask your child's doctor to arrange for your child's situation to be discussed at the tumor board. Many parents seek a second opinion at the time of diagnosis, but it is better not to do this in secret. Explain to your child's pediatric oncologist that, before proceeding, you would like an additional viewpoint. To allow for a thorough analysis, arrange to have copies of all records, test results, and pathology slides sent ahead to the doctor who will give the second opinion.

Personally, I feel there is nothing wrong with getting a second opinion from another major center. If you like and feel comfortable with your current team, that's great, but I definitely do not like when a doctor tells us there's "no reason" to go elsewhere, that "they can't do anything we don't do," and so forth. Many people travel great distances to get treatment at another facility whose treatment philosophy they prefer. And, granted, that is their choice. Now, your second opinion doctor may look at your child's records and say, "Your team is doing exactly the right things; stick with them," or he may tell you something totally different and then you can make your own decision on what to do.

Doctors informally seek second opinions all the time. For example, residents confer with their fellows about complicated situations. Fellows confer with the attending when unusual drug reactions or responses to treatment occur. Also, attendings call colleagues within other specialties and at other institutions. Thus, parents should feel free to ask their child's physician whether he has conferred with other staff members to gain additional viewpoints.

Brent developed a seizure disorder after a rare drug reaction, so he was on anticonvulsants as well as chemotherapy for two years. We worried about the interaction of all the drugs, as well as the advisability of his continuing on the more aggressive arm of the protocol. We asked the fellow to arrange a care conference, and she met with us, the clinic director, and Brent's neurologist to discuss how best to manage his case.

Conflict Resolution

Conflict is a part of life. In a situation where a child's life is at risk, the heightened emotions and constant involvement with medical bureaucracy guarantee conflict. Clashes will happen, so resolving them is very important. A speedy resolution may result if you adopt Henry Ford's motto, "Don't find fault; find a remedy." Following are some suggestions from parents about how to resolve problems:

• Treat the doctors with respect and expect respect from them.

I always wanted to be treated as an intelligent adult, not someone of lesser status. So I would ask each medical person what they wished to be called. We would either both go by first names or both go by titles. I did not want to be called mom.

• Expect a reasonable amount of sensitivity from the staff.

Soon after my daughter began treatment, I was walking by the open door of the residents' room, which was directly across from the nurses' station. Written in large letters on the blackboard were the words "Have a blast of a day!" with a picture of a smiling leukemia blast drawn below. I felt like I had been punched in the stomach. I was too upset to say anything, but I always regretted not complaining.

- Treat the staff with sensitivity. Recognize that you are under enormous stress, and so are the doctors and nurses. Do not blame them for the disease or explode in anger. Be an advocate, not an adversary.

- If a problem develops, state the issue clearly and without accusations—then suggest a solution.

- Recognize that although it is hard to speak up, especially if you are not naturally assertive, it is very important to solve the problem before it grows and poisons the relationship.

- Most large medical centers have social workers and psychologists on staff to help families. One of their major roles is to serve as mediators between staff and parents. You can ask for their advice about problem solving.

- Monitor your own feelings of anger and fear. Be careful not to act inappropriately toward the staff. On the other hand, do not let a doctor or nurse behave unprofessionally toward you or your child. Parents and staff members all have bad days, but they should not take it out on each other.

> During our little boy's first procedure, I was very emotional, and wondered out loud if he could feel or hear what was going on even though he was sedated. The nurse caught me completely off-guard by banging loudly on the side of the transport bed without getting any reaction from him. "See, he's out," she said. I was too startled then, but I wished I had told her how much that bothered me.

- Do not fear punishment for speaking up. It is possible to be assertive without being aggressive or argumentative. If you are worried, you can practice what you have to say with a trusted listener before approaching the treatment team.

- There are times when no resolution is possible, but expressing one's feelings can be a great release.

> My son and I waited in an exam room for over an hour for a painful procedure. When I went out to ask the receptionist what had caused the delay, she said that a parent had brought in a child without an appointment. When the doctor finally came in, an hour and a half later, my son was in tears. The doctor did not explain the delay or apologize, he just silently started the procedure. After it was finished, I went out of the room, found the doctor, and said, "This makes me so angry. You just left us in here for hours and traumatized my son." He told me that I should have more compassion for the other mother because her life was very difficult. I replied that he encouraged her to not make appointments by dropping everything whenever she appeared. I added that it wasn't fair to those parents who played by the rules; she was being rewarded for her irresponsibility. After we had each stated our position, we left without resolution.

Changing Doctors

Facing childhood cancer is one of life's greatest struggles. A skilled doctor you trust, who communicates easily and honestly with you, can greatly ease this struggle. If the doctor adds to your family's discomfort rather than reducing it, you may have to change doctors. Changing doctors is not a step to be taken lightly, but it can be a great relief if the relationship has deteriorated beyond repair. It is a good policy to exhaust all possible remedies before separating and to examine your role in the relationship to prevent the same problems from arising with the new doctor. Mediation by social service staff and improved communication can often resolve the issues and prevent the disruption of changing doctors.

Although there are many valid reasons for changing doctors, some of the most common are:

- Grave medical errors being made.
- Poor communication skills or refusal to answer questions.
- Serious clash of philosophy or personality; for example, a paternalistic doctor and a parent who wishes to be informed and share in decision making.

Many parents, fearing retribution, stay with a doctor in whom they have no confidence. But children may actually suffer more from the added family stress caused by a poor doctor–parent relationship than from changing doctors. Although there may be lingering bitterness or anger between parents and doctors if you change doctors at the children's hospital, the child will continue to benefit from the best-known treatment.

> *Early in my daughter's treatment, we changed doctors. The first was aloof and patronizing, and the second was smart, warm, funny, and caring. He was a constant bright spot in our lives through some dark times. So every year during my daughter's treatment, she and her younger sister put on their Santa hats and brought homemade cookies to her doctor and nurse. This year was the first time she was able to walk in, and she looked them in the eye and sang, "We Wish You a Merry Christmas." Her nurse went in the back room and cried, and her doctor got misty-eyed. I'll always be thankful for their care.*

Once the decision is made to change doctors, parents must be candid. They should give an explanation for the change, either verbally or in writing, and make a formal request to transfer records to the new doctor. Doctors are legally required to transfer all records upon written request.

We've had wonderful docs, mediocre docs, and one who made a terrible mistake. We've had warm, compassionate docs, ho-hum docs (on a good day they're nice, on a bad day they're neutral), and we've met a couple of world-class jerks. Sounds pretty much like a slice of humanity, right?

Parents hold doctors to a different standard because the stakes are so high—our kids' lives. But the reality is they are usually overworked, exhausted, and deal with newly diagnosed families on an almost daily basis, day after day, week after week, year after year. I can't even begin to imagine the emotional toll that must take.

I tell my kids all human relationships are like a goodwill bank. If you make lots of deposits, an occasional withdrawal won't be so noticeable. I tell my docs and my kids' docs whenever things go right. I like to write, so I send many thank-you notes. When our pediatrician went on sabbatical, he took me into his office and showed me every Christmas card my kids had created and sent him lined up on the back of his messy desk.

I also have been known to bring in brownies for the office staff. We did this on my daughter's last day of radiation and several people brushed away tears when they saw the thank-you note she drew—a picture of herself holding a Snow White and the Seven Dwarves audiotape. She listened to that during every radiation session because I'd promised that day's radiation treatment would be over before the dwarves appeared.

I recently asked one of my favorite doctors (a pediatric oncologist who has incredible compassion) how many thank-you notes she had received from parents over the years. She said she could count them on two hands. I asked how many complaints, and she said, "You wouldn't want to know."

So, while I think docs should be called out for bad behavior and bad medicine, I also think we should continually acknowledge good medicine and good behavior. I'd like to encourage the good ones to stick around—new little innocents keep getting cancer every day.

Chapter 11

Hospitalization

"Every day is a journey, and the journey itself is home."
— Matsuo Basho

THERE ARE FEW THINGS in life more uncomfortable than rising from a lumpy pull-out couch to face another day of your child's hospitalization for leukemia. Hospitals are noisy bureaucracies that run on a time schedule all their own. Staff members wake children in the middle of the night to draw blood or check temperature, pulse, and blood pressure. Groups of doctors at all levels of training drop in unannounced.

For a child, being hospitalized means being separated from parents, brothers, sisters, friends, classmates, pets, and the comfort and familiarity of home. A child's hospitalization can rob both parent and child of a sense of control, leaving them feeling helpless. But with a little ingenuity, you can make the most of the facilities, liven up the atmosphere, and even have some fun on the good days.

The Room

Because kids on chemotherapy are at increased risk of infection, many hospitals give them private rooms. This means more space for the child, the parents, and visitors; it also means much more freedom to personalize and decorate the room. Covering the walls with big, bright posters of interest to your child can brighten up the room immensely.

> *The first thing we put up in Meagan's room was a huge poster of* The Little Engine That Could *saying, "I think I can, I think I can."*

Cards can be displayed on the walls, hanging from strings like a mobile, or taped around the windowsills. You can display pictures of your child engaged in her favorite activities and add photos of her friends. Most hospitals do not allow flowers on oncology floors because they can grow a fungus that can make children sick; but it's fun to have bouquets of plastic balloons bobbing in the corners (children's hospitals do not allow latex balloons). Younger children may be greatly comforted by having a favorite stuffed animal, blanket, or quilt on their bed. If your child likes certain scents, you can make the room smell good with aromatherapy oils.

> *I bought a travel bag on wheels. It is so much easier than trying to carry several handle bags when Zach is admitted. It has several pockets to carry stuff. I love it and wished I had done it two years ago when we started this! I take these things to the hospital: flavored creamer for my coffee (a little treat for me); a book for us to read together so I don't go crazy from Cartoon Network (we are reading the Narnia series, and Zach begs me to read to him. I snuggle up with him in his bed while we read); his favorite pillow from home; little airplanes and parachuters to drop from the third floor at night when the lobby is empty (if he's feeling well enough); my thermometer so I can check his temp any time I want to; lots of Legos®; phone numbers of friends; canned ravioli; toaster strudels; audio books (Adventures in Odyssey®); and music DVDs with earphones.*

To personalize visits, some parents bring a guestbook for people to sign. Others put up a medical staff sign-in poster, which must be signed before examinations begin or vital signs are taken. Another variation of the sign-in poster is to have each staff member or visitor outline his or her hand and write his or her name within the handprint. Children can use a digital camera or smartphone to take pictures of the many staff members who come into the room.

> *In my position as a parent consultant, I suggest that a journal (possible titles are* Book of Hope, Book of Sharing, My Cancer Experience, *and* Friends Indeed) *be kept in the child's room for any visitor, family member, or medical caregiver to write in at any time. Leaving a message if the child is sleeping or out of the room for procedures can be a nice surprise. Later, a surviving child and her family, or the family of a child who has died, have a memory book of those who have touched their lives.*

Bringing music and a portable music player with small speakers will help block out some of the hospital noise and can help everyone relax. A portable sound machine that has relaxing sounds such as ocean waves, falling rain, or white noise can be played while the child sleeps. An iPod® or other portable audio device with headphones and the child's favorite music or audio books can also make the time pass more quickly.

> *My daughter's preschool teacher sent a care package. She made a felt board with dozens of cutout characters and designs that provided hours of quiet entertainment. She also included games, drawings from each classmate, coloring books, markers, get well cards, and a child's tape player with earphones. Because we had run out of our house with just the clothes on our backs, all of these toys were very, very welcome.*

Many children's hospitals have in-room or portable DVD players available. You can check out DVDs from the hospital media library or bring a favorite funny movie or DVD of a television show. Humor helps, so joke books and things that make kids laugh (such as Silly String®) are great items to pack. Most hospitals have Wi-Fi, so children and teens can use social media, play games online, and stream movies and television shows.

> *A friend brought in a bag from the local dollar store. He included a water pistol, Play-Doh®, a Slinky®, checkers, dominos, bubbles, a book of corny jokes, and puzzles.*

The Floor

It helps to have a floor tour as soon as possible after admission. During the tour, you will find out whether a microwave and refrigerator are available, what the approved parent sleeping arrangements are, and whether showers are available for parents. You can also ask about a hospital handbook. These booklets often include information about billing, parking, discounts, and other helpful items.

> *Either my husband or I stayed with Delaney the entire time she was in the hospital (with AML that is not a small number of nights). To improve the comfort of the fold-out chair that the hospital provides for the sleep-in parent, we used an inflatable camping mat. When it is rolled out, it self-inflates with a one-way valve. The straps can be used to secure it to the vinyl chair. It makes the chair much more comfortable and allows your muscles to relax. When it is not in use, it can be rolled up with straps and set in the corner.*

Although many hospitals provide colorful smocks for young patients, some children and teens prefer to wear their own clothing. This can pose a laundry problem, so find out whether the hospital has laundry facilities for families to use.

> *Our entire family stayed in the hospital for most of the six months when my 4-year-old daughter was treated for AML—me, my husband, and our three children, ages 4, 2, and 9 months. A few months in, we learned that the guest bathroom on the floor just below was much better than ours. So I'd take the baby down, strapped in a little umbrella stroller, to shower. The girls were very good about staying in the room alone—one time I came back and found a nurse playing hide and seek with them. The nurses were wonderful to us. Nurse Jesse even came in on Christmas morning to tell the kids that she saw Rudolph's glowing nose the night before.*

Food

Buying meals day after day in the hospital cafeteria is expensive. Check with the hospital social worker to find out whether the hospital has food discount cards or free meals for parents. Some hospitals deliver meals to families via a meal cart or provide sandwiches in a family lounge at meal times. You can do an internet search or staff members can give you directions to the grocery store nearest the hospital to purchase fresh food and healthy snacks. Also check to see whether the floor has a refrigerator for parents' food and stock it with your favorite items.

> Our hospital provides vouchers for the cafeteria that can be used instead of ordering food for the room. For us, they have been a godsend. The food on the tray is much worse than what is in the cafeteria. Also, oncology patients have no spending cap on the vouchers, so we can get a few extras. When our son is not able to go to the cafeteria, we go down and bring the food back to his room.

Many hospitals have cooking facilities for families where they can cook or microwave favorite meals brought from home. Family and friends can bring food when they visit, and some parents order extra items for their child's tray. Ordering out for dinner can also be a nice change of pace for you and your child. As long as there are no medical restrictions, food from local restaurants can usually be delivered to your child's hospital room. Check with the nurses to see whether they have menus from local restaurants or recommendations.

> Just the smell of food nauseated my daughter. I'll never forget taking the tray out in the hall and gobbling the food down myself. I always felt so guilty, and thought that the staff viewed me as that parent who ate her kid's food. But it saved money and prevented her meals from going to waste. I also did not want to leave her side for the few minutes it took to go to the cafeteria although, in hindsight, the walk would have done me some good.

Parking

Many parents of children with cancer have unpleasant memories of driving around in endless loops looking for a parking space while their child was throwing up in a bucket in the back seat (or even worse, when the bucket was left at home). Some hospitals charge patients to park and some do not. The hospital might have both long-term and short-term parking arrangements. If your hospital charges for parking, the nurses or the patient advocate can tell you whether parking passes are available or where the cheapest parking is located. Some hospitals have valet parking, which may be as cheap as self-parking for a short appointment.

> I had no idea that the hospital gave out free parking passes to their frequent customers. Now I tell every new parent to check as soon as possible to see if they can get a parking pass. It will save them lots of money that they would have spent on meters and parking tickets, and time that they would have spent running out to move the car out of the emergency parking spot.

The Endless Waiting

Everything seems to take forever in the hospital. Parents must learn the art of waiting patiently or they will always be frustrated. For example, the nurse might tell you not to go to the playroom because someone will be "right up" to take your child for an echo-cardiogram. "Right up" can easily mean two hours or more. Many parents find them-selves getting nervous or angry while waiting for the doctors to appear during rounds each morning (when the attending physicians, fellows, residents, and interns move from room to room in a large group), then feeling let down when the visit lasts only a few moments. If you have questions to ask the doctors, you can write them down and tell the doctors when they come in that you would like a moment to discuss concerns or ask questions.

> *You don't have to go too crazy. Make sure you watch the videos or eat the popcorn or flirt with the nurses or taunt the residents or leave notes for the cleaning lady or chat with the security guard or make coffee for all the parents or pretend you like puking or show the nurses how to hack into the hospital mainframe or paint your face with butt paste. Or, all of the above, if you like. Just do something.*

It helps for both the parent and child to be prepared for long waits each time they come to the hospital. Some well-supported institutions have iPads®, DVDs, video games, books, and toys available, but you might need to bring your own entertainment, such as favorite card games, board games, computer games, drawing materials, and books. Some children will take comfort from having a favorite blanket or pillow with them for a day in the clinic or during a hospitalization. If your child is scheduled for surgery, you can bring a good book, a model airplane project, your holiday card list, or a jigsaw puzzle that several people can work on together—anything portable that can keep you occupied.

> *Our emergency bag had two sides. The most important was mine, because our hospital provided nothing for parents. I would pack deodorant (plus an extra set of clothes), a book I had not read (I survived on romance novels that I bought at the used bookstore, four for a dollar), decent lighting, a soft sweatshirt top and bottom to wear at night, paper and pen for taking notes, and clean socks. You might laugh, but I can deal with a scared, irritable kid for a L-O-N-G time as long as I have clean, soft socks!*

> *On Matthew's side was an art kit with Play-Doh®, crayons, pencils, markers, scissors, glue, finger paints, clay, and reams of paper. It also had plastic cutlery, and some cookie cutters for the Play-Doh®. I always brought the game Trouble®, since it's self-contained and the dice are enclosed in the little bubble. The pieces fit nicely in a plastic sandwich bag (or medication bag). The lifesaver was video games. They provided hours of enjoyment. We also brought a Lego® table with blocks. Since Matthew is usually neutropenic, or in isolation for some mysterious complication, we bring our own games. Monopoly® and Battleship® are both games that can take*

an entire morning to play. We always bring Matthew's special blanket on any clinic or ER visits. I cannot imagine trying to have him in the hospital without it. He does not carry it around, but it is always there at bedtime.

I also kept a box of stuff for me to do in case of incarceration at Club Children's. In particular, the box had pictures and photo albums. One nurse remarked how organized I was, but I pointed out that the album I was putting together was of Matthew's first birthday. He was almost six at the time.

Working with the Staff

There are wonderful and not-so-wonderful people employed by hospitals. It helps to remember that working in the pediatric oncology field is extremely stressful and that most of the staff are dedicated to the children. Even the tiniest effort on your part to ease their burden or empathize with their circumstances will go a very long way toward establishing a cooperative and friendly relationship. For example, if parents help change soiled bedding, take out food trays, and give their child baths, it can free up overworked nurses to take care of medicines and IVs. If you are making a run to the coffee shop, ask whether you can bring them something, too. Simply remembering to thank them every day will make a big difference. Chapter 10, *Forming a Partnership with the Medical Team*, contains suggestions for how to develop a positive relationship with the staff.

I always made a point of introducing myself to my daughter's nurse and resident for each shift. I told them my child's name and which room we were in. I told them that I would be there the whole time and that I would help as much as I could. I tried to talk to them about non-hospital matters to give them a break from their routine, as well as to get to know them. I thanked them for any kindnesses and told them I appreciated how hard their jobs were. Although I wasn't angling for favors, I found that they soon came to like me and helped me out whenever any difficulty arose. Although there were a few that I didn't care for, on the whole I found the staff members to be warm, caring, dedicated people.

• • • • •

We've spent 144 days in the hospital so far, and I don't mince words about foolish things that make life hard in there. I'm not easily intimidated and I use common sense. My daughter wears a pull-up diaper at night, so when nurses come in to check the restroom for pee, I tell them to leave because she wears a pull up. When they turn on the overhead light in the middle of the night, I turn it off and tell them to go get a flashlight. Most of the time, they are fine with that.

Having cancer strips children of control over their bodies. To help reverse this process, parents can take over some of the nursing care. Children may prefer to have their parents help them to the bathroom or clean up their diarrhea or vomit. Making the bed, keeping the room tidy, changing dressings, and giving back rubs helps your child feel more comfortable and lightens the burden on the nurses. However, some children and teens may feel better if the nurses provide these services.

Parents should not have to worry about helping the staff or whether the staff is stressed. They have enough on their plate to worry about. But families often feel like they're so helpless, and they think, "What can I do, how can I get in control of this situation?" Many parents find comfort in changing the bed; they very often feel so completely overwhelmed, because they can't give the medicines, and they can't make the cancer go away. So they do what they can do for their child. Look at the staff as a team. You are part of that team. But no one can be your child's parent but you.

In addition, parents and staff can help children regain some control by encouraging choices whenever possible. Older children should be involved in discussions about their treatments, while younger children can decide when to take a bath, which arm to use for an IV, what to order for meals, what position their body will be in for procedures, what clothes to wear, and how to decorate their room. Some children request a hug or a handshake after all treatments or procedures.

Our son is almost six. He prefers to talk first with the nurse or technician about fun stuff, like his trains, before he allows any kind of IV or blood draw. Most good techs don't mind; they try to do that anyway. He definitely prefers it when I step back, stay quiet, and let him lead.

It helps to learn about the shift changes on the oncology floor. If you need to leave during the day or night, do not leave a request with one nurse if another will be coming on duty soon. If you have a request or reminder, you can post it on your child's door, on the wall above the bed, or on the chart.

It also helps to find out whether there are support groups for parents, children with cancer, and siblings. These groups help family members of newly diagnosed children better understand the diagnosis and treatment, and provide much-needed support.

Staying with Your Child

Hospitals can be frightening places for children. Fear can be prevented or lessened if parents are there to provide comfort, support, and advocacy for their child. Most pediatric hospitals are quite aware of how much better children do when a parent is allowed to sleep in the room. Some rooms contain small couches that convert into beds, or parents can use a cot provided by the hospital.

Whenever my husband couldn't be at the hospital at bedtime, he would bring in homemade tapes of him reading bedtime stories. Our son would drift off to sleep hearing his daddy's voice.

Of course, sometimes it isn't possible to stay with your child if you are a single parent or if both parents work full time. Many families have grandparents, older siblings (older than age 18), or close friends who stay with the hospitalized child when the parents cannot be present. Older children and teenagers may not want a parent in the room at night, but they may need an advocate there during the day just as much as preschoolers.

> We were always there with her in the hospital, and one of us was always with her for treatments. However, she did not want us going back with her into the examining room, so we respected those wishes. Her doctor was very kind in always coming out and talking to us. He showed her complete respect as a 15 year old and also took time to meet our needs. She has always kept up with her own medical reports and concerns. Although her father and I have always been there with her and for her in the background, she has been much more knowledgeable about the whole cancer experience than we have in her treatments, medications, etc. She loves being in charge of her medical needs.

· · · · ·

> Our son was 3 years old when our 14-month-old daughter Emi was diagnosed with AML. Our daughter was in the hospital almost full time for six months. First, I tried to keep him with us at the hospital during the day, but he was pushing buttons and running around, so that was difficult. The hospital had a sibling space where they had lots of games and activities, but it isn't for full time day care. So, we were so grateful when one of the moms at his preschool offered to watch him during the weekdays when my husband was at work. My husband would pick him up, and bring him to the hospital so he could see me and Emi for an hour or two. I stayed every week day at the hospital, and my husband and I alternated nights. We never left her alone. We had relatives who drove up to do round-the-clock weekend hospital duty so that we had time at home with our son and each other.

In contrast, other families find staying at the hospital day and night to be too stressful. An oncologist made the following suggestion:

> When people are subject to stress, some people cope by focusing on all the details. For these people, being there all the time reduces their stress level. In other words, they would be more stressed if they were at home or work because they would be worrying all the time. Other people cope with stress by blocking out the details and trying to make life normal. I think that you need to think about how your family can best cope with this process and make your decisions based on that. Have a family meeting to sort out these issues, and don't feel bad if you decide what is best for your family is different from what other people say you should do.

Preventing Mistakes

Everyone makes mistakes and hospital workers are no exception. You can help by checking before any medications or blood transfusions are given. For instance, check that the name of the drug and the dose match what the protocol says should be given; if you were not given a summary of the protocol (sometimes called the roadmap), you can ask your nurse or doctor for a copy. You should feel free to ask questions or point out any deviations from prescribed treatment. Parents are the last line of defense against mistakes.

> In the beginning I didn't feel comfortable voicing my opinion, but I got over that, thank goodness. I used to be a people pleaser and worried about stepping on people's toes. But now, I recommend trusting your instincts and never doubting that you know your child best. For instance, when a nurse was putting a new dressing on my daughter's line, I saw a hole in the dressing right over the site. It felt like an out of body experience. I pointed out the hole and the nurse said, "Oh, my goodness!" and she fixed it. I've learned not to second guess myself about things that bother me. I've always been naive thinking that doctors and nurses always know what they are doing. But, now I realize it's been empowering for me as a mom that I know when things are wrong. Although I wish I was learning that lesson in a different way.

Whenever a family member isn't present, children who are old enough should have a charged cell phone or be taught to use the phone in the room. Tape a phone number nearby where a parent can be reached and tell your child to call if anyone tries to do procedures that are unexpected. The hospital staff should be informed that any changes in treatment (except emergencies) need to be authorized by a parent.

> Brian was 12 and could have stayed alone, but we never left him for more than five minutes to run down the hall for coffee, bathroom, etc. Someone—my husband, me, a grandparent, an aunt or uncle—was always there. If we had needed them, church members and friends had also volunteered, as Kevin (the younger brother) was only 2 at the time. With my husband rotating days at work and the hospital, and me rotating home and hospital, somehow we managed. A caring employer is essential.
>
> Also, Brian became very familiar with all his drugs, allergies, reactions, and doses. Several times he corrected the staff even before I could. We also had errors and near-errors, as I'm sure everyone does, but many fewer, I'm sure, because of the constant presence and watchful eyes. Operating room doctors and nurses accessed his line without first swabbing with alcohol. Someone wanted to give ibuprofen for fever. Non-oncology nurses were working the pediatric oncology floor and knew less than we did. Our hospital is now greatly improved, but things like this happen everywhere.

Playing

Children need to play, especially when hospitalized. The hospital probably has a recreation therapy or child life department that has toys, books, dolls, and crafts. The specialists in these departments use therapeutic play to help children express fears or concerns about what is happening to them.

> *Sometimes you can create your own fun with just a little imagination. On one particular occasion, Matthew was feeling especially bored. With a little ingenuity, we soon discovered that four unused IV poles and as many blankets as we could "steal" from the linen cart made for one pretty cool tent. We then used the mattress from a roll-away cot, and spent the night "camping" in his hospital room. He had a wonderful time.*

The fun-filled activities and smiling staff people in the child life or recreation therapy department are a cheerful change from lying in a hospital bed. If your child is too ill or if her counts are too low to go to the play area, arrangements can be made for a bundle of toys, games, and books to be brought to the room. Some hospitals host bingo games and silly variety shows on closed circuit TV so children who aren't able to go to the playroom can be included in the fun. Music and art therapists may also come to the bedside. A therapy dog and his human may visit to provide some canine love and comfort. These visits allow parents time to go out to eat or take a walk.

> *When I wanted to have a conference with the oncologist about Katy's protocol, I called recreation therapy and they sent two wonderful therapists to the clinic. The doctor and I were able to talk privately for an hour, and Katy had a great time making herself a gold crown and decorating her wheelchair with streamers and jewels.*

Exercise is important, too. For kids strong enough to walk, exploring the hospital can be fun. Even if they can't walk, you can wheel them around or pull them in a wagon if they feel up to it. (This is also a great workout for you.) Plan a daily excursion to the gift shop or the cafeteria. Go outside and walk the entire perimeter of the hospital if weather and the neighborhood permit. Don't feel limited by an IV pole; it can be pushed or pulled and will feel normal after a while. Many children stand on the base of the IV pole with a parent pushing them down the hall at a good clip. Physical and occupational therapists can help your child incorporate exercise into his daily routine.

> *At our hospital, there was a large metal tricycle with a huge metal basket on the back. I would cap off Kenny's IV, toss him in the back, then we would pedal all over the hospital. There is one part of the hospital called "the tunnel" that connects the children's hospital with Emory Hospital. It is about a mile-long tunnel—all downhill. Man, we would fly—laughing and screaming. Of course, coming back up was pure hell.*

Any action that parents, family members, and friends take to support and advocate for the child with cancer buoys the spirit.

In our hospital photos, I have several of a grinning 4 year old, hooked up to an IV, in a hospital bed, with the head raised waaaaaaayyyy up, as she'd slide down to the bottom. Of course I was doing guard duty at the door, to alert the happy child when a nurse was coming and she needed to "cease this unsafe behavior immediately!" Sometimes you have to make memories while you can, wherever you are.

Chapter 12

Central Venous Catheters

"Do what you can, with what you have, where you are."

— Theodore Roosevelt

MOST CHILDREN WITH LEUKEMIA require intensive treatment, including chemotherapy, intravenous (IV) fluids, IV antibiotics, transfusions, frequent blood sampling, and sometimes IV nutrition. Central venous catheters provide a very effective way to allow entry into the large veins for intensive therapy. They eliminate the difficulty of finding veins for peripheral IVs (commonly just referred to as IVs) and allow drugs to be put directly into the bloodstream, where they are rapidly diluted and spread throughout the body. Most important, they reduce stress and discomfort for the child by getting rid of the need for hundreds of needle sticks.

The three most common types of central venous catheters are external catheters, subcutaneous ports, and peripherally inserted central catheters (PICC). Other names for a central venous catheter include venous access device, right atrial catheter, implanted catheter, indwelling catheter, central line, Hickman®, Broviac®, PORT-A-CATH®, and Medi-port®.

This chapter first describes external, implanted, and PICC catheters—what they look like, how they are placed, the care they need, and their risks. Because some institutions allow families to choose the type of catheter, a section is included about making a decision. The chapter ends with descriptions of the types of adhesives that can be used to secure the lines in place.

External Catheter

An external catheter is a long, flexible tube with one end located in the right atrium of the heart and the other end outside the skin of the chest. The tube tunnels under the skin of the chest, enters a large vein near the collarbone, and threads inside the vein to the heart (see Figure 12-1). The tube that channels the fluid is called a lumen. Some external catheters have two channels (called double lumens).

Because chemotherapy drugs, transfusions, and IV fluids are put in the end of the tube hanging outside the body, the child feels no pain when blood is drawn out or medications are put in. Blood can be drawn from the end of the catheter for various blood tests. Central lines may be temporary or may stay in for months or years.

How it's put in

External catheters are usually put in while the child is under general anesthesia. Once the child is anesthetized, the surgeon or interventional radiologist makes two small incisions. One incision is near the collarbone over the spot where the catheter will enter the vein, and the other is in the area on the chest where the catheter exits the body. To prevent the catheter from slipping out, it may be stitched to the skin where it comes out of the chest (see Figure 12-1). There is a plastic cuff around the catheter right above the exit site (under the skin) into which body tissue grows. This tissue growth further anchors the catheter.

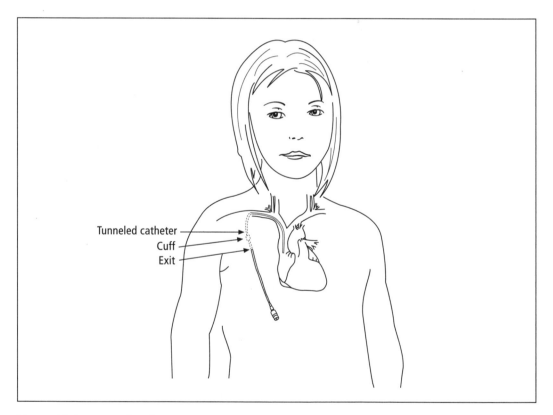

Figure 12-1: External catheter

Daily care

An external catheter requires careful maintenance to prevent infection or the formation of blood or drug clots. The site where the catheter exits the body needs to be cleaned often and a dressing applied. Procedures and schedules for cleaning and dressing vary from one institution to another. No matter what the care schedule is, the site should be checked daily for redness, swelling, and drainage, and you should contact your child's medical team if any of these are present.

To prevent clots in the catheter, parents or older children are taught to flush the line with a medication called heparin. Each institution uses its own flushing schedule, and nurses at the hospital teach parents and children how to care for the catheter. Both parent and child should be given lots of time to practice with supervision and should not be discharged until they are comfortable with the entire procedure. At discharge, parents can arrange for home nursing visits to provide further help, if needed.

> We were very grateful for Matthew's Hickman® line. Like a lot of children, he was terribly afraid of needles. The maintenance that was necessary to keep his line working properly became second nature to me. After his diagnosis, and again after his relapse, he had a Hickman® implanted. In total, he had his external catheter for more than four years.

Risks

The major complications of using an external catheter are infections—either in the blood or at the insertion site—and the formation of clots in the line. Rare complications include kinking of the catheter, the catheter moving out of place, or breakage of the external part of the catheter.

Infections. Even with the best care, infections still occur in children with external catheters. Children who have low white blood cell counts for long periods of time are at risk for developing infections anyway, and each time the line is flushed or cleaned there is a chance of contamination. It's important that all procedures are followed as closely as possible to decrease this risk.

> The surgeons inserted a tube—called a Broviac®—into 4-year-old Trevor's chest. This enabled Trevor to receive his chemotherapy treatment without getting a new IV put in each week. My husband and I were responsible for cleaning and flushing the Broviac® tube daily. Throughout the whole thing, Trevor was so strong and brave. After he had completed all his treatments, we were told that the catheter needed to stay in for a few more weeks. However, soon after treatment ended, Trevor was admitted back to the hospital when his catheter became infected. The doctors treated

him with antibiotics and decided to remove the Broviac® a little early. The Broviac®
prevented a lot of unnecessary pain, and we were grateful that he had it.

If your child develops a fever higher than 101° F (38.5° C), redness or swelling at the insertion site, or pain in the catheter area, you should suspect an infection. This is a life-threatening situation, so call the doctor immediately. To determine whether bacteria are present, blood will be drawn from the catheter to culture (i.e., grow in a laboratory for 24 to 48 hours). Treatment with antibiotics will start whenever an infection is suspected and may end if the culture comes back negative and your child does not have a low ANC. If the culture is positive, treatment usually continues for 10 to 14 days. Some doctors require that the child be hospitalized for antibiotic treatment, while others allow the child to receive treatment at home. If the infection doesn't respond to treatment or is a certain type of bacteria or fungus, the catheter may need to be removed.

> *We used the IV infusion ball when Joseph needed a vancomycin infusion because he didn't have to sit chained to a pump. The IV infusion ball is cool because if you have a sweatshirt with front pockets, you can make a tiny hole in the back of the sweatshirt to put the tubing through and stash the ball in the pocket so you can go about your business while your IV is infusing and no one has to know a thing! It's handy for pain meds, too. He even used it at school, as long as I was there with him. An awesome invention—brilliantly simple. Here's the website that describes it: www.halyardhealth.com/solutions/iv-therapy/homepump-infusion-systems.aspx*

Clots and blockages. Even with excellent daily care, some external catheters develop blockages or clots. If the catheter becomes blocked with a blood clot, it will be flushed with a drug that dissolves the clot, such as alteplase, urokinase, or streptokinase. These medications are given in the clinic or hospital, and the child usually needs to remain nearby for one to four hours. Rarely, the catheter becomes blocked by solidified medications, which can occur if two incompatible drugs are given simultaneously. In those cases, a diluted hydrochloric acid solution may be used to dissolve the blockage.

> *Two months before the end of Kristin's treatment, her line plugged up. We tried several maneuvers at home unsuccessfully. We had to bring her in for the IV team to work on it. I think the bumpy ride to the hospital loosened it because at the hospital they were able to dislodge the clot just by flushing it with saline.*

Kinks. Rarely, a kink develops in the catheter due to a sharp angle where the catheter enters the neck vein. In such cases, the fluids may go in the catheter but it is hard to get blood out. Parents and nurses are often able to work around this problem by trying different positions for the child when blood is drawn. The nurse may ask your child to take a deep breath, cough, stretch, laugh, or bear down as if having a bowel movement.

My son is 16, and his Hickman® was giving the nurses problems, so they planned to do a dye study. They didn't even have to inject the dye; the x-ray showed the line had come out and was clear across the opposite side of his chest and kinked! I don't think it had been out of place long, but it was a little scary to think that chemo may be going everywhere. They did a procedure where they go in and pull the catheter back into place. We are all so happy they got it fixed without surgery.

Catheter breakage. Breaks in the line do happen, but they are extremely rare. If a break or rupture of the line inside the body occurs when the line is not in use, only heparin will leak into surrounding tissues. If the break occurs when chemotherapy drugs are flowing through the catheter, they may leak and cause damage to surrounding tissue. However, the risk of an internal line leaking is far lower than the chance of leakage from a peripheral IV.

When the Hickman® was first put into our 1-year-old daughter, it leaked and chemo went into her chest. Her entire chest was bruised. They took that line out and we ended up using a series of PICCs for the next six months. She has tiny and hard-to-access veins, so the PICC lines were inserted under general anesthesia with the use of ultrasound.

The external portion of the catheter can also break. If this occurs, clamp the line between the point of breakage and the chest wall, cover the break in the line with a sterile gauze pad, and notify the doctor immediately. In most cases, the line can be repaired. Many treatment centers send a catheter repair kit home with parents so they can put on a temporary patch until a new line can be inserted.

I think it is important for parents to obtain clamps from the treating institution to carry with them. The preschool or school the child attends should also have one, in case something happens to the external line above the clamps that exist on the catheter. Younger children should wear a snug tank top that helps hold the catheter in place. Pinning it to the shirt is not the best solution for an active or young child.

Other factors to consider

The proper care and maintenance of an external catheter requires concentration and organization. The site needs to be cleaned and dressed frequently using sterile technique. If your child's skin is quite sensitive, or if he cries when tape or Band-Aids® are removed from his skin, the external line may not be the best choice, because the dressing must be taped to the skin.

One of my most difficult times was learning to change the dressing for Ben's catheter. I am totally freaked out by syringes, and anything like that, and we were given a 10-minute demonstration in the hospital and an instruction book and that was it. I was petrified of doing something wrong to hurt my son. I went into panic mode the first week home from the hospital. I felt like the most inadequate mother in the whole world. We called a home health agency and they sent a nurse. Kathy was the most wonderful person on earth. She told me that she perfectly understood my fears. She had me watch her over and over again until I was comfortable enough to do it with her watching, and then finally on my own. She also talked to our insurance company numerous times to explain why she had to change the dressing instead of the family, and they ended up paying for her services! It was totally amazing.

The external line is a constant reminder of cancer treatment and can cause changes in body image. Both parent and child need to be comfortable with the idea of seeing and handling a tube that emerges from the chest. It is noticeable under lightweight clothing and bathing suits, but not under heavier clothing such as sweaters or coats.

Some types of treatment (e.g., stem cell transplants) require double lumen access, and the external catheter is the only option for this.

My son had a double-lumen catheter, a long tube with two ends that came out of his chest just above his right nipple. When not in use, it was curled and taped against his skin. I hated this thing. It made him Borg-like. I had to clean it every day for more than a year, and flush both ends of the tube. This hated thing, however, was what kept my son from having to be stuck with needles several times a week. It was direct access to his blood supply, for tests, medication administration, and chemo- therapy. One day he told me he had "made friends with his tubies." They had names, "The red one was Ralph, and the white one was Henry." He liked his tubies, he said, because they kept him from getting "ouchies." I was speechless. His matter-of-fact example showed me that the sooner I made friends with Ralph and Henry, the better off I'd be.

Children with external catheters sometimes have restrictions about playing contact sports, swimming, using hot tubs, bathing, and showering. Your child's medical team will tell you about any restrictions.

Subcutaneous Port

Several types of subcutaneous (under the skin) ports are available. The subcutaneous port differs from the external catheter in that it is completely under the skin. A small metal chamber with a rubber top is implanted under the skin of the chest. A catheter threads from the metal chamber (portal) under the skin to a large vein near the collarbone, and then inside the vein to the right atrium of the heart (see Figures 12-2 and 12-3). Whenever the catheter is needed for a blood draw or an infusion, a needle is inserted by a nurse through the skin and into the rubber top of the portal. Usually a topical numbing agent such as EMLA® is used to make the needle insertion less painful.

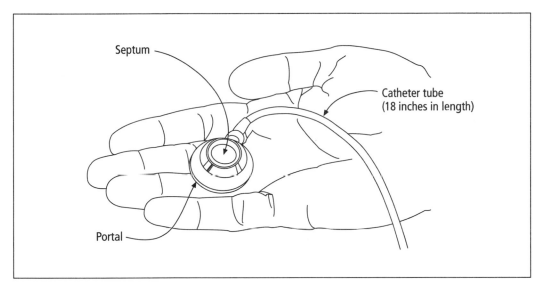

Figure 12-2: Parts of the subcutaneous port

How it's put in

The subcutaneous port is implanted under general anesthesia; the procedure generally takes less than an hour. The surgeon or interventional radiologist makes two small incisions: one in the chest where the port will be placed, and the other near the collarbone where the catheter will enter a vein in the lower part of the neck. First, one end of the catheter is placed in the large blood vessel of the neck and threaded into the right atrium of the heart. The other end of the catheter is tunneled under the skin where it is attached to the portal. Fluid is injected into the portal to ensure the device works properly. The portal is then placed under the skin of the chest and stitched to the underlying muscle. Both incisions are then stitched closed. The only evidence that a catheter has been implanted are two small scars and a bump under the skin where the portal rests.

Christine had her port surgery late at night. The resident gave her some premedication, then the chief resident ordered him to give her more. She felt so silly that she looked at me, giggled, and said, "Mommy has a nose as long as an elephant's." I asked the surgeon if I could be in the recovery room when she awoke, and he said, "Sure."

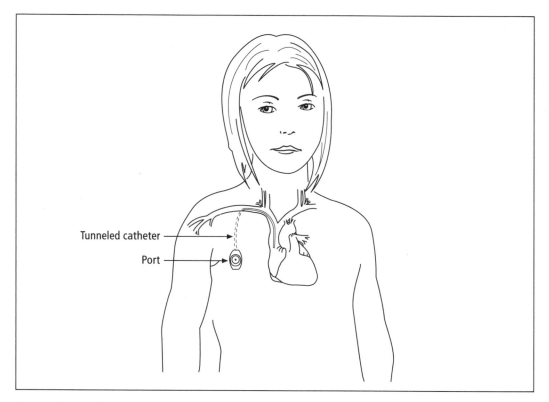

Tunneled catheter

Port

Figure 12-3: Subcutaneous port

How it works

Because the entire subcutaneous port is under the skin, a needle is used to access it. The skin is thoroughly cleansed with antiseptic, and then a special needle is inserted through the skin and the rubber top of the portal. The needle is attached to a short length of tubing that hangs down the front of the chest. A topical anesthetic cream can be applied one hour before the needle poke to anesthetize the skin (see Chapter 9, *Coping with Procedures*). Subcutaneous ports have a rubber top (septum) that reseals after the needle is removed. It is designed to withstand years of needle insertions, as long as a special "non-coring" needle is used each time.

If your child is in a part of treatment that requires using the line every day, the nurse will attach the tubing to IV fluids or will close the end off with a sterile cap after flushing the line with saline solution. A transparent dressing will be put over the site where the needle enters the port. The port can remain accessed in this way for up to seven days. After that time, to avoid the risk of infection, the needle should be removed and the port reaccessed when necessary. If the needle and tubing are to be left in place, it is important to tape them securely to the chest to avoid accidents.

> Molly (3 years old) hated tape removal, so we did not secure the IV tubing to her stomach or chest. On one of her many trips to the potty, we accidentally tugged on the tubing and caused a very small tear in the skin around the needle. It became infected. We did home antibiotics on the pump and felt very fortunate that we were able to clear the line with antibiotics. We were glad our doctor was not too quick to remove the line, but it did require two weeks off chemotherapy.

Care of the port

The entire port and catheter are under the skin, so no daily care is required. After insertion, once the skin over the port heals it can be washed just like the rest of the body. Frequent visual inspections are needed to check for signs of infection, including redness, swelling, pain, drainage, or warmth around the port. Fever, chills, tiredness, and dizziness may also indicate that the line is infected. You should notify the doctor immediately if any of these signs are present or if your child has a fever above 101° F (38.5° C).

> My son had a PORT-A-CATH® for 3 years, from age 14 to 17. During that time, he played basketball, football, softball, and threw the shot put in track. His port was placed on his left side just below his armpit. For football, I worked with the trainer and we developed a special pad that went into a pocket I sewed into some T-shirts. That way the port had a little extra padding. We also found shoulder pads that had a sidepiece that covered the area. He never had any problems or soreness from the port.

The subcutaneous port must be accessed and flushed with heparin at least once every 30 days, which might coincide with clinic visits or blood draws. Ports don't require maintenance by a parent.

> Nico completely flips out when his port is accessed now (since a really bad experience in-patient). So the child life specialist always comes in and tries to help and offer suggestions. Today she said something that reminded me of a book that I absolutely love called Happiest Toddler on the Block. The basic idea is that you validate their feelings by repeating their feelings, and if you do this enough, they calm down. For example, to calm Nico who was hitting, kicking, and screaming after the port access, the child life specialist said, "Nico is really mad." She said it several

times and eventually he just stopped screaming/crying. Then he started yelling that he wanted to go home and she just said, "I bet you really do want to go home." He calmed down to this whereas my "We can go home later" was only making him more upset. The book basically explains that if kids (or really anyone) does not feel that their feelings are recognized, they will escalate behaviors that communicate the feelings.

Risks

The risks for a subcutaneous port are similar to those for an external catheter: infection, clots, and, rarely, kinks or rupture. If the needle is not properly inserted through the rubber septum, or if the wrong kind of needle is used, fluids can leak into the tissue around the portal.

Brent (8 years old) has had a PORT-A-CATH® for 33 months with absolutely no problems. He uses EMLA® to anesthetize it prior to accessing. He hates finger pokes so much that he has his port accessed every time he needs blood drawn.

Infection. Most studies show that the infection rate for subcutaneous ports is lower than that of external catheters. If the subcutaneous port does become infected, it is treated the same way an infected external catheter is treated.

When my daughter had a line infection, I wanted to use the antibiotic pump at home. It was hard, though. It took two hours per dose, three doses per day, for 14 days. I would get up at 5 a.m. to hook her up, so that she would sleep through the first dose. The second dose I would give while she watched a TV show in the early afternoon. Then I would hook her up at bedtime so she would sleep through it. I had to wait up to flush and disconnect, so I was very tired by the end of the two weeks.

Kinks, clots, and ruptures. These events rarely occur with a subcutaneous port. If they do occur, they are treated as described in the external catheter section.

When we got to the clinic for weekly chemo, no matter what gravity-defying positions we tried (raising arms, lying down, standing up), our nurse couldn't get the line to flush. The port was clogged. Luckily, they were able to clear the line with an injection of streptokinase, although it meant entertaining her in the clinic for more than an hour while we waited for it to work. They did tell us that if this didn't work we'd have to go in overnight for slow infusion of chemo, but the line cleared, and we did chemo outpatient.

Peripherally Inserted Central Catheter

A peripherally inserted central catheter is also referred to as a PICC line. This type of catheter is placed in the antecubital vein (a large vein in the inner elbow area) and is threaded into a large vein above the right atrium of the heart (see Figure 12-4). The PICC line can remain in place for many weeks or months, avoiding the need for a new IV every few days. It can be used to deliver chemotherapy, antibiotics, transfusions, and IV nutrition. When the PICC line needs to be used for an infusion, IV tubing is connected to the end of the catheter. When it's not in use, the IV tubing is disconnected and the catheter is flushed.

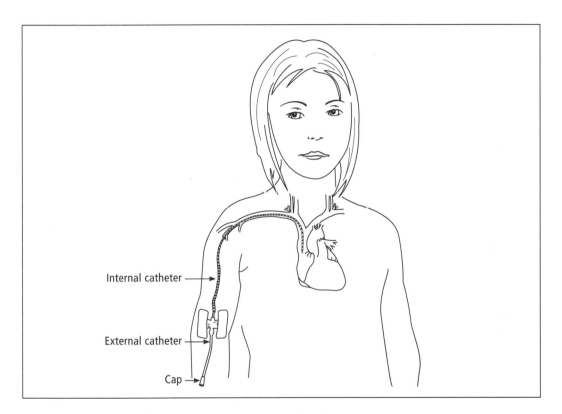

Figure 12-4: Peripherally inserted central catheter (PICC) line

How it's put in

The PICC line may be inserted in your child's hospital room or in an operating room or interventional radiology room by a nurse or doctor. Many children receive sedation medications to help stay relaxed and still during the procedure. Your child will be positioned on a flat surface, and he will need to keep his arm straight and motionless during the procedure. An injection to numb the area is given to decrease discomfort during insertion. A special needle is used to place the PICC line into the arm vein. The catheter is then threaded through the needle. Once the line is in place, a chest x-ray is taken to ensure it is positioned properly.

> Brian had his Hickman® pulled when he started maintenance, but two weeks later he developed pancreatitis and needed total parenteral nutrition. Since he was still on active treatment, he was given the choice of another Hickman® or a PICC, which he decided to try. It was inserted right in our room with no anesthetic other than the morphine pump he was already on for the pancreatitis pain. He pushed his PCA button (the control that allows patients to administer their own doses of pain medication) moments before it was inserted because he was not sure what to expect. The procedure was uncomfortable, but not terribly painful. They did an x-ray to make sure that it was in the right place.

Care of the PICC line

The PICC line, like the external catheter, requires care to prevent problems. A nurse will teach you how to change the dressing, flush the line, change the injection cap, and inspect the site for possible signs of infection if your child will be going home with it. The line must be flushed after every use, or at least every day. You should get plenty of practice under the supervision of a nurse until both you and your child are comfortable with caring for the line. The care required for your child's PICC line may be slightly different from what has been described in this section, because institutional preferences vary.

> Kelsey had a PICC line in her right arm, and she would not straighten it out, but kept it a little bent. I definitely think she was protecting it, and also I think when she tried to straighten it, it pulled on the suture and on the dressing in an uncomfortable way that could have been painful, so she just wouldn't try. I had to do a heparin flush every day and change the dressing twice a week. She could not tolerate Tegaderm®, so we used another kind of porous adhesive bandage, and doused it with Detachol®, which dissolved the adhesive within a few minutes, allowing us to get the bandage off quite easily. The Detachol® was a godsend for her, as removing the adhesive was a source of unnecessary pain. (For more information about Detachol®, see the section "Adhesives" later in this chapter.)

Several companies make colorful sleeves to cover PICC lines. A web page that describes several types of them can be found at *https://themighty.com/2017/08/picc-line-covers*.

Risks

The problems associated with a PICC line are similar to those of any external catheter. Veins may become irritated, infection can occur, or the line can be accidentally torn or moved.

Irritated veins. Within the first few days of insertion, the vein where the catheter is located may become irritated. Signs of irritation include swelling or pain in the area. Often, the discomfort can be eased by placing a warm cloth on the vein. Elevating the arm on a pillow is also sometimes helpful.

Infection. Meticulous care using sterile techniques is extremely important to reduce the risk of infection. The dressing over the exit site should be changed every week or if it becomes wet, soiled, or peels up. Injection caps must also be regularly changed using sterile techniques when the line is not in use, and the line must be flushed on a regular basis. Signs of infection include redness, swelling, pain, drainage, or warmth around the exit site. Fever, chills, tiredness, and dizziness may also indicate that the line has become infected. You should notify the doctor immediately if any of these signs are present or if your child has a fever above 101° F (38.5° C).

Torn catheter. Accidents sometimes happen, and a hole or tear in the line can occur. Careful handling of the catheter can help prevent these accidents. You should suspect a torn catheter if fluid leaks out of the line, especially during an injection. If a tear is found, you should try to find the hole, fold the line above the tear, tape it together, cover it with sterile gauze, and immediately notify your child's doctor.

Displaced catheter. As with other external catheters, a PICC line must be securely taped to prevent movement. Signs of a displaced catheter include chest pain, burning or swelling in the arm above the exit site or in the chest, fluid leaking around the catheter, or pain when fluid is injected into the line.

Choosing Not to Use a Catheter

Many doctors automatically schedule surgery for catheter implantation as soon as a child is diagnosed with leukemia. A few, however, do not recommend using central venous catheters in their pediatric patients. If your child's doctor recommends not using one, ask why and discuss it thoroughly if you are uncomfortable with the options presented.

> *Stephan (6 years old) has no catheter. Sometimes I wish he had one. It seems like it would be easier. We were told he didn't need it. He is running out of usable veins and it is getting harder and harder.*

Some children and teens prefer IVs to an implanted catheter.

> *My son had a port for a very short time, and due to frequent fevers (with no evidence of infection) and because he had a blood clot form in his heart, they pulled the port. He had IVs for the remainder of treatment and was much happier with the IVs than with what he called "that foreign object in my chest."*

Making a Decision

After getting information about your options, talk with the doctor about the merits of each type of catheter and ask for his opinion. Talk about the pros and cons with your child, if she is old enough. You can ask parents and children which type of catheter they chose and why. You will probably hear many opinions about the benefits and drawbacks of each type of catheter. In some cases, you won't have a choice.

> *The doctor told us that the cytogenetics results would determine whether my son got a port or a Hickman®. If he was very high risk, they preferred to use a double-lumen Hickman®, but if he was high risk, they would implant a port. In the meantime, they put in a PICC line and started chemo. When the cytogenetics results came back several days later, they pulled the PICC line and put in the port.*

· · · · ·

> *We didn't have a choice. Nico had a fever for a while after he was diagnosed. We were told if it was from an infection, there was a risk the port would just end up infected. So a PICC was placed after he'd been fever-free for a month. Personally, we hated the PICC. It required daily flushing and Nico could smell/taste the flush. He screamed every time. Bathing made me nervous. It was hard to ensure it wouldn't end up submerged, so he got sponge baths. The PICC also required weekly sterile dressing changes. He was only two years old and we had to hold him down to change the dressing. We were glad to be rid of it.*

The nurses in the clinic and on the unit are another source of valuable information. They will have seen dozens (or hundreds) of children with catheters, and they can give excellent advice. There is no right or wrong choice, just different options for each unique child.

> *My 4-year-old daughter Christine loved ballet and was extremely interested in her appearance. Her younger sister was very physical, and we were worried that if we chose the Hickman® her toddler sister would grab and pull on the tubing. We chose the PORT-A-CATH® so that Christine could wear her tutus without reminders of cancer, and so the children could play together without mishap.*

· · · · ·

> *We chose the Hickman® for Shawn because we didn't want any needles coming at him. He spent almost the whole first year in the hospital, so it saved him from so many pokes. The line was a blessing. He went 3 years and 3 months with no infections. We thought it was just a beautiful thing.*

· · · · ·

> *We didn't get a choice when my daughter needed a stem cell transplant. They needed to put in two Broviac® lines to accommodate all of the meds, fluids, and TPN [total*

parenteral nutrition] she needed for the procedure. I remember seeing six bags hanging up at once. I did the dressing changes, and we didn't have any trouble with the lines throughout her recuperation.

Adhesives

Whether your child has a subcutaneous port, external catheter, or PICC line, dressing changes will be needed. Some children don't mind having the Tegaderm® or tape pulled off. For others, it is very difficult. The hospital may have rules about use of certain products, but following are suggestions from parents about ways to make dressing changes easier for children and teens.

- To cover EMLA®, try plastic wrap cut into a square and use paper tape or tape with perforations. If you turn the ends back of the paper tape to form tabs, you won't have to pick at the corners when it needs to be pulled off.

    Our daughter, diagnosed with T-cell ALL at age 5, is allergic to almost every adhesive and has developed horrible PTSD from tape removal. We can't even use plastic wrap over EMLA, and we need to bring our own brand of Band-Aids®. We tried everything, and what works best is using Mepitac®, a soft brown spongy tape used for preemies and Brava®, a spray adhesive remover.

- Don't use Tegaderm® if it bothers your child or reddens the skin.
- Try Hypafix®, a dressing retention material that looks like gauze with a sticky side. Usually, several sterile 2x2 gauze pads are put over the needle entry site, and then Hypafix® is applied to hold them in place.

    I like Hypafix® because when it's time to take it off, you can use the adhesive dissolver where it's stuck to the skin, and even without the dissolver, it comes off more easily and gently than the Tegaderm®. The nurses at our oncology clinic use this all the time. Our local clinic and hospital do not use Hypafix®, so I bought a roll and take it with me whenever we have to go locally for a port access so we don't have to use the Tegaderm®.

- Use an adhesive remover such as Detachol® (an orange-colored product made by Eloquest Healthcare—*www.eloquesthealthcare.com/detachol*).

    My 4-year-old daughter hated shots and had very sensitive skin. Any Band-Aids® or dressing changes were really difficult. For EKGs, we'd ask them to clip the lines so we could pull off the stickies when she was sleeping. The nurses used adhesive dissolver for dressing changes, but it was still hard and left her skin raw. We did the bravery beads. Now, at 11 years old, she doesn't remember what each of the beads mean except the round green ones—for dressing changes. While she doesn't remember what exactly a dressing change was, she remembers that they hurt and that she didn't like them.

- Ask for expert advice.

Apryl has had skin tears and reactions from the adhesives as a result of using Tegaderm®. We were using Primapore® dressings for a while, but after a year she started having the same reaction. When she had her line replaced, I asked for a consultation with the skin care nurse. She recommended All-Dress®. It is a waterproof dressing with non-stick gauze in the center surrounded by Hypafix® tape. Apryl changes hers once every three days, whether it gets wet or not. She also has this pink tape that has zinc oxide in the adhesive to protect the skin. These two materials have worked out great.

Using adhesive dissolver (which involves peeling off tape millimeter by millimeter) takes a bit of time, but it works. It has to soak in and takes some time to dissolve the sticky stuff. Once you find a routine that works well, work with the nurses to help determine what works for your child and is within the institution's policies and procedures.

I know the nurses are really busy, so I deal with this by always being the one to get the Tegaderm® off. I try to make a joke of it: "I have a deal with my kid that I'm taking off the Tegaderm®. It might take a while and I wouldn't want you to fall asleep waiting on us—how about if I holler out the door when it's off and we're ready?" That way they don't have to stand around and wait, and you don't feel like you need to hurry your child.

Catheters are usually removed when treatment ends; this process is explained in Chapter 24, *End of Treatment and Beyond.*

When Scott (age 3) was diagnosed, his doctor gave us a choice of which central line we could use. He showed us a mannequin with a Broviac® and a PORT-A-CATH®. He also told us the pros and cons of each type, then asked us to decide. We chose the Broviac®, and feel it was the best decision for Scott. The day it was installed was the end of a lot of unnecessary pain (from needle sticks) for Scott.

Scott finished all his treatments three months ago, and yesterday he had his Broviac® removed. It went extremely smoothly. And to think I fretted and worried about the removal all week! He has lots and lots of energy. His hair is coming back in and he actually has color in his face. He looks so healthy! I love it!

Chapter 13

Chemotherapy and Other Medications

"The first wealth is health."
— Ralph Waldo Emerson

THE WORD CHEMOTHERAPY IS DERIVED from a combination of the words "chemical" and "therapy." Chemotherapy drugs are used individually or in combination to destroy or disrupt the growth of cancer cells without permanently damaging normal cells.

This chapter explains how chemotherapy drugs work, how they are given, and how dosages for children and teens are determined. It then describes the most common drugs used to destroy leukemia cells, as well as medications used to prevent infections, treat nausea, and decrease pain. Numerous stories are included to show the range of responses to different chemotherapy drugs. This chapter ends with a brief discussion of complementary and alternative treatments.

Reading about chemotherapy's potential side effects can be disturbing. However, by learning what to expect from the various drugs, you may be able to recognize symptoms early and report them to the doctor so swift action can be taken to make your child more comfortable. On rare occasions, side effects may be life threatening and some can persist throughout life. However, most side effects are unpleasant and subside soon after treatment ends.

How Chemotherapy Drugs Work

Normal, healthy cells divide and grow in a well-established pattern. When these cells divide, an identical copy is produced. The body only makes the number of normal cells it needs at any given time. As each normal cell matures, it loses its ability to reproduce. Normal cells are also preprogrammed to die at a specific time. In contrast, cancer cells reproduce uncontrollably and grow in unpredictable ways. They invade surrounding tissue and can travel in blood or lymph to lodge in other parts of the body.

All chemotherapy drugs work in some way to interfere with the cancer cells' ability to live, divide, and multiply.

How Chemotherapy Drugs Are Given

The five most common ways to give drugs during treatment for childhood leukemia are:

- **Intravenous (IV):** Drugs are delivered directly into the bloodstream through a venous catheter in the chest or an IV in the arm or hand. IV medicines can be administered in a few minutes or as an infusion over a number of hours.

- **Oral (PO):** Drugs—taken by mouth in liquid, capsule, or tablet form—are absorbed into the blood through the lining of the stomach and intestines.

- **Intramuscular (IM):** Drugs that need to seep slowly into the bloodstream are injected into a large muscle such as the thigh or buttocks.

- **Intrathecal (IT):** Doctors perform a spinal tap and inject the drug directly into the cerebrospinal fluid (the fluid surrounding the brain and spinal cord).

- **Subcutaneous (Sub-Q):** Drugs are injected into the soft tissues under the skin of the upper arm, thigh, or abdomen.

- **Sublingual (SL):** Several drugs are available as lozenges that dissolve quickly when placed under the tongue.

Dosages

Dosages vary by protocol, but most are based on your child's weight or body surface area (BSA). BSA is calculated from your child's weight and height, and it is measured in meters squared (m^2). Your child's doses should be recalculated by the doctor at the start of each new phase of treatment. If your child has significant weight gain or loss (more than 10% of initial weight), more frequent recalculating of doses will be needed.

> My son's protocol required that his height and weight be measured each time chemotherapy was to start. When we would arrive in the clinic, the nurses would take his measurements, then calculate his body surface area using those figures. His weight fluctuated considerably over the course of his treatment, so the actual dosage of the drugs that he received was never quite the same.

You don't need to do the calculations, but it is important to know the right dosage for each drug given at home and how you should give it to your child. Most families write the dosages on a calendar and cross them out after each dose has been given to make sure they don't forget a drug or accidentally repeat a dose.

Different Responses to Medications

Children's bodies have a wide range of responses to medications, some of which are due to their genes. Some children inherit genes that don't allow them to break down (metabolize) certain drugs, or that cause them to metabolize the drugs very slowly. In these children, the drug can build up in the body and cause excessive toxicity.

In addition, the cancer cells in individual children vary greatly in how they respond to different chemotherapy drugs. The cancer cells in one child's body might be extremely sensitive to a certain chemotherapy drug, while the cancer cells in another child's body can be very resistant to that same drug. As a result, the combined variability in children's ability to metabolize drugs and how sensitive their cancer cells are to certain drugs causes a big range in the effectiveness of standard doses of medications. How much of this variability is due to genetics is not well understood.

However, researchers are finding ways to test children's ability to metabolize certain drugs and are tailoring treatments based on that genetic information. This area of science is called pharmacogenetics. Here are three examples of genetic characteristics that are used by doctors to tailor treatments to a child's unique genetic makeup.

Thiopurine-S-methyltransferase (TPMT)

Some children are not genetically coded to make an enzyme called TPMT, which is involved in breaking down (metabolizing) two chemotherapy drugs used to treat leukemia—thioguanine (6-TG) and mercaptopurine (6-MP). One way to identify how children can metabolize these drugs is a type of testing called genotyping.

Around 1 in 400 people cannot metabolize 6-TG and 6-MP at all and are called "TPMT poor metabolizers." When children with this genetic variation are given standard doses of these drugs, the drugs quickly build up to toxic levels. In these children, the numbers of red cells, white cells, and platelets drop dramatically putting the child at risk for anemia, infections, and bleeding. Children who are poor metabolizers are given only about 10% of the standard dose of 6-MP.

Ten out of every 100 people are able to slowly metabolize 6-TG and 6-MP and are called "TPMT intermediate metabolizers." Children with this genetic makeup need lower doses of 6-TG and 6-MP to prevent big drops in blood counts. Guidelines from the Clinical Pharmacogenetics Implementation Consortium recommend a starting dose of 30 to 70% of the standard dose.

> Josh has not been on full doses of 6-MP for over a year now. It did take the doctors a long time to realize that they needed to increase Josh's 6-MP slowly. For months they would drop the dose to 50%, and in two weeks his counts were okay. Not great, but high enough to increase the dose, so they would. Another two weeks at 75% and he

would crash. Finally, they did the TPMT test and sure enough he does not metabolize the 6-MP normally. I remember them telling me that 10% of the population has this enzyme deficiency and you would never know unless you had to take 6-MP.

The remainder of the population (approximately 90%) can break down these medications at the normal rate and are started on the standard dose. Some treatment centers test all children with leukemia for their genetic ability to metabolize 6-TG and 6-MP before they give them either drug. Other institutions test children if their blood counts drop dramatically after getting the first doses of these drugs. Genotyping identifies the majority of children with a decreased ability to metabolize 6-MP or 6-TG.

Even if the TPMT genotype test comes back normal, some children have high or low levels of other enzymes that affect how 6-MP and 6-TG are metabolized. In these cases, tests of 6-MP metabolites (called 6-MMPN and 6-TGN) are sometimes done.

If liver enzymes are up, it may be due to 6-MP metabolites. 6-MP is metabolized into 6-MMPN, which is liver toxic and has no anti-leukemic properties (the bad one) and 6-TGN, which is anti-leukemic (the good one). In my son's case, his liver enzymes went up but were still well below the protocol guidelines for when to worry about liver toxicity. But he was having problems with hypoglycemia and looked ill. So they checked his metabolites just to be safe. Well, everyone was surprised because his 6-MMPN was outrageously high—should be less than 5,700 but was almost 45,000. His 6-TGN was on the low side. When the results came back, our oncologist notified us the same day and told us to take him off chemo immediately. We ended up inpatient within a week.

CYP2D6

Another genetic variation involves the CYP2D6 gene, which affects the metabolism of codeine. About 10% of people do not get pain relief from codeine because they are genetically unable to metabolize codeine into morphine. Recently, the U.S. Food and Drug Administration released a statement that codeine should not be given to children younger than age 12. Some institutions test all children with leukemia who are older than 12 for this genetic variation so the right pain medications can be prescribed.

In contrast, some people metabolize codeine very rapidly because they have extra copies of the CYP2D6 gene. This results in symptoms of opiate overdose—sleepiness, confusion, shallow breathing. Teens with this genetic variation should be given pain medications that don't contain codeine. For more information on this topic, visit the National Institute of Health webpage called "Codeine Therapy and CYP2D6" at *www.ncbi.nlm.nih.gov/books/NBK100662.*

Methlyenetetrahydrofolate reductase (MTHFR)

A genetic variation called MTHFR C677T may increase some children's sensitivity to methotrexate, resulting in liver toxicity, very low blood cell counts, and other side effects. Some institutions test children who have these reactions while receiving methotrexate for this genetic variation.

> My daughter was on standard treatment for standard risk B-cell ALL with good cytogenetics. However, she didn't tolerate the chemo well—she developed grade 3 neuropathy from the vincristine and liver problems from the methotrexate (her liver enzymes were off the chart). She had many delays in treatment and reductions of doses. After delayed intensification, she was on a 3-month chemo hold because her counts crashed and did not come back up. One of the moms on an online support group suggested that she be tested for the MTHFR gene to see if she was unable to metabolize methotrexate. The staff oncologist I initially discussed the test with resisted, but I insisted. It turns out that she is homozygous for MTHFR, and so she got only about 15% of the normal dose of that drug for the rest of treatment. She also needed the rescue drug, leukovorin, after getting intrathecal methotrexate. I gave the leukovorin every six hours for the 24 hours after every spinal tap. She got the medicine her body needed and has been in complete remission seven years now.

• • • • •

> Our facility did not test for MTHFR or TPMT until after my daughter was in her second year of long-term maintenance. Her blood counts were continually bottoming out and she had elevated bilirubin. It was at my request that the tests were administered. The tests showed that she is homozygous (has two copies) of MTHFR C677T; however the tests show normal ability to process 6-MP. With that said, she has spent an enormous amount of time off chemo with elevated liver enzymes and/or counts that have bottomed out. She currently is off chemo again. This will be her fourth week with no 6-MP or methotrexate. When she is on chemo, she takes 25% of the standard amount of methotrexate and 50% of 6-MP. This just goes to show how very different each child is, and why we must continue working toward protocols that are tailored to individuals and standardizing testing which helps to identify these types of anomalies at the beginning of treatment.

Questions to Ask the Doctor

Before giving your child any drug, you should be given answers to the following questions:

- What is the dosage? How many times a day should it be given?
- Should the drug be given at a particular time of day or under specific conditions (e.g., on an empty stomach or before bed)?
- What are the common and rare side effects?

- What should I do if my child experiences any of the side effects?
- Will the drug interact with any over-the-counter drugs (e.g., Tylenol®), foods (e.g., grapefruit), or supplements (e.g., folate)?
- What are both the brand and generic names of the drug?
- Is it okay to use the generic version?
- What should I do if I forget to give my child a dose?
- Will you counsel my teen about the risks associated with drinking alcohol, smoking cigarettes or marijuana, or getting pregnant while using this drug?

Guidelines for Calling the Doctor

Sometimes parents are reluctant to call their child's oncologist with questions or concerns, so here are some general guidelines about when you should call:

- A temperature above 101° F (38.5° C)
- Shaking or chills
- Shortness of breath
- Severe nausea or vomiting
- Unusual bleeding, bruising, or cuts that won't heal
- Pain or swelling at a chemotherapy injection site
- Pain, swelling, or redness around the central line site
- Any severe pain that cannot be explained
- Exposure to chicken pox or measles
- Severe headache or blurred vision
- Constipation lasting more than two days
- Severe diarrhea
- Severe headaches
- Painful urination or bowel movements
- Blood in urine

Parents should not hesitate to bring their child to the hospital if she is ill and her blood cell counts are low, as this can be a life-threatening emergency. Any time your child is sick and you are concerned, call the oncologist or nurse practitioner.

Chemotherapy Drugs and Their Possible Side Effects

This section contains not only common and infrequent side effects of anticancer drugs, but also parent and survivor experiences and suggestions. You may be overwhelmed by reading about all the potential side effects of each drug. Please remember, each child is unique and will handle most drugs without major problems. Most side effects are unpleasant, not serious, and subside when the medication stops. The parent experiences included here may provide insight, comfort, and suggestions should your child have an unusual side effect. If you have any concerns after reading these descriptions, consult your child's oncologist. (Appendix C, *Books, Websites, and Support Groups* contains resources for obtaining information about drugs not covered here.)

Remember to keep all chemotherapy drugs in a locked cabinet away from children and pets.

Chemotherapy Drugs

Drugs used to treat children with cancer are known by various names, which can get very confusing. You may hear the same drug referred to by its generic name, an abbreviation, or one of several brand names, depending on which doctor, nurse, or pharmacist you talk to. The list below provides the generic name of the most commonly used chemotherapy drugs and some of the most common brand names.

Drug name	Brand name(s)
Allopurinol	Zyloprim®, Lopurin®, Aloprim®
Arsenic trioxide	Trisenox®
Asparaginase L-Asparaginase ASP PEG-asparaginase Erwinia asparaginase	Elspar® Oncaspar®
Bosutinib	Bosulif®
Busulfan	Busulfex®, Myleran®
Cyclophosphamide	Cytoxan®, Neosar®
Cytarabine Cytosine arabinoside ARA-C	Cytosar-U®, Tarabine PFS®, Cytosar®
Dasatinib	SPRYCEL®
Daunorubicin Daunomycin	Cerubidine®
Dexamethasone DEX	Decadron®, Hexadrol®, and multiple other brand names

Drug name	Brand name(s)
Doxorubicin	Adriamycin®, Rubex®
Etoposide VP-16	VePesid®, Toposar®, Etopophos®
Filgrastim	Neupogen®, Granix®, Zarxio®
Fludarabine	Fludara®
Hydrocortisone	Cortef®, Hydrocortone®, Hydrocortone Phosphate®, Solu-Cortef®, and multiple other brand names
Idarubicin	Idamycin®
Ifosfamide	Ifex®
Imatinib	Gleevec®
Isotretinoin 13-cis-retinoic acid	Accutane®, Amnesteem®, Claravis®, Sotret®
Melphalan	Alkeran®
Mercaptopurine 6-MP	Purinethol®, Purixan®
Methotrexate MTX	Otrexup™, Rasuvo®, Rheumatrex®, Trexall™
Mitoxantrone	Novantrone®
Mycophenolate mofetil	CellCept®
Nilotinib	Tasigna®
Ponatinib	Iclusig®
Prednisone	Deltasone®, Liquid Pred®, Meticorten®, Orasone®
Thioguanine 6-TG	Tabloid®
Tretinoin Cis-retinoic acid All-trans retinoic acid ATRA	Vesanoid®
Vincristine	Oncovin®, Vincasar PFS®

This section lists the drugs most commonly used to treat children newly diagnosed with leukemia. It explains how the drugs are given, how they work, and the most common side effects. To learn about less common side effects, visit *http://chemocare.com/ chemotherapy/drug-info*.

Allopurinol (al-o-PUR-in-all)

How given: Pills by mouth; IV infusion

Common side effects:

- Rash
- Diarrhea
- Nausea
- Liver toxicity

Arsenic trioxide (AR-sen-ick try-OX-ide)

How given: IV injection or infusion over several hours

Precaution: Arsenic trioxide is associated with a serious condition known as APL differentiation syndrome. This complication is characterized by breathing difficulties, lung and heart problems, fluid retention, and weight gain.

Common side effects:

- Nausea and vomiting
- Cough
- Fatigue
- Dizziness
- Headache
- Rapid heartbeat
- Swelling of arms, hands, feet, and lower legs
- Rash or itching
- Fever
- Swelling at the injection site
- Insomnia
- Numbness or tingling
- Itching
- Diarrhea

> *We worked out a system with the hospital and home health company to give most of the arsenic doses at home. We'd go to the hospital on Mondays where they would access the port and give the first dose (2-hour infusion). Then, we'd go home and a*

home health nurse would bring the next four doses to us, each in a little container that looked like a grenade. Every day, one of these would be hooked to the line from his port, and he could just carry it around in his pocket while it infused. After his Friday dose, we'd deaccess the port.

L-Asparaginase (L-a-SPARE-a-jin-ase)

How given: IM injection

Types: The three types of L-asparaginase are E. coli asparaginase, Erwinia asparaginase, and pegylated asparaginase (also called PEG- or PEG-L-asparaginase).

Precautions: Occasionally a child will have a severe allergic reaction to L-asparaginase. It is important that the drug be given by trained medical personnel who have emergency equipment available. The child should be monitored at the clinic for 20 to 30 minutes after receiving the drug in case a reaction occurs. If a child has a reaction to one type of asparaginase, one of the other forms of this drug may be tried. If the child reacts to all forms of asparaginase, use of the drug is usually stopped.

Common side effects:

- Nausea and vomiting
- Fever and chills
- Loss of appetite and weight
- Fatigue
- Headaches
- Sleepiness
- Stomach or abdominal cramps
- Allergic reaction, including swelling, difficulty breathing, and rash

> *Meagan had no problem with the L-asparaginase other than that the shots in her thigh were painful. I'd recommend that parents put EMLA® on two hours before the shot to reduce the pain.*

> • • • • •

> *A couple of hours after Preston's third dose of L-asparaginase his leg began to swell up around the injection site. His leg grew to three times its normal size. The doctors switched him to a different kind of L-asparaginase for all subsequent doses, and he had no further problems.*

Bosutinib (boe-SUE-ti-nib)

How given: Pill by mouth

Precaution: Do not chew, crush, or break the pills; avoid grapefruit and grapefruit juice.

Common side effects:

- Diarrhea
- Nausea and vomiting
- Abdominal pain
- Low platelet count
- Rash

Busulfan (byoo-SUL-fan)

How given: Pills by mouth

Precaution: Children should have lung function tests for early detection of possible toxicities.

Common side effects:

- Low blood counts, which may increase risk of infection or bleeding, and cause weakness, fatigue, and paleness
- Patchy darkening of the skin
- Nausea, vomiting, and diarrhea (usually mild)
- Loss of appetite

Hints for parents: Giving your child busulfan at bedtime may decrease nausea and vomiting. Schedule your child's pulmonary function tests the week before starting a new cycle of therapy so test results will be available for your child's doctor to review.

Cyclophosphamide (sye-kloe-FOSS-fa-mide)

How given: IV injection or infusion

Precautions: The child should drink lots of water or be given large amounts of IV fluids while taking cyclophosphamide to prevent bladder damage. A drug called mesna is also given to prevent bladder damage. Antinausea drugs should be given before and for several hours after this drug is given.

Common side effects:

- Low blood counts, which may increase risk of infection or bleeding, and cause weakness, fatigue, and paleness
- Nausea and vomiting
- Loss of appetite
- Temporary hair loss

> *Christine breezed through the Cytoxan® infusions. She would go to Children's in the afternoon, they would give her lots of IV fluids, and then ondansetron a half hour before the Cytoxan®. She would sleep through the night with absolutely no nausea, because they were so good about giving her the ondansetron all night and the next morning. It was hard on me because I had to wake up every two hours to change her diaper so that the nurse could weigh it to make sure she was passing enough urine.*

Cytarabine (sye-TARE-a-been)

How given: IV infusion; intrathecal injection; subcutaneous injection

Common side effects:

- Low blood counts, which may increase risk of infection or bleeding and cause weakness, fatigue, and paleness
- Nausea and vomiting
- Loss of appetite
- Mouth sores
- Headache

> *I told my daughter's oncologist how happy I was that she had not had any severe nausea after her first few doses of ARA-C (cytarabine). His only reply was, "It's cumulative." Within an hour, on the long drive home, she was vomiting constantly. We became ensnared in a 2-hour traffic jam. She ran out of clean clothes, so for two hours, I repeatedly carried her to the side of the road, a naked, bald, 25-pound 4-year-old with tubing hanging from her chest, and supported her as she dry-heaved. The people in the cars around us were in tears and kept asking if there was anything they could do to help. I just focused on comforting her, and getting her home to that vial of ondansetron in our fridge.*

Dasatinib (da-SA-ti-nib)

How given: Pills by mouth

Precaution: Do not chew, crush, or break the pills.

Common side effects:

- Low blood counts, which may increase risk of infection or bleeding and cause weakness, fatigue, and paleness
- Diarrhea
- Headache
- Fatigue
- Muscle and bone pain
- Rash
- Slowed growth
- Fever
- Fluid in legs and around the eyes

Daunorubicin (daw-no-ROO-bi-sin)

How given: IV injection or infusion

Precautions: Daunorubicin causes urine to turn red; this discoloration is normal. This drug can injure the heart muscle, so heart function must be monitored during and after treatment. If daunorubicin leaks into the tissue surrounding the injection site, it can cause localized tissue damage.

Common side effects:

- Low blood counts, which may increase risk of infection or bleeding and cause weakness, fatigue, and paleness
- Nausea and vomiting
- Hair loss
- Mouth sores

> *My son didn't have any problems from daunorubicin, but I sure worried about heart damage. I went to a conference and learned that the cut-off dose was below what he had on the protocol. I requested an echocardiogram, and his heart function was normal, but I know we need to follow this for life.*

Dexamethasone (dex-a-METH-a-zone)

See **Prednisone**

Doxorubicin (dox-o-ROO-bi-sin)

How given: IV injection or infusion

Precautions: Doxorubicin causes urine to turn red; this discoloration is normal. This drug can injure the heart muscle, so heart function must be monitored before starting the drug and throughout treatment. If doxorubicin leaks out into the tissue surrounding the injection site, it can cause localized tissue damage.

Common side effects:

- Low blood counts, which may increase risk of infection or bleeding and cause weakness, fatigue, and paleness
- Nausea and vomiting
- Hair loss
- Mouth sores

> The Adriamycin® (doxorubicin) just burned right through my son. He never got mouth sores, but he sure had problems at the other end. They had him lie on his stomach with the heat lamp on his bare bottom. His whole bottom was blistered so badly that it looked like he'd been in a fire. They used to mix up what they called "Magic Butt Paste," and I'll never forget the recipe: one tube Nystatin® cream, one tube Desitin®, and Nystatin® powder. It was like spackle that they would just slather on. He had a lot of gastrointestinal bleeding, too, so he was continuously getting platelets. That's when they decided that he wouldn't have the delayed intensification phase.

· · · · ·

> Other than red urine and the expected low counts, hair loss, and nausea, Christine had no problems from her many doses of doxorubicin. She is now 29 and has an EKG (electrocardiogram) and echocardiogram every two years. So far, no problems.

Etoposide (e-TOE-poe-side)

How given: IV injection or infusion; pills by mouth

Precautions: This drug interacts with several common drugs and herbs, such as aspirin, cyclosporine, and St. John's wort. Etoposide may cause birth defects if taken during pregnancy. It can also irritate the vein where it is injected or damage nearby tissue if it leaks out of the vein.

Common side effects:

- Low blood counts, which may increase risk of infection or bleeding and cause weakness, fatigue, and paleness
- Loss of appetite
- Nausea and vomiting
- Temporary hair loss

Filgrastim (fil-GRA-stim)

How given: Subcutaneous injection; IV infusion

What it is: Filgrastim is a colony stimulating factor that stimulates the production of white blood cells (WBCs). This medication does not treat cancer; it helps increase WBC counts after chemotherapy.

Common side effects:

- Nausea and vomiting
- Low platelet counts, which may increase risk of bleeding
- Fever
- Bone pain

Fludarabine (flew-DARE-a-bean)

How given: IV injection or infusion

Precautions: This drug can cause infertility. If the child needs a blood transfusion while taking fludarabine, the blood must be irradiated to minimize the chance of an autoimmune reaction.

Common side effects:

- Low blood counts, which may increase risk of infection or bleeding and cause weakness, fatigue, and paleness
- Weakness
- Nausea and vomiting
- Loss of appetite
- Fever, with or without chills
- Cough

Idarubicin (eye-dah-ROO-buh-sin)

How given: Slow IV injection

Precautions: Idarubicin causes urine to turn red; this discoloration is normal. This drug can injure the heart muscle, so heart function must be monitored before starting the drug and throughout treatment. If idarubicin leaks out into the tissue surrounding the injection site, it can cause localized tissue damage.

Common side effects:

- Low blood counts, which may increase risk of infection or bleeding and cause weakness, fatigue, and paleness
- Nausea and vomiting
- Temporary hair loss
- Abdominal cramps and diarrhea
- Decreased appetite
- Mouth sores

Ifosfamide (eye-FOSS-fah-mide)

How given: IV infusion

Precautions: The child should be given extra fluids by mouth or IV during infusion. Mesna, a drug that protects the bladder, should also be given.

Common side effects:

- Low blood counts, which may increase risk of infection or bleeding and cause weakness, fatigue, and paleness
- Temporary hair loss
- Nausea and vomiting
- Loss of appetite
- Blood in the urine

Hints for parents: Have your child drink plenty of fluids, if possible, prior to treatment. This drug is usually given over three to five consecutive days, so make sure you have an adequate supply of antinausea medicine at home for your child. This drug may cause the kidneys to lose important substances, such as calcium and phosphorus, and your child may need to take oral supplements.

Imatinib (im-AT-in-ib)

How given: Pills by mouth, taken with food and water

Precautions: This drug causes birth defects if taken during pregnancy. It also interacts with many other medications and with grapefruit juice. Tell the doctor about all medications your child takes and avoid grapefruit and grapefruit juice.

Common side effects:

- Low blood counts, which may increase risk of infection or bleeding and cause weakness, fatigue, and paleness
- Nausea and vomiting
- Swelling of face, feet, and hands
- Muscle cramps and bone pain
- Bone pain
- Diarrhea
- Skin rash
- Fever

Isotretinoin (eye-soe-TRET-i-noin)

See **Tretinoin**

Melphalan (MEL-fa-lan)

How given: Pills by mouth; IV infusion

Common side effects:

- Low blood cell counts, which may increase risk of infection or bleeding and cause weakness, fatigue, and paleness
- Nausea and vomiting

Mercaptopurine (mer-kap-toe-PYOOR-een)

How given: Pills by mouth

Precautions: Certain drugs, including allopurinol and sulfa-based antibiotics, can worsen side effects of mercaptopurine or depress blood counts. Mercaptopurine can raise blood levels of uric acid, resulting in kidney damage.

Note: See earlier section in this chapter called "Different Responses to Medications" to review the genetic tests that determine whether and how quickly your child might metabolize this drug.

Common side effects:

- Low blood counts, which may increase risk of infection or bleeding and cause weakness, fatigue, and paleness

- Liver toxicity

- Loss of appetite

- Nausea and vomiting

> *My son was diagnosed with B-cell ALL. He is currently in long-term maintenance and doing very well. During interim maintenance he had a severe drop in all counts. This was labeled as pancytopenia. His marrow shut down. When this first happened all counts were at rock bottom, and they thought he had relapsed. He was tested for TPMT, and we found out the full dosage of 6-MP was poisoning him. He is currently being treated at 50% of the standard dose and being monitored through bimonthly CBCs [complete blood counts]. The doctor will slowly increase the dosage to maintain a desired ANC if needed.*

Methotrexate (meth-o-TREX-ate)

How given: Pills by mouth; IV infusion; IT or IM injection

Precautions: Children should not be given extra folic acid in vitamins or the methotrexate will not be effective. Several drugs can cause methotrexate to stay in the system too long or worsen its side effects. Some of these drugs include aspirin, non-steroidal anti-inflammatory drugs, penicillin, Bactrim®, Septra®, and several anti-seizure drugs. Children taking methotrexate are very sensitive to the sun and should always wear protective clothing and sunscreen.

Common side effects:

- Low blood counts, which may increase risk of infection or bleeding and cause weakness, fatigue, and paleness

- Extreme sun sensitivity

- Diarrhea

- Skin rashes

- Mouth sores

- Headaches, tingling pain down legs, and spinal irritation (when given by IT injection)
- Neurotoxicity that can cause learning disabilities (depends on dose and child's age)
- Redness at the site of previous radiation ("radiation recall")

Hints for parents: Most of the common side effects of this drug are temporary and reversible. Mouth sores can be quite painful, and your child may not eat or drink well when she has them. Always remember to have your child use sunscreen (SPF 30 or higher) when playing outside. Minor skin rashes can be treated effectively with over-the-counter cortisone cream. When given as high-dose therapy, methotrexate requires administration of a reversing agent (antidote) called leucovorin. It is critical that your child begin the leucovorin at the correct time to prevent serious, possibly irreversible, side effects.

> My daughter had serious problems with rashes during maintenance. The doctors thought she had developed an allergy to the weekly methotrexate. She often would be covered with rashes that looked like small, red circles with tan, flaky skin inside. They were extremely itchy and unattractive. We spent hundreds of dollars at the dermatologist trying various prescription remedies. None worked. In desperation, I went to our local herbalist and asked if she had anything totally nontoxic, which would help the rash but not affect her chemotherapy. She sold me a small tub of salve made from olive oil, vitamin E oil, and calendula flowers. We checked with my daughter's oncologist before using it. It totally cured the rash after two days and worked each time that the rash reappeared. What a relief!

· · · · ·

> Carl was on an experimental IV high-dose methotrexate protocol funded through the National Institutes of Health. Side effects ranged from nausea and vomiting to diarrhea, sore bones, mood swings, and disorientation.

· · · · ·

> My son developed learning disabilities from his high-dose methotrexate protocol. He received tutoring through high school and is doing extremely well in college.

Mitoxantrone (mye-TOX-an-trone)

How given: IV injection

Precautions: Mitoxantrone can injure the heart muscle, so heart function must be monitored before starting the drug and throughout treatment. If mitoxantrone leaks out into the tissue surrounding the injection site, it can cause localized tissue damage.

Common side effects:

- Low blood counts, which may increase risk of infection or bleeding and cause weakness, fatigue, and paleness
- Nausea and vomiting
- Fever
- Liver toxicity

Mycophenolate mofetil (MYE-koe-FEN-oh-late MOE-fe-til)

How given: Pills by mouth

Precautions: Do not chew, crush, or break the pills; take on an empty stomach.

Common side effects:

- Anxiety
- Back pain
- Constipation or diarrhea
- Headache
- Nausea and vomiting
- Trouble sleeping

Nilotinib (nye-LOE-ti-nib)

How given: Pills by mouth

Precautions: Do not chew, crush, or break the pills; avoid grapefruit and grapefruit juice.

Common side effects:

- Low blood counts, which may increase risk of infection or bleeding and cause weakness, fatigue, and paleness
- Rash

- Headache
- Itching
- Nausea and vomiting
- Cough
- Diarrhea
- Constipation
- Fatigue
- Muscle and bone pain
- Slowed growth

Ponatinib (poe-NA-ti-nib)

How given: Pills by mouth

Precautions: Do not chew, crush, or dissolve the pills; avoid grapefruit and grapefruit juice.

Common side effects:

- Low blood counts, which may increase risk of infection or bleeding and cause weakness, fatigue, and paleness
- High blood pressure
- Rash
- Increased blood sugar
- Abdominal pain
- Constipation
- Fatigue and weakness
- Headache
- Dry skin
- Fever
- Joint pain
- Decreased appetite
- Liver toxicity

Prednisone (PRED-ni-zone) and dexamethasone (dex-a-METH-a-zone)

These two steroids are grouped together because they are closely related chemically and have similar action and side effects. The biggest difference in side effects appears to be the increased risk of avascular necrosis (death of bone due to decreased blood supply) from dexamethasone. Dexamethasone is given in high doses as a chemotherapy drug and in low doses to prevent nausea. To see the side effects of dexamethasone when it is used as an antinausea drug, look under "Antinausea Drugs Used During Chemotherapy" later in the chapter.

How given: Pills or liquid by mouth; IV or IM injection

Precautions: Every parent who contributed stories for this book described problems that their child had while on prednisone or dexamethasone. The side effects ranged from mild to severe, but were universal. At high doses, steroids create major behavioral problems in children, which gradually subside after the drug is stopped.

Common side effects:

- Mood changes, from extreme irritability to rage
- Increased appetite and food obsessions
- Increased thirst
- Weight gain
- Heartburn
- Fluid retention
- Round face and protruding belly
- Sleeplessness and nightmares
- Nervousness, restlessness, hyperactivity
- Muscle weakness with loss of muscle mass
- Hypersensitivity to lights, sound, and motion
- Muscle cramps or pain
- Swelling of feet or lower legs
- High blood pressure
- High blood sugar

> *Judson was a hyper, high-strung child who became extremely hyperactive when he was on prednisone. My recommendation for other parents dealing with this difficult side effect is to run—don't walk—to your nearest library or bookstore and get some books on hyperactive behavior in children. It is important that parents understand this problem and learn to deal with it in a loving way. Remember, too, that this side*

effect will go away when the prednisone is out of the child's system. Judd would be hyperactive for the entire two weeks, desiring to eat every 15 minutes or so, making noises constantly, itching all over, sleeping less, having a terrible temper, and losing his fine motor and concentration skills.

During this time he would develop bad behavior because we could not parent him the way we would normally. A few days after his prednisone ended, we would become very firm and structured in our parenting, and he would return to his normal behavior patterns. My son has been in remission 10 years, has never exhibited abnormal hyperactivity since ending chemotherapy, and is a well-adjusted teen and an excellent student.

• • • • •

Meagan is very emotionally labile after only two doses of prednisone. She is very frustrated, quick to anger, hits, screams. For those five days we try to stay home, and this helps to decrease the stimulation. We plot it out on the calendar in advance so that we can plan accordingly. I think the kids deserve some tender, loving care while taking prednisone. Of course, I don't allow the hitting, but I do try hard not to aggravate the situation when she is on prednisone. I can see how she is uncomfortable being out of control, but she just can't help it.

• • • • •

Prednisone sends Stephan into a whirlwind of emotions. Sometimes he seems especially happy, and the rest of the time he is in tears at the drop of a hat. We explained to Stephan that the pill can make him feel this way, and it's okay to tell us, "I'm grumpy and I need to be alone for awhile." He gets physical side effects, too. He takes prednisone five days a month, and, like clockwork, on Day 6 he gets itchy, on Day 7 he aches all over, on Day 8 he has severe back, chest, arm, and leg pain, and on Day 9 he starts to feel better.

• • • • •

Preston didn't act out while on prednisone; instead he became depressed and too compliant. He spent most of his time moodily cooking himself food and eating. We bought a second wardrobe of sweat pants with elastic waists so that he would be comfortable.

• • • • •

Rachel had a dual personality on prednisone. She would be fine one minute and then fly into a rage. One time, she literally had an argument with herself. She asked to watch a tape, and then for 20 minutes she argued with herself over whether she should watch the tape. It was painful to watch.

• • • • •

Prednisone and dexamethasone were the worst drugs for Katy. When she was on steroids for a month straight, she hallucinated horrible things. She'd scream that *boys were chasing her or that her heart had stopped beating. She'd sob that I was melting and would disappear. She'd dig her fingers into my arm begging me to help her. She sometimes did this all night, and nothing consoled her. She slept very little while taking steroids. She spent day after day and night after night in my arms while I rocked her in the rocking chair, only leaving my arms to eat huge amounts of food. She would eat an entire loaf of bread, and always asked to have "butter spread on it like icing on a cake." She has never once said that since ending treatment.*

· · · · ·

Elke is currently in long-term maintenance for ALL. After one particularly bad steroid pulse, I told her oncologist about how heart-rending it was to watch a 3-year-old repeatedly wail, "I'm so sad!" while lying despondently on the couch. Her doctor prescribed potassium supplements to counteract the severe depression and mood swings caused by the dexamethasone. She starts the potassium a couple days before she begins the steroid pulse, and ends a couple of days after. Although she is by no means even-tempered during her pulses, she no longer seems despondent. The potassium has also greatly decreased the muscular pain she always suffered from the steroids.

· · · · ·

Jeremy never slept well when he was on prednisone. He had nightmares of doctors chasing him through the hospital halls. He had a lot of night sweats and was hungry all night and day. He slept with a loaf of bread, and when we would go places, he always carried a can of Campbell's® chicken soup and a can opener. He desperately needed to make sure that he would never be without food.

· · · · ·

When you add steroids to a teen boy's already hyped up emotional level, you get ignition. My son was ages 14 to 19 when taking steroids. It helped to talk to him about how it would change how he feels and thinks. After a while, he could describe how he was becoming more agitated and wanted to stay in his room alone. He really didn't like being crabby and angry and would voluntarily isolate himself. I suggested ways for him to control his environment while on the steroids so things wouldn't irritate him as much. He also knew that rules of behavior did not change just because he was on steroids.

· · · · ·

Jody just seemed a little high while on prednisone. He was crazy for food but didn't have any behavior problems. He had lots of energy.

Thioguanine (thigh-oh-GWAN-neen)

How given: Pills taken by mouth on an empty stomach

Precaution: In some cases, thioguanine (6-TG) has caused liver problems. If your child's abdomen rapidly enlarges, call your doctor immediately.

Note: See earlier section in this chapter called "Different Responses to Medications" to review the genetic tests that determine whether and how quickly your child might metabolize this drug.

Common side effects:

- Low blood counts, which may increase risk of infection or bleeding and cause weakness, fatigue, and paleness
- Nausea and vomiting
- Mouth sores
- Headaches
- Loss of appetite
- Liver toxicity
- Swelling of the legs, hands, and feet

> *Tay's abdomen slowly began to enlarge and then it suddenly went from a little bloated to huge. He looked pregnant and his abdomen was rock hard. He gained 10 pounds in one day—from 55 to 65 pounds. It affected his white, red, and platelet counts. Tay was taken off all meds. He was given potassium by mouth, albumen by IV, and several blood and platelet transfusions. It was very scary! He also ran a fever off and on, and we were in the hospital for days. Once his abdomen shrank and his counts stayed steady we went home.*

Tretinoin (TRET-in-oin) and Isotretinoin (iso-TRET-in-oin)

How given: Capsules taken by mouth; do not crush, chew, or dissolve capsules

Precautions: These medications interact with several antibiotics and other classes of drugs. People using these drugs should avoid taking vitamin A or any multivitamins containing it, as this vitamin can cause toxic levels to build up in the body.

Common side effects:

- Low blood counts, which may increase risk of infection or bleeding and cause weakness, fatigue, and paleness
- Headaches

- Fever
- Dry skin
- Bone and joint pain
- Rashes
- Nausea and vomiting
- Flu-like symptoms
- Swelling of feet and ankle
- Abdominal pain
- Liver toxicity

Vincristine (vin-CRIS-teen)

How given: IV injection or infusion

Precautions: Care should be taken to prevent leakage of vincristine from the IV site because it will damage tissue. Before taking the first dose of vincristine, your child should be started on a program to prevent constipation.

Note: The side effects of vincristine are most obvious during induction and consolidation, when it is given weekly. It is generally better tolerated during maintenance when it is given monthly.

Common side effects:

- Severe constipation
- Temporary hair loss
- Nausea and vomiting
- Pain (may be severe) in jaw, face, back, joints, and/or bones
- Foot drop (child has trouble lifting front part of foot)
- Numbness, tingling, or pain (may be severe) in fingers and toes
- Extreme weakness and loss of muscle mass
- Drooping eyelids
- Pain, blisters, and skin loss if drug leaks into tissues
- Abdominal cramps
- Changes in taste

Hints for parents: Start your child on a stool softener at the beginning of treatment with this drug (do not wait!) and give it consistently. Joint pain (in the jaw, wrists, elbows, and knees) is a temporary side effect, but it is often severe enough to warrant strong pain medications. Watch your child's gait and strength, especially going up and down stairs and performing fine-motor activities, such as coloring, writing, or buttoning clothes. Report problems in these areas promptly, because your child's doctor may choose to alter the dose. Sometimes medications (e.g., gabapentin, also known by the brand name Neurontin®) and physical therapy are needed to counteract this drug's side effects.

Erica (diagnosed at age 1) once had a vincristine burn on her arm at the IV site. It was red when we went home from the clinic, but by the second day it was badly burned. She developed a blister as big as a half dollar, which left a bad scar. It hurt and was sensitive for a long time. She also developed severe foot drop (she could not lift up the front part of her foot) and fell a lot.

• • • • •

Preston (diagnosed age 10) had an awful time from vincristine. He would develop cramping in his lower legs, and would just curl up in bed, in great pain. It would start a couple of days after he received the vincristine, and would last a week. I would massage his legs, use hot packs, and give him Tylenol®. I would have to carry him into the clinic, because he couldn't walk. I did some research and discovered that when the bilirubin is high, the child can't excrete the vincristine and therefore the toxicity is increased. We lowered his vincristine dose and got him into physical therapy.

• • • • •

Vincristine incapacitated Katy. She couldn't walk, lift her head, or open one eyelid. She had trouble swallowing and stayed in bed for weeks during induction and consolidation. I read the package insert for vincristine and discovered that the manufacturer recommended that vincristine be given at least 12 to 24 hours before asparaginase to minimize toxicity. Katy's protocol required that both drugs be given at the same time. I negotiated with the doctors and had her schedule changed so that these two drugs were given on different days. She was soon back on her feet, but still, after a year off treatment, she has generalized muscle weakness and problems with balance.

• • • • •

My daughter Elke (age 2½ at diagnosis of ALL) is very sensitive to the neuropathic effects of vincristine. During induction she developed breathing and swallowing issues due to vocal cord paresis, had severe jaw and leg pain, and could not walk. Her doctors quickly started her on Neurontin® (generic name: gabapentin) to combat the neuropathy. She is currently in long-term maintenance and taking Elavil® for the same purpose. Although these are off-label uses of these medications, they are fairly effective at alleviating some of the pain caused by the vincristine. Since the damage done by vincristine can be long-term and cumulative, it is important to be proactive in addressing its side effects. Elke may not be able to run yet but she can walk, thanks to the continuous use of these medications and the willingness of her doctors to withhold or reduce her dosages of vincristine when warranted.

• • • • •

Soon after diagnosis at age 5 ½, Robby became so weak in the hospital that he stopped walking. He did not walk for at least a week, maybe more. When Robby did walk, he was up on his toes. I kept asking the doctors about it, and they poohpoohed it, saying it was just the vincristine. Finally, I took Robby to the pediatrician, who was horrified at how bad his feet had gotten. We immediately started daily physical therapy and got traction boots for him to wear at night.

Prophylactic Antibiotics

Children and teens on chemotherapy take antibiotics two to three days each week to prevent pneumocystis pneumonia (PCP). They usually keep taking the antibiotics a few months to a year after treatment ends. The antibiotic of choice for PCP prevention is a combination drug containing sulfamethoxazole and trimethoprim; it is sold under the brand names Bactrim® and Septra®. This antibiotic can cause gastrointestinal upset, skin rashes, sun sensitivity, and low blood counts. If a substitute is needed, one of the following is used:

• Pentamidine is administered by IV once a month, as an aerosol, or through a nebulizer. Use of the nebulizer can be difficult for children because it takes 20 minutes to administer and it smells and tastes bad.

• Dapsone® is a pill given once a day.

> *The oncologist explained it this way. Bactrim® is the best prophylactic antibiotic for PCP (pneumocystis), but it can affect counts. Pentamidine IV can affect counts, but nebulizer treatments (once a month) usually don't. Dapsone® can be used, but it can cause anemia. We just started the Dapsone® because Katie was starting to buck the nebulizer treatment because it smells and tastes horrible. The Bactrim® costs about $3/month, the Dapsone about $7/month, and the pentamidine nebulizer treatment is about $300/month!*

Colony-stimulating Factors

Colony-stimulating factors (CSFs) are not generally used for children with ALL, unless they suffer persistent and drastically reduced blood counts. They are sometimes used for children with acute myeloid leukemia (AML) or for those who have stem cell transplants. High-dose chemotherapy reduces the number of white blood cells used by the body to fight infections. The administration of CSFs, such as granulocyte colony-stim-ulating factor (G-CSF, also known by the brand name Neupogen®) and granulocyte-macrophage colony-stimulating factor (GM-CSF, also known as sargramostim, or by the brand name Leukine®), can reduce the severity and duration of low white blood counts, lessening the chance of infection. G-CSF may be given by IV or by subcutaneous injec-tion. GM-CSF must be administered by subcutaneous injection.

Kenny was only two years old when he was receiving G-CSF, so he was too young to understand why he needed the shots. He would cry and beg us not to hurt him—that he was sorry. My heart would break, but I would have to give him the shot. We finally developed a really good system. Right before being discharged after a round of chemo, we would put EMLA® on Kenny's arm and then have the nurse place an insulflon. It was a small catheter that Kenny didn't even notice was in his arm. It was good for 7 to 10 days, which was the duration of his G-CSF for the entire month. We would draw up the amount needed for injection, then place it in the insulflon and inject it very slowly. Kenny never felt it and no longer begged us not to do the G-CSF. Oh, how I wished we had done this from the beginning! Kenny's counts would usually start to decline about four days after his chemo. At about Day 10 the G-CSF would kick in, and his counts would skyrocket.

· · · · ·

Katie had G-CSF (brand name is Neupogen®) after each high-dose cytarabine. But it is in her protocol to give it to her after her other chemotherapy if low counts caused a delay of over seven days in treatment—and we were pretty close a few times. She's had no side effects from Neupogen® that I can recall. The worst thing about it for us was giving the shots at home. They're subcutaneous, so the needle is short, but Katie still said they hurt, even with EMLA®.

Antinausea Drugs Used During Chemotherapy

Antinausea drugs, also referred to as antiemetics, make chemotherapy treatments more bearable, but they can cause side effects. This section lists the most commonly used antinausea drugs. Other less commonly used drugs to prevent nausea are not described here.

Antinausea drug list

As with chemotherapy drugs, several names can be used to refer to each antinausea drug. The list below will help you find detailed information about each drug on the following pages.

Drug name	Brand name(s)
Aprepitant	Emend®
Dexamethasone	Decadron®
Diphenhydramine	Benadryl®
Granisetron	Granisol®, Kytril®, Sancuso®
Lorazepam	Ativan®
Ondansetron	Zofran®
Prochlorperazine	Compazine®
Promethazine	Phenergan®

Aprepitant (a-PREP-it-ant)

How given: Capsule by mouth; IV infusion

When given: Capsule is taken one hour before chemotherapy. IV infusion is given over a 15-minute span, starting 30 minutes before chemotherapy.

Precaution: This drug interacts with many drugs, so make sure the pharmacist knows about every drug your child takes.

Common side effects:

- Fatigue
- Dizziness
- Constipation
- Diarrhea
- Hiccups
- Heartburn
- Itching
- Loss of appetite

Dexamethasone (dex-a-METH-a-zone)

How given: IV injection, usually given in combination with other antinausea drugs

Common side effects: Side effects are different than those experienced when it is given in high doses for long periods of time. When dexamethasone is used to treat nausea, side effects include:

- Euphoria
- Restlessness
- Confusion

Diphenhydramine (die-fen-HIGH-dra-meen)

How given: Liquid, pills, or caplets by mouth; IV injection

When given: Usually given every six to eight hours.

Common side effects:

- Drowsiness
- Dizziness
- Impaired coordination
- Dry mouth
- Excitability (in young children)
- Low blood pressure

Granisetron (gran-ISS-eh-tron)

How given: IV injection; pills by mouth; patch on the skin (called Sancuso®)

When given: Granisetron is usually given 30 minutes prior to the start of chemotherapy infusion. Doses may be repeated every 12 to 24 hours.

Common side effects:

- Headaches
- Diarrhea
- Constipation

> *Sarah got Zofran® at first, then the clinic switched to liquid Kytril®. Sarah usually hates liquid meds (she much prefers pills), but she loves Kytril®. She thinks it's really yummy. And it works, too!*

Kytril® is an antinausea pill. It is incredibly expensive but brilliant in treating chemo-related sickness. It sometimes takes a bit of juggling to get the timing right; Michael used to take it an hour before taking the pills at bedtime. None of the other antiemetics worked for him nearly as well.

Lorazepam (lor-AZ-a-pam)

How given: Pills or liquid by mouth; sublingual (pill dissolved under the tongue); subcutaneous, IV, or IM injection.

When given: This tranquilizer is generally given in combination with other antinausea drugs.

Precaution: This drug interacts with several other drugs, so parents should tell the doctor about everything else their child is taking, including over-the-counter drugs.

Common side effects:

- Drowsiness and sleepiness
- Poor short-term memory
- Impaired coordination
- Low blood pressure
- Excitability (in young children)

Ondansetron (on-DAN-se-tron)

How given: IV injection; liquid by mouth; pills by mouth; or sublingual (pill dissolved under the tongue).

When given: Usually given 30 minutes prior to chemotherapy drugs, then every four to eight hours until nausea ends. It can be given in a higher dose once a day.

Note: Ondansetron comes in flavored oral solutions; 1 teaspoon = 4 mg. You can mix the dose in a small amount of a drink your child likes.

Common side effects:

- Headache with rapid IV administration
- Diarrhea
- Constipation

After Jeremy had his first inpatient treatment, he was allowed to go on an outpatient basis, wearing a cad pump at home. He felt fine, but every couple hours he would vomit for no reason. The next morning, when his oncologist asked him how it had gone, Jeremy was hesitant to tell him about the vomiting. When he did, the doctor asked us if the Zofran® hadn't helped. I gave him a confused look and asked him what a Zofran® was. I can laugh about it now, but it was an oversight. Everyone thought someone else had taken care of it! We rarely had any problems with nausea after that.

• • • • •

The absolute best for me were the Zofran® lozenges: simply dissolve on or under the tongue for instant relief. The prescription must state lozenges. You'll love those "melty pills."

• • • • •

Ondansetron works great for Ethan. He does have late nausea after chemo, so he takes it once a day for 10 days afterwards, and hasn't vomited or felt nauseated.

Prochlorperazine (pro-chlor-PAIR-a-zeen)

How given: Pills, long-acting capsule, or liquid by mouth; IM or IV injection

When given: Used when mild nausea is expected.

Common side effects:

- Drowsiness
- Low blood pressure
- Nervousness and restlessness
- Uncontrollable muscle spasms, especially of jaw, face, and hands
- Blurred vision

Promethazine (pro-METH-ah-zeen)

How given: Pills or liquid by mouth; IM or IV injection

When given: Usually given every four to six hours.

Common side effects:

- Drowsiness
- Dizziness
- Impaired coordination
- Fatigue
- Blurred vision
- Euphoria
- Insomnia

Drugs Used to Relieve Pain

As with other medicines, drugs used for pain relief can be given by various methods and can cause side effects. This section lists some drugs commonly used to relieve pain. Many other drugs are used to relieve pain in children, including acetaminophen, nalbuphine, fentanyl, hydrocodone, and others.

Pain medication list

Several different names can be used to refer to each of the pain medications. You may hear the same drug referred to by its generic name, an abbreviation, or one of several brand names, depending on which doctor, nurse, or pharmacist you talk to. The list below provides the generic name of several commonly used pain medications and some of the most common brand names.

Drug name	Brand name(s)
Codeine	Codrix®
Hydromorphone	Dilaudid®
Meperidine	Demerol®, Mepergan®
Morphine	Astramorph PF®, Avinza®, Duramorph®, Infumorph®, Kadian®, MS Contin®, Oramorph SR®, Roxanol®
Oxycodone	Percocet®, Percodan®, Oxycontin®, Roxicet®, Roxilox®, Roxycodone®, M-Oxy®, Oxyfast®, OxyIR®, ETH-Oxydose®, Tylox®

Codeine

How given: IM injection; IV injection or infusion; subcutaneous injection; pills or liquid by mouth

Note: People who cannot metabolize codeine get no pain relief from this drug (see section earlier in this chapter called "Different Responses to Medications"). Codeine should not be given to children younger than age 12.

Common side effects:

- Light-headedness
- Dizziness
- Sedation
- Euphoria
- Constipation

Hydromorphone

How given: IV injection or infusion; pill by mouth; subcutaneous injection

Precaution: It can cause slowed breathing.

Common side effects:

- Dizziness and light-headedness
- Sedation
- Nausea and vomiting
- Excessive sweating
- Euphoria and other mood alterations
- Headaches
- Constipation
- Slowed breathing

Meperidine

How given: IV, IM, or subcutaneous injection; liquid or pill by mouth. It is not as effective if taken by mouth.

Common side effects:

- Sedation
- Constipation
- Dizziness
- Nausea and vomiting
- Dry mouth
- Flushing or sweating

Morphine

How given: IV injection or infusion; pill by mouth (long-acting or short-acting); liquid by mouth

Common side effects:

- Euphoria
- Nausea and vomiting
- Sedation

- Dry mouth
- Headaches
- Drowsiness
- Constipation

Oxycodone

How given: Pills or liquid by mouth

Common side effects:

- Light-headedness
- Dizziness
- Sedation
- Constipation
- Nausea and vomiting

Topical anesthetics to prevent pain

Several products are commonly used to prevent pain from injections, finger pricks, and IV insertions. Most fall into two categories, which are described below. Use of these drugs is also discussed in Chapter 9, *Coping with Procedures.*

Topical anesthetizing creams

Examples: EMLA®, ELA-Max®, and many other brand names

How given: Each product has slightly different instructions. In general, they are applied to the skin 30 to 90 minutes before a procedure. Some must be covered with an airtight dressing.

How they work: These creams contain the topical anesthetic lidocaine. ELA-Max® uses lidocaine alone; EMLA® uses lidocaine in combination with prilocaine.

Notes: It may take longer than an hour to achieve effective anesthesia in dark-skinned children. When using EMLA®, the blood vessels sometimes constrict, making it harder to find a vein. To prevent this problem, it helps to apply a warm damp cloth right before the injection.

We use EMLA® for everything: finger pokes, accessing port, and shots. I even let her sister use it for shots because it lets her get a bit of attention, too. Both of my children have sensitive skin that turns red when they pull off tape, so I cover the EMLA® with plastic wrap held in place with paper tape. I also fold back the edge of each piece of tape to make a pull tab so the kids don't have to peel each edge back.

Vapocoolant sprays

Examples: Fluori-Methane Spray® and Fast Freeze®

How given: These aerosol sprays are applied to the target area right before the procedure. They can also be applied by spraying the solution into a medicine cup for 10 seconds, then dipping a cotton ball into the solution and holding it on the site for 15 seconds right before the procedure.

How they work: Most vapocoolant sprays use the refrigerant ethyl chloride to numb the area before an injection or infusion.

Note: If the spray is applied for too long, it can cause frostbite. Spray just until skin begins to turn white (3 to 10 seconds). The spray can should be held between 3 to 9 inches away from the skin.

Complementary Treatments

In recent years, increasing research has been done on mind–body medicine and its effect on coping with the side effects of illness. Complementary (also called adjunctive) therapies are those that can be expected to add something beneficial to the treatment. For example, visualization and music therapy are widely used to help children and teens prepare for or cope with medical procedures. Other helpful complementary therapies are acupuncture, aromatherapy, biofeedback, relaxation, massage, mindfulness meditation, prayer, and Reiki.

Christine was terrified of needles, and it was a nightmare every time we went in to get her port accessed or blood drawn. We went to a psychologist who specialized in methods to cope with pain. She taught my daughter visualization. They made an audiotape of an underwater snorkeling trip. It included watching all of the colorful fish and feeling the soothing warm water. She would listen to it in the clinic, or visualize the trip without the tape. It really helped her develop a technique to cope with accessing the port.

Alternative Treatments

Alternative treatments are defined as either:

• Treatments that are used in place of conventional medical treatments, or

• Treatments that may have unknown or adverse effects when used in addition to conventional treatments.

Sometimes alternative treatments are illegal or unavailable in the United States or Canada, and families travel to other countries to obtain them.

Alternative treatments are usually based on word-of-mouth endorsements, called anecdotal evidence. Medical treatments are based on scientific studies using data collected from large groups of patients. In treating childhood cancer, these large clinical trials have resulted in dramatic increases in survival rates over the past three decades.

It is extremely important that any alternative therapy that involves ingestion or injection into the body (e.g., herbs, vitamins, oils, special diets, enemas) only be given with the oncologist's knowledge. The oncologist's involvement is needed to prevent you from giving something to your child that could lessen the effectiveness of the conventional chemotherapy or cause added toxicity. For instance, folic acid (a type of B vitamin) replaces methotrexate in cells and reduces or eliminates its effectiveness, allowing cancer cells to flourish. The oncologist will be much more knowledgeable about these potential conflicts than a parent, herbalist, or health food store salesperson.

Never inject any alternative product into a central line. Children have developed life-threatening infections and have died from this.

If you want to evaluate claims made about alternative treatments, check the National Institutes of Health's National Center for Complementary and Integrative Health to see whether any scientific evidence or warnings exist about the treatment that interests you. This information is available online at *https://nccih.nih.gov*.

Take all the information you gather to your child's oncologist to discuss any positive or negative impacts the alternative treatment may have on your child's current medical treatment. Do not give any alternative treatment or over-the-counter drugs to your child in secret. Some treatments prevent chemotherapy from killing cancer cells, and other substances, such as those containing aspirin or related compounds, can cause uncontrollable bleeding in children with low platelet counts. If the alternative treatment is made from plant materials, it may contain bacteria or fungi that could make a child with low blood cell counts very ill.

At one point, we decided to try some alternative therapies with our son. Our plan was to use it in conjunction with his conventional treatment. I scheduled a meeting with his oncologist and discussed the alternatives with him. I wouldn't dare attempt to start anything, not even vitamin supplements, without first talking it over with the doctor, because I was scared that I would cause my child more harm than good. I was grateful that the oncologist was willing to listen to what I had to say and offer his opinion.

We both agreed that the alternative therapy we had in mind wouldn't do any damage or interfere with the chemotherapy my son was receiving. Two months later, we decided that it was doing absolutely nothing for him, so we stopped. I figured the money would be better spent at the toy store than on a useless therapy. I learned a valuable lesson from that experience. I'm much more skeptical now than I used to be. My new motto is "show me the proof."

· · · · ·

I gave my son echinacea when he received chemotherapy. I checked with his doctor first. He didn't think it would hurt but didn't think it would help, either. Still, all the nurses in emergency swore by the stuff. We got good results, too. We started the echinacea after lots of treatment, and it was the first time that he didn't have to be readmitted three days after chemo for febrile neutropenia. I'm convinced that it helped him during the recovery period when his counts would bottom out.

If, after thorough investigation, you feel strongly in favor of using an alternative treatment in addition to conventional treatment and your child's oncologist adamantly opposes it, listen to her reasoning. If you still disagree, get a second opinion from another oncology specialist. Remember, your child's health should be everyone's priority.

My daughter Meagan was diagnosed with average-risk ALL seven years ago. She had many chemotherapy-related side effects, including severe high blood pressure and ongoing liver problems. We were constantly adjusting her doses or taking her off chemo altogether. I was so obsessed about it that the doctor took me aside and told me that it's easier to treat leukemia than liver failure, and he just had to take her off her medications. He told me I had to stop worrying, but I couldn't. When her hair fell out again during maintenance, I just worried more. I realized that every child seemed to have something that went wrong, but I was amazed at how many different "somethings" there were. Now she has a head full of gorgeous hair. She was just chosen for the select soccer team and is quite an accomplished skier. She has no long-term effects and is healthy and happy.

Chapter 14

Common Side Effects of Treatment

"In the depths of winter I finally learned there was in me an invincible summer."

— Albert Camus

CHEMOTHERAPY DRUGS AND RADIATION THERAPY INTERFERE with cancer cells' ability to grow and reproduce. Because cancer cells divide frequently, they are more susceptible to chemotherapy and radiation than most normal cells. Unfortunately, healthy cells that multiply rapidly can also be damaged by chemotherapy and radiation. These normal cells include those of the brain, bone marrow, mouth, stomach, intestines, hair follicles, and skin.

This chapter explains the most common side effects of treatment for childhood leukemia and explores ways to deal with them. It also covers different types of rehabilitation services and questions about owning pets when your child is receiving chemotherapy. Chemotherapy and radiation therapy side effects that prevent good nutrition are discussed in Chapter 22, *Nutrition*. The most common side effects of treatment are listed in alphabetical order below.

Bed Wetting

Bed wetting can be a very upsetting side effect of cancer treatment, particularly for older children and teens. It might happen because:

- Some chemotherapy drugs increase thirst and others disrupt normal sleep patterns, both of which make bed wetting more likely.

- Intravenous (IV) fluids at night cause the bladder to fill with urine.

- Anything that disturbs sleep (e.g., steroids, anxiety, nightmares, post-traumatic stress) increases the likelihood of bed wetting.

When the bed wetting is caused by drugs or IV fluids, time will cure the problem. If bed wetting continues beyond an expected length of time, or there is pain involved, you can request a consultation with a urologist to rule out any ailments or damage that might require treatment.

> My teenaged son wet the bed whenever he was given antinausea medicine prior to high doses of chemotherapy. He was so embarrassed. He was so groggy that even if he woke up in time, I had to help him out of bed and support him while he stood, half asleep, to use the urinal.

There are also psychological reasons for bed wetting during treatment. The trauma of cancer treatment causes many children to regress to earlier behaviors such as thumb sucking, baby talk, temper tantrums, and bed wetting. Punishment for these behaviors only adds to the child's distress and rarely solves the problem. Following are parents' suggestions:

- Adopt an attitude that lets your child know bed wetting is "no big deal." There should be no shaming or punishment.
- Use disposable, absorbent underwear.
- Change sleeping arrangements.

> Prednisone and dexamethasone caused my daughter to have nightmares and frequent bed wetting. I felt if she could sleep through the night, the bed wetting might stop. I told her she could sleep with me during that round of chemo, but when the round of chemo was over she would move back into her own bed. It calmed her to sleep with me. The nightmares and bed wetting decreased, and she moved back into her own bed without complaint when the time came.

- Put down a plastic liner covered by fitted and flat sheets, and then put another plastic liner with a fitted and flat sheet on top. During the night, simply pull off the wet top sheets and plastic and there are fresh and dry sheets below. Or purchase absorbent fitted sheets, which can be washed, are softer than plastic, and don't make the noise that plastic sheets do.
- Keep a pile of extra-large towels next to the bed. Cover the wet spot with towels and save the bed change for the morning.
- Give the last drink two hours before bedtime so your child can go to the bathroom right before bed.
- If your child is bothered by bed wetting, ask whether he wants you to set the alarm for the middle of the night so he can get up and go to the bathroom.
- Give extra love and reassurance.

> When my daughter started bed wetting, I didn't think it was the drugs. I thought long and hard about any additional worries that she might have, and I realized that

because her dad had emotionally withdrawn from her during her illness, she might be worried that I would do the same. So I told her one night, "You know, I just realized that every day I tell you how much I love you. But I've never told you that no matter how hard life gets and no matter how mad we get at each other, I will always love you. I love you now as a child, I will love you as a teenager, and I will love you when you are all grown up." She started to sob and hugged and hugged me. She has never wet the bed again.

Changes in Taste and Smell

Chemotherapy can cause changes in the taste buds, altering the brain's perception of how food tastes. Meats often taste bitter, and sweets can taste unpleasant. Even foods that children crave can taste bad. The sense of smell is also affected by chemotherapy, heightening smells that other family members do not notice and sometimes causing nausea in the child on chemotherapy.

Both the senses of smell and taste can take months to return to normal after treatment ends. During chemotherapy and radiation treatment, it is best to avoid favorite foods that do not taste the same; that way, when treatment ends, these foods can be enjoyed once again.

Once Katy begged me to make her my special double chocolate sour cream cake. Surprisingly, it smelled really good to her as it baked. She took a big bite, spit it out all over the table, and ran back to her room sobbing. She cried for a long time. She told me later that it had tasted "bitter and horrible."

Constipation

Constipation means a decrease in a child's normal number of bowel movements or dry, hard stool that is painful to pass. Some drugs, such as vincristine, slow the movement of stool through the intestines, causing constipation. Pain medication, decreased activity, decreased eating and drinking, and vomiting can all affect the normal rhythm of the intestines. Following are parents' suggestions for preventing and/or coping with constipation:

- Encourage your child to be as physically active as possible.
- Urge your child to drink plenty of liquids every day. Prune juice is very helpful.
- Serve high-fiber foods such as raw vegetables, beans, bran, graham crackers, whole-wheat breads, whole-grain cereals, dried fruits (especially prunes, dates, and raisins), and nuts.
- Check with the doctor before using any medications for constipation. He may recommend a stool softener such as Colace®. If the doctor suggests liquid Docusate®, be

aware that many children don't like the taste. Senokot®, another frequently prescribed stool softener, comes in a tablet form, chocolate-flavored liquid, and granules that can be mixed into yogurt or ice cream. Metamucil® and Citrucel® increase the volume of the stool, which stimulates the intestines. Milk of Magnesia®, magnesium citrate, and MiraLax® help the stool retain fluid and remain soft.

> Vincristine constipation resulted in horrible screaming, bottom itching, constant trips to the bathroom with no luck, for days at a time. It is absolutely frustrating! We now have a preventative routine so that never happens again. Beginning the morning of a vincristine injection, I give one Peri-Colace® (stool softener plus laxative) each morning and evening until things improve—which is usually after about a week or so. Then, I taper down to one a day until things seem to be getting on the too soft side, then stop. The Peri-Colace® is manufactured in a brown "soft-gel" thing, and the liquid inside it tastes horrible. If at any time during our Peri-Colace® phase there are two consecutive days with no bowel movements, I give bisacodyl in the evening of the second day, and things usually get straightened out the next morning. Unfortunately, if it's a school day, I have to keep him home until mid-morning, as the prednisone diet and laxatives lead to a very busy morning in the bathroom.

Do not give enemas or rectal suppositories. These can cause anal tears that can be dangerous for a child with a weakened immune system. When your child feels the need to have a bowel movement, sipping a warm drink can help the feces come out.

> My 4-year-old daughter either had diarrhea or severe constipation for the entire eight months of intensive treatment. Her bowel habits returned to normal during maintenance. When constipated, she would just sob and try to hold it in. This made her stool even harder and more painful. One time she cried, "Why is my anus round and my poop square?" We ended up just putting her in a bathtub full of warm water, gave her warm drinks, and let her go in the bathtub.

Dental Problems

Both cranial radiation and chemotherapy can cause changes in the mouth, teeth, and ability to salivate. Awareness of the potential problems, combined with good preventive care, can help maintain oral health during treatment. Ask your child's oncologist and dentist for advice about tooth care when white blood cell counts are very low. Often parents are advised to use a sponge or damp gauze to gently wipe off their child's teeth after meals instead of brushing.

During treatment, plaque can build up rapidly on your child's teeth, increasing the likelihood of cavities and gum infections. Take your child to the dentist for a cleaning and check-up every three to four months, as long as her blood counts are high (an absolute neutrophil count [ANC] of more than 1,000 and platelets of more than 100,000).

Children with a central venous catheter should be given antibiotics before and after each visit to the dentist.

> *My daughter had problems with thick yellow saliva during the entire time she was treated. It coated her teeth and formed a lot of plaque. I brought her to an excellent pediatric dentist every three months to have the plaque removed. She took antibiotics half an hour before treatment and then again six hours afterward. He also put sealants on all of her molars and, even though there were many weeks when her teeth could not be brushed, she never got a cavity.*

Some parents report delays in the arrival of their child's permanent teeth. Children who receive chemotherapy or cranial radiation therapy may also have poorly developed or absent permanent teeth and short tooth roots.

Diarrhea

Because chemotherapy destroys cells that are produced at a rapid rate, such as those that line the mouth, stomach, and intestines, it can cause diarrhea, ranging from mild (frequent, soft stools) to severe (abundant quantities of liquid stool). Diarrhea during chemotherapy can also be caused by some antinausea drugs, antibiotics, and intestinal infections. After chemotherapy ends and immune function returns to normal, the lining of the digestive tract heals and the diarrhea ends. Following are parents' suggestions for coping with diarrhea:

• Do not give any over-the-counter medicine to your child without approval from the oncologist. She might want to test your child's stool for infection prior to treating the diarrhea. Frequently recommended drugs for diarrhea are Kaopectate®, Lomotil®, and Immodium®.

• It is very important that your child drink plenty of liquids. The liquids will not increase the diarrhea, but they will replace the lost fluids.

> *My 3 year old had stopped drinking from bottles months before her diagnosis. When she first began her intensive chemotherapy, she had uncontrollable, frequent diarrhea. Liquid would just gush out without warning. One night she said in a small voice, "Mommy, would it be okay if I drank from a bottle again?" I said, "Of course, honey." It was a great comfort to her, and she took in a lot more fluids that way.*

• Hot or cold liquids can increase intestinal contractions, so give your child lots of room-temperature clear liquids (e.g., water, Gatorade®, ginger ale) or mild juices such as peach juice or apricot nectar.

• Diarrhea depletes the body's supply of potassium, so give your child foods high in potassium, such as bananas, oranges, baked or mashed potatoes without the skin, broccoli, halibut, mushrooms, asparagus, tomato juice, and milk or yogurt (if tolerated).

- Low potassium can cause irregular heartbeats and leg cramps. If these occur, call the doctor.

- Do not serve foods high in fiber, such as bran, fruits (dried or fresh), nuts, beans, or raw vegetables.

- Do not serve greasy, fatty, spicy, or sweet foods. Instead, give your child bland, low-fiber foods such as bananas, white rice, noodles, applesauce, unbuttered white toast, creamed cereals, cottage cheese, fish, and chicken or turkey without the skin.

> *In the middle of maintenance, my son had severe diarrhea for a week. He had large amounts of liquid stools 20 times a day. I felt so sorry for him. The doctor cultured a stool specimen, but they never identified a cause. It cleared up after a week of the BRAT diet (bananas, rice, applesauce, toast). He had a problem with diarrhea almost weekly throughout his treatment.*

- If your child's anus is sore, check with the doctor before using any non-prescription medicine. He may recommend using Desitin®, A&D ointment®, or Bag Balm® after each bowel movement.

> *While taking ARA-C my daughter had a terribly sore rectum. It hurt to have bowel movements, she'd cry and have to squeeze our hands to go, then the urine would run back and burn. She was also very itchy. We carried around bags with Q-tips® and every known brand of rectal ointment—A&D®, Preparation H®, Desitin®, and Benadryl®. Thank goodness this cleared up quickly on maintenance.*

- Call the doctor if your child has significant pain with bowel movements, especially if your child has low blood counts.

Fatigue and Weakness

Fatigue, a feeling of extreme tiredness, is an almost universal side effect of cancer treatments. General weakness, although different from fatigue, is also caused by cancer treatment. Fatigue and weakness may be constant throughout therapy or may come and go. They can be minor annoyances or totally debilitating. Fatigue and weakness are usually caused by one, or a combination, of the following:

- Radiation therapy
- Your child's body working overtime to heal tissues damaged by treatment and to rid itself of dead and dying cancer cells
- Medications to treat nausea or pain
- Mineral imbalances caused by chemotherapy, diarrhea, or vomiting
- Malnutrition caused by nausea, vomiting, loss of appetite, or taste aversions
- Anemia (low red blood cell count)

- Infections
- Emotional factors such as anxiety, fear, sadness, depression, or frustration
- Disruption of normal sleep patterns (common when hospitalized or when taking some chemotherapy drugs)

> My son is almost 19 and is just beginning his third year of maintenance for ALL. He is a quiet and studious young man, has never dated, and does not go about partying and the like. The last three months, he appears to be all right, but he is, in his own words, always "exhausted." In college and living in the dorm, he can get up in the morning at 6 a.m., but if he has two classes in a row, he is quite likely to fall asleep during the second class. He's too tired to concentrate on homework for more than an hour at a time. Before diagnosis, a 50-mile bike ride was nothing to him. Even six months ago he could ride 30 miles, although he did feel some fatigue. Now, his beloved bike rests gathering dust. It breaks my heart that my son cannot feel the exuberance of young adulthood that I experienced at his age, but I am so very thankful that the treatment for leukemia has saved his life. I hope that when he is off treatment he will finally feel good again.

Following are suggestions from parents about ways to deal with fatigue and weakness:

- Make sure your child gets plenty of rest. Naps or quiet times spaced throughout the day help.

> Erica took a 2 ½ hour nap every afternoon throughout therapy. She's 4 now and off treatment, but her endurance is low and she still tires easily.

- Limit visitors if your child is weak or fatigued.

> While in the hospital, my daughter was very weak. She had too many visitors, yet didn't want to hurt anyone's feelings. We worked out a signal that solved the problem. When she was too tired to continue a visit, she would place a damp washcloth on her forehead. I would then politely end the visit.

- Serve your child well-balanced meals and snacks, but don't get upset if he doesn't eat them (see next point about stress).
- Parents and children should try to avoid physical and emotional stress, whenever possible.
- Encourage your child to pursue hobbies or interests, if able. For example, if your child is too weak to play on an athletic team, let her go cheer the team on.

> My eighth-grade daughter was a fabulous athlete prior to her diagnosis. When she went back to school after missing a year, she wasn't very competitive, but she managed the softball team and dressed for basketball. So she was still part of the social scene and was able to do things with the teams.

Some children go through treatment without fatigue or weakness, but other children are not so lucky. The following stories describe two common experiences.

> Before Brent was diagnosed at age 6, he was exceptionally well coordinated and a very fast runner. During treatment, he slowed down to about average. He played soccer and T-ball throughout, and was very competitive.

· · · · ·

> Jeremy has had some major, persistent problems with weakness and loss of coordination. When he was 9 years old, a year off therapy, he still could not catch a ball. When he ran, he was like a robot, and the trunk of his body stayed straight. Some kids made fun of him, and he got very frustrated with himself. He had lots of physical therapy, and now, three years off treatment, his skills have improved, but he still has to work harder than the other kids. We put him into martial arts in hopes of further increasing his motor skills and his confidence.

Hair Loss

Because hair follicle cells reproduce quickly, chemotherapy causes some or all body hair to fall out. The hair on the scalp, eyebrows, eyelashes, underarms, and pubic area may slowly thin out or fall out in big clumps. Hair regrowth usually starts one to three months after maintenance starts or intensive chemotherapy ends. The color and texture may be different from the original hair. Straight hair may regrow curly; blond hair may grow back brown. Sometimes during maintenance, some children's hair begins to thin or fall out again. Here are a few tips from parents:

- When hair is thin or breaking, use a brush with very soft bristles. When hair is wet, use a wide-toothed comb, not a brush.
- Once hair loss begins, consider a very short hair cut to ease the transition to complete hair loss.
- A flannel blanket placed on the pillow at night will help collect hair that falls out.
- Recognize that coping with hair loss is difficult for almost all children, but it is especially hard on teenagers.
- Emphasize to your child that the hair loss is temporary and that it will grow back.

> During the first year after Belle was diagnosed (and lost her hair), her brother and I found some Barbie® hats/bandanas with wigs attached at the local dollar store. So the Barbies® whose heads were shaved had something to wear while their hair grew out! Belle also made numerous outfits for "chemo Barbie®" out of supplies at the hospital: napkins, masks, various kinds of tape.

- Allow your child to choose a collection of hats, scarves, or cotton turbans to wear. These are tax-deductible medical expenses and may be covered by insurance.

- To order several styles of reversible, all-cotton head wear for girls and teens, contact Just in Time Soft Hats® at (215) 247-8777 or online at *www.softhats.com*. Another company called Hip Hats with Hair® sells hats with human hair, which are soft, comfortable, and fun to wear. Visit its website at *www.hatswithhair.com*.

- If your child expresses an interest in wearing a wig, take pictures of her hairstyle prior to hair loss. Also, cut snippets of hair to take in to allow a good match to the original color and texture. The cost of the wig may be covered by insurance if the doctor writes a prescription for a "wig prosthesis" and includes the medical reason for the wig, such as "alopecia due to cancer chemotherapy." The American Cancer Society, (800) ACS-2345, and some local cancer service organizations offer free wigs in some areas.

- Advocate that school-aged children be permitted to wear hats or other head coverings in school. Use a 504 Plan, described in Chapter 20, *School*, if necessary.

- Separate your feelings about baldness from your child's feelings. Many parents rush out to buy wigs and hats without discussing with their child how he or she wants to deal with baldness. Allow your child to choose whether to wear head coverings or not. Let it be okay to be bald. A pediatric oncologist comments:

> *Consider whether hair loss bothers your child. If it bothers him, then you should pursue things to hide or resolve the problem. If it bothers you but not him, then focus your efforts on trying to deal with your concern and anxiety. Think of this as an opportunity to teach him that it is what is on the inside that counts. In today's culture that places so much emphasis on outward appearance and conformity, this is a valuable lesson. It has been my experience that kids who have visible late effects after cancer treatment can adjust quite well to external differences if they are given a lot of support at home. As a parent, if you let him know he is a great kid, he will believe it.*

The amount of hair loss varies among children being treated for leukemia. Some children lose some of their hair, some have hair that thins out, and some quickly lose every hair on their head.

> *Preston never completely lost his hair, but it became extremely thin and wispy. When he was first diagnosed, a friend bought him a fly-fishing tying kit, and he became very good at tying flies. He even began selling them at a local fishing shop. When his hair began to fall out, we would gather it up and put it in a plastic bag. He started tying flies out of his hair, and they were displayed in the shop window as "Preston's Human Hair Flies." He was only 11, but the shop owner hired him to help around the shop. He became very popular with the clientele, because everyone wanted to meet the boy who tied flies from his own hair. He really turned losing his hair into something positive.*

Three-year-old Christine's hair started to fall out within three weeks of starting chemo. She had beautiful curly hair, but she never talked about losing it, and I thought it didn't bother her. Occasionally she would wear a hat or the hood of a sweatshirt, but most of the time she went bald. One day, I learned how she really felt. We were talking about the different colors of hair in our family, and she began shouting, "I don't have brown hair! I'm bald, just like a baby."

The chemo greatly affected Meagan's hair. During maintenance, it came back in lush and curly, then after a few months it began falling out again. This was very upsetting. She hasn't gone completely bald again, but it remains very thin and unhealthy hair, while others in the same stage of treatment have beautiful hair back again.

My daughter, Katie (age 11), cut and dyed her hair bright fuchsia as soon as she realized she had cancer. It made her hair seem less hers than something to play with. Then, when she started receiving chemo, she asked that it be cut and shaved really short like some of her boy friends in her class. Our local coach came over and shaved it for her. It was only about a quarter of an inch long at that point. Then when it fell out a week later, it was no big deal for her, because she had already taken it off. That was her way of controlling the situation.

Now we celebrate her baldness by painting henna designs on her head and using face paints to paint fancy designs whenever we go somewhere special, or visit the hospital. On July 4th, we painted stars and rockets in red, white, and blue. On our last visit to the hospital, we painted a floral vine with flowers and lightning bolts above her ears to show she's hot stuff. She even had her sisters add two eyes at the back of her head—to watch the doctors and nurses when her back is turned. Everyone loves to check out her head when she comes in the hospital, and she receives tons of attention as a result of it. She also loves to dress up her head with funny wigs and masks. Last week she was dancing in the front yard with a black/blue fright wig, monster ears, a Grateful Deadhead shirt and black platform heels. She literally stopped traffic! It was a riot. She absolutely refuses to talk to most of her doctors and nurses, and is extremely shy, but this is her silly way of poking fun at them and the whole situation with her cancer.

Learning Differences

Some children who have been treated for leukemia are at risk of developing learning disabilities as a consequence of their treatment. Those at highest risk include children younger than age 5 who receive radiation to the brain and/or certain chemotherapy drugs, especially high-dose methotrexate. Much is known about the types of learning difficulties caused by treatment for childhood cancer (see Chapter 20, *School*).

Low Blood Cell Counts

Bone marrow—the spongy material that fills the inside of the bones—produces red blood cells (RBCs), white blood cells (WBCs), and platelets. Chemotherapy drugs can damage or destroy the cells inside the bone marrow and can dramatically lower the number of cells circulating in the blood. Frequent blood tests will be done to determine whether your child needs a transfusion. Many children treated for leukemia require transfusions of RBCs and sometimes platelets. When the number of infection-fighting WBCs is low, your child is in danger of developing serious infections.

Absolute neutrophil count (ANC)

The ANC provides an indication of a child's ability to fight infection. Generally, an ANC of 500 to 1,000 provides children with enough protective neutrophils to fight off infection caused by bacteria and viruses. When your child's ANC is this high, you can usually allow her to attend all normal functions such as school, athletic events, and parties. However, it is wise to keep close track of the pattern of the rise and fall of your child's ANC. If you know the ANC is 1,000, but is on the way down, it will affect which activities are appropriate for your child. The activities of families of children with cancer usually revolve around the sick child's WBC count and, specifically, the ANC.

When your child has an abnormally low level of neutrophils (WBCs) in the blood, it is called neutropenia. Your child will be deemed neutropenic when he has a low ANC (below 500).

When a child has blood drawn for a complete blood count (CBC), one section of the lab report will state the total WBC count and a "differential." The differential lists each type of WBC as a percentage of the total. For example, if the total WBC count is 1500 mm³, the differential might look like this:

WBC type	Percentage of total WBC
Segmented neutrophils (also called polys or segs)	49%
Band neutrophils (also called bands)	1%
Basophils (also called basos)	1%
Eosinophils (also called eos)	1%
Lymphocytes (also called lymphs)	38%
Monocytes (also called monos)	10%

The ANC is calculated by adding the percentages of segmented and band neutrophils, and then multiplying by the total WBC. Using the example above, the ANC is 49% + 1% = 50%; 50% of 1,500 (.50 x 1500) = 750; so the ANC is 750.

Erica ran a fever whenever her counts were low, but nothing ever grew in her cultures. They would hospitalize her for 48 hours as a precaution. She was never on a full dose of medicine because of her chronically low counts. She's two years off treatment now and doing great.

How to protect a child with a low ANC

Every hospital has different guidelines concerning activities for children with low ANCs, but here are parents' suggestions for ways to prevent and detect infections:

- Insist on frequent, lengthy (at least 1 to 2 minutes), and thorough hand washing for every member of the family. Use plenty of soap and warm water, lather well, and rub all portions of the hands, including between all the fingers and under the fingernails. Children and parents need to wash before preparing meals, before eating, after playing outdoors, after petting an animal, and after using the bathroom.

  We always had antibacterial baby wipes in our car. We washed Justin's hands, and our own, after going to any public places such as parks, museums, or restaurants. They can also be used to wipe off tables or high chairs at restaurants.

- Make sure all medical personnel at the hospital or doctor's office thoroughly wash their hands before touching your child.

  Nurses and doctors frequently come into the room and don't wash their hands. I make them wash their hands, change their gloves, or squirt Purell® on them. I always had a bottle of Purell® with me. They would say that they washed their hands before they came into the room. I tell them, "Well, you just touched the doorknob and you have to wash them again." I had a situation like this with our oncologist. He washed his hands, and then right before starting my daughter's spinal, his cell phone rang and he answered it. He started to proceed, and I stopped him and told him to wash his hands again because he touched the cell phone. He was taken aback for a second, and then agreed.

- Whenever your child needs a needle stick, make sure the technician washes his hands and then cleans your child's skin thoroughly with both betadine and alcohol.

- If your child gets a small cut, wash it with soap and water, rinse it with hydrogen peroxide, and cover it with a small bandage.

- When your child is ill, take her temperature every two to three hours. Call the doctor if your child's temperature is 101° F (38.5° C) or above.

- Do not permit anyone to take your child's temperature rectally (in the anus) or use rectal suppositories, as these may cause anal tears and increase the risk of infection and bleeding.

Believe it or not, we once stopped the nursing assistant from doing a rectal temp during an inpatient admission. When we had a room on the pediatric oncology side, this never happened. But for that admission those rooms were full, and we were on the other side of the floor.

- Do not use a humidifier, as the stagnant water can become a reservoir for bacteria.

- Apply sunscreen whenever your child plays outdoors. The skin of children taking certain chemotherapy drugs or who have recently received radiation therapy is sensitive to the sun, and a bad sunburn can easily become infected.

- Your child should not receive routine immunizations while on chemotherapy. Your child's doctor or nurse can complete medical exemption forms for your child's school. Siblings should not be given the live polio virus (OPV); they should get the killed polio virus (IPV). Verify that your pediatrician is using the appropriate vaccine for the siblings.

  Christine was diagnosed just a week after her younger sister, Alison, had been given the live polio vaccine. Because there was a small risk that Alison could infect any immunosuppressed child with polio, she was not allowed to visit the oncology floor of the hospital.

- If your child's ANC is low, an infected site may not become red or painful.

  My daughter kept getting ear infections while on chemotherapy. They would find them during routine exams. I felt guilty because she never told me her ears were hurting. I told her doctor that I was worried because she didn't complain of pain, and he reassured me by telling me that she probably felt no pain because she didn't have enough white cells to cause swelling inside her ear.

- Never give aspirin for fever, because aspirin and drugs containing aspirin interfere with blood clotting. Ibuprofen may be given if approved by your child's oncologist. If your child has a fever, call the doctor before giving any medication.

- Call the clinic if any of the following symptoms appear: fever above 101° F (38.5° C), chills, cough, shortness of breath, sore throat, severe diarrhea, bloody urine or stool, and pain or burning while urinating.

  Some people choose to keep their kids away from everything and everyone during treatment, while others restrict their activities when they're neutropenic or receiving a particularly heavy dose of chemo. You will learn how to trust your instincts and your doctor's advice, and also learn how to take your cues from your child. For us, we try to walk a fine line between keeping Hunter's life as normal and stimulating as possible, while not taking any foolish risks with his health. When he's neutropenic (ANC below 500), when he's in a particularly heavy round of chemo, or when there're illnesses going around we keep him at home. When he's doing well then we take him out a bit more, but sensibly: no shopping malls on Saturdays, no contact with anyone who's sick, and limited contact with other kids. During the week, I will take him with me to the grocery store, or to see his grandparents or cousins, provided everyone is healthy. When he's feeling well we also go to the park, ride our bikes, and do normal kid stuff. I carry around antibacterial hand wipes with me so I can keep him clean after visiting playgrounds.

Mouth and Throat Sores

The mouth, throat, and intestines are lined with cells that divide rapidly and can be severely damaged by chemotherapy drugs. This damage is more common for children on very intensive protocols and for those having stem cell transplants. The sores that develop in the mouth, throat, and intestines are extremely painful and can prevent eating and drinking. Check your child's mouth regularly for sores, and if any are present ask the oncologist for advice. Following are some suggestions from parents:

- To prevent infection, the mouth needs to be kept as clean and free of bacteria as possible. After eating, have your child gently brush teeth, gums, and tongue with a soft, clean toothbrush.

  We use Biotene® to prevent mouth sores. It is a little minty, foams a bit, and is alcohol-free, so it does not burn. Our nurse practitioner swears by it. She told us that it is the only thing that she has seen that seems to prevent mouth sores. We suspected Nico had sores in his throat after the high-dose methotrexate based on drooling, complaining of pain, and refusing to eat or drink without pain medication, but he never had visible sores in his mouth. We use Biotene® religiously when we are inpatient. We apply it with an oral sponge or an extra soft toothbrush. One warning though, Nico does not enjoy it.

- If your child is old enough, the doctor may recommend a rinse to decrease the amount of bacteria in your child's mouth, which helps prevent mouth sores.

  When David was told to use Peridex®, I asked the doctor if we could substitute 0.63% stannous fluoride rinse. He said yes. As a dentist, I knew Peridex® kills bacteria and lasts up to eight hours, but it tastes terrible and stains teeth. Children do not like using it. The 0.63% stannous fluoride has the same bacteria-killing properties and also lasts up to eight hours, but has a better taste and does not stain as badly. The fluoride also helps prevent cavities and makes the teeth less sensitive. It comes in a variety of flavors like mint, tropical, and cinnamon. It is a prescription drug that a lot of dentists dispense. To prepare, mix ⅛ ounce of concentrate with warm water, making one ounce. A measuring cup comes with the bottle. I have David swish with half the mixture for one minute. (Time it, because it's longer than you think!) This rinse can only be used by kids who are old enough not to accidentally swallow it. Six-year-old David has no problem doing this once a day before he goes to bed. If and when he starts developing mouth sores, he will use it morning and evening. It's important not to eat or drink for 30 minutes after rinsing. That is why David rinses before bedtime, after he has taken his meds and brushed his teeth.

- Serve bland food, baby food, or meals put through the blender.
- Use a straw with drinks or blender-processed foods.

Preston got bad mouth sores every time he was on high-dose methotrexate. He could not swallow, but we were supposed to be forcing fluids to flush the drugs out. The only thing that felt good on his throat was guava nectar. It was very expensive and hard to find, and he would drink several quarts a day. Unfortunately, my daughter and husband both developed a liking for it, too. At one point we cornered the market on guava nectar at three grocery stores in our neighborhood.

Several prescription products are available to treat mouth sores. One common product is called "magic mouthwash," which contains an antibiotic, antihistamine, antifungal, and antacid. Some formulations add dexamethasone. More information about this product is available at *www.mayoclinic.com/health/magic-mouthwash/AN02024*. If your child has painful mouth sores, ask the oncologist for a prescription. Because large amounts of lidocaine can numb the back of the throat and cause difficulty swallowing, this medication should be used at a dose recommended by the oncologist.

Glutamine, a nutritional supplement available at most drug and health food stores, may help prevent or minimize mouth sores in some children. If your child is receiving chemotherapy with a high probability of causing mouth sores, you may want to try glutamine as a preventive measure. The powder can be mixed in juice and should be started one or two days before your child starts a cycle of chemotherapy. Be sure to get your oncologist's approval before giving glutamine.

Nausea and Vomiting

The effects of anticancer drugs vary from person to person and dose to dose. A drug that makes some children violently ill often has no effect on other children. Some drugs produce no nausea until several doses have been given, but others cause nausea after a single dose. There is no relationship between the amount of nausea and the effectiveness of the medicine. Because the effects of chemotherapy are so variable, each child's treatment for nausea must be tailored to her individual needs.

Antinausea medications help prevent or minimize the amount of nausea and vomiting associated with chemotherapy. Many children eat normally and never exhibit any signs of nausea while on chemotherapy because of the effectiveness of the antinausea medications. For a discussion of drugs used to prevent nausea and vomiting, see Chapter 13, *Chemotherapy and Other Medications*.

Following is a list of suggestions for helping children and teenagers cope with nausea and vomiting:

- Give your child antinausea medications as prescribed. Nausea is easier to keep under control than to get control of, so never miss a dose.

  During Christine's treatment, nausea was a big problem at first. I made a point to work with the staff to address this, and this is the plan we came up with: Christine would be given the maximum tolerated dose of Zofran® the first time chemo was administered, then four hours later she'd get the regular dose, then we would give the regular dose every six hours.

- Have your child wear loose clothing, because it is both more comfortable and easier to remove if soiled.
- Try to have at least one change of clothes for your child in the car.
- Keep large zip-lock plastic bags in the car. They are an easy-to-use and highly effective container if your child gets sick. They can be sealed and disposed of quickly and neatly, ridding the car of unpleasant odors that could make your child's nausea worse.
- Carry a bucket, towels, and baby wipes in the car in case of vomiting.
- Try to keep your child in a quiet, well-ventilated room after chemotherapy.
- Try not to cook in the house when your child feels nauseated. If possible, open windows to provide plenty of fresh air. Smells can trigger nausea.
- Use a covered cup with a straw for liquids if your child is nauseated by smells.
- Do not serve hot foods if the odor aggravates your child's nausea.
- Serve dry foods such as toast, pretzels, cereal, or crackers in the morning or whenever your child is feeling nauseated.
- Serve several small meals rather than three large ones.
- Have your child keep his head elevated after eating. Lying flat can make nausea worse.
- Provide plenty of clear liquids such as water, Gatorade®, and ginger ale.
- Avoid serving sweet, fried, or very spicy foods. Instead, stick with bland foods such as potatoes, cottage cheese, soup, bananas, applesauce, rice, or toast when your child feels nauseated.
- Watch for any signs of dehydration, including loose or dry skin, dry mouth, sunken eyes, dizziness, and decreased urination. Call the doctor if your child appears dehydrated.
- Have your child rinse her mouth with water or a mixture of water and lemon juice after she vomits to help remove the taste.
- Let your child chew gum or suck on ice pops if he develops a metallic taste in his mouth; it may help alleviate the taste of metal.

- Consider trying acupuncture, aromatherapy, massage, or meditation to help alleviate symptoms.

> *Meagan has always had problems in every phase of treatment with stomachaches, especially in the morning. She will often vomit once and then be over it. She is frequently soothed with just rubbing her tummy or laying a hot towel on it.*

If antinausea medications do not work well for your child, investigate the U.S. Food and Drug Administration-approved Relief Band®. This wrist band gives an electrical stimulation (too faint to feel) to an point on the wrist that affects the portion of the brain that controls nausea. Information about this band is available at *www.reliefband.com*. A similar product that works well is the Sea-Band® (*www.sea-band.com*).

Osteonecrosis

Osteonecrosis, also called avascular necrosis (AVN), is a condition caused by the death of small blood vessels that nourish the bones and joints. In children and teens treated for leukemia, AVN is caused by the use of steroids. It is more commonly caused by dexamethasone than prednisone (except when prednisone is given in high doses for long periods of times, such as for children who relapse or who are treated with stem cell transplants). AVN is much more common in children older than age 10; however, on protocols that use dexamethasone exclusively, it is being seen in younger children more often. The course of AVN is variable. Some children and teens have the condition for years with only minor problems with pain and movement, but others require one or more surgeries soon after the condition is diagnosed.

> *At the beginning of long-term maintenance (COG trial AALL0331 augmented therapy), my 6-year-old daughter, Emilie, said that her arms hurt at night, so we did some research and learned quite a bit about AVN from the ALL-KIDS list on www. acor.org. Our nurse practitioner is very good, but we had to push to get an x-ray done. When substantial AVN was confirmed in Emilie's left shoulder, she had an MRI of both shoulders and finally a nuclear bone scan of her entire body to see if it was in any of the other joints. The bone scan did not show any damage to other joints, but Emilie's knees hurt after an active day, so it may be starting there as well. Our oncologist took her off the steroids, and I had to get my head wrapped around that, which was hard for me. But, he believed her body had probably had enough and he was not concerned regarding her prognosis. We met with an orthopedic surgeon and he recommended a procedure called small-diameter percutaneous decompression be done on both shoulders. She had the surgery two months ago. Within two weeks her symptoms disappeared in both shoulders and the x-rays six weeks later showed stabilization, so it was very effective. I am so glad that we did it.*

Rehabilitation

Rehabilitation services include physical therapy, occupational therapy, and recreational therapy. Children and teens who need these services often start receiving them while they are in the hospital (e.g., for vincristine neuropathy). Then, at discharge, the oncologist will write orders for home services. Various rehabilitation services are available either privately (paid for by insurance, if covered) or through the school system.

Physical therapy

Physical therapy involves using exercise and motion to improve the body's strength and movement. If an arm or leg is not moving at all, the physical therapist moves the limb through the entire range of motion to prevent the muscles from tightening during recovery. When the arm or leg begins to recover, the physical therapist devises strengthening exercises for the affected limb. Physical therapy uses equipment such as tilt tables, stationary bicycles, and treadmills. Therapy in a pool (also called aquatic therapy) is another form of physical therapy used to strengthen affected limbs.

> William's vincristine neuropathy is pretty bad. He didn't get much physical therapy for the seven months we were inpatient, nor during the stay for his BMT [bone marrow transplant]. He is getting lots of help now. He has the half boot orthotics and also wears orthotics in his shoes. His arch completely dropped. He has both nerve and strength issues.

Occupational and recreational therapy

Occupational therapy focuses on recovering or maintaining the ability to participate in activities of daily life. For example, occupational therapists help children regain the fine motor skills needed to tie shoes, hold a pencil, eat, and dress themselves. They also evaluate the child's need for any special equipment to maximize independence, such as an adaptive holder to help the child write with a pencil or a computer if writing by hand is not a realistic goal.

Recreational therapy also works on activities of daily living, as well as on social and cognitive functioning, developing coping skills, and integrating children back into community settings. Examples of methods used by recreational therapists are creative arts (e.g., painting, dance, drama), sports, and leisure activities.

Accessing therapies in school

Rehabilitation helps many children make a full, or near full, recovery. Your child may be able to get rehabilitative services at school, because schools are required to provide educationally relevant therapies (e.g., physical therapy and occupational therapy). For information about therapies provided by schools, see Chapter 20, *School*.

Our son had some physical therapy as soon as he could tolerate it in the hospital. He was under 3 and eligible for early intervention services (which are available to all children younger than school age who have the potential for delayed development) because of his diagnosis, so we asked for and received some physical therapy from them for a period of time after he was discharged from the hospital.

Serious Illnesses

Two illnesses that are especially dangerous for children during treatment are pneumonia and chicken pox.

Pneumonia

Pneumonia is inflammation of the lungs caused primarily by bacteria, viruses, or other organisms. The symptoms of pneumonia are rapid breathing, chills, fever, chest pain, cough, and bloody sputum. Children with low WBC counts can rapidly develop a fatal infection and must be treated quickly and aggressively. Most cancer centers recommend an annual influenza (flu) shot to help prevent pneumonia.

My son received his high-dose methotrexate and vincristine injection just days before he was scheduled to go to cancer camp. His ANC was 1,200 and he looked so sick, but he begged to go and I let him. It was early in his treatment, and I didn't realize the pattern of his blood counts. They called me from camp on Friday to say he had a temperature of 103° and needed to go to the hospital. He was very weak and feverish; his WBC was 140, and his ANC was 0. Both lungs were full of pneumonia. I was furious at the doctor for giving him permission to go to camp and at myself for not paying closer attention to how quickly his counts dropped. I'm sure he had the pneumonia before he even went to camp. They started him on five different antibiotics, and his fever went up to 106° that night. We didn't know if he would live or die. He started to improve the next morning and was completely recovered in a week.

• • • • •

Erica complained that her back hurt for two days. Then she woke up in the night crying, and she couldn't move because it hurt her too badly. She was blazing with fever, and screamed if I touched her. Her x-ray showed that her left lung was half full of fluid. They put her on antibiotics, and within 24 hours she was on the mend.

Children taking steroids (e.g., prednisone, dexamethasone) are at increased risk for contracting serious and potentially life-threatening lung infections. See section called "Prophylactic antibiotics" in Chapter 13, *Chemotherapy and Other Medications*.

Chicken pox

Chicken pox is a common childhood disease (although less so than it used to be because of the vaccine) caused by a virus called varicella zoster. The symptoms are headaches, fever, and tiredness, followed by eruptions of pimple-like red bumps that typically start on the stomach, chest, or back. The bumps rapidly develop into blister-like sores that break open, then scab over in three to five days. Any contact with the sores can spread the disease. Children are contagious up to 48 hours before breaking out.

Chicken pox can be a fatal disease for children with low ANCs, so extreme care must be taken to prevent exposure. You will need to educate all teachers and friends so they will vigilantly report any outbreaks. Your child should not go to school or preschool until the outbreak is over.

Chicken pox can be transmitted through the air or by touch. Exposure is considered to have occurred if a child is in direct contact or in a room for as little as 10 minutes with an infected person. If an immunosuppressed child is exposed to chicken pox, call the doctor immediately. If the doctor gives a shot called VZIG (varicella zoster immune globulin) within 72 hours of exposure, it may prevent the disease from occurring or lessen its effects.

> We knew when Jeremy was exposed, so he was able to get VZIG. He did get chicken pox, but only developed a few spots. He didn't get sick; he got bored. He spent two weeks in the hospital in isolation. We asked for a pass, and we were able to go outside for some fresh air between doses of acyclovir.

If a child develops chicken pox while on chemotherapy, the current treatment is hospitalization or, if possible, home therapy for IV administration of acyclovir, a potent antiviral medication that has dramatically lowered the complication rate of chicken pox.

> Kristin broke out with chicken pox on the Fourth of July weekend. Our hospital room was the best seat in the house for watching the city fireworks. She did get covered with pox, though, from the soles of her feet to the very top of her scalp. We'd just give her gauze pads soaked in calamine lotion and let her hermetically seal herself. They kept her in the hospital for six days of IV acyclovir; then she was at home on the pump (a small computerized machine that will administer the drug in small amounts for several hours) for four more days of acyclovir. She had no complications.

A child who has already had chicken pox may develop herpes zoster (shingles). If your child develops crusty bumps similar to chicken pox that are in lines (along nerves), call the doctor. The treatment for shingles is the same as that for chicken pox.

Kristin also got a herpes zoster infection, this time on Thanksgiving. It looked like a mild case of chicken pox, limited to her upper right arm, her upper right chest, and her right leg. They kept her overnight on IV acyclovir and then let her go home for nine more days on the pump.

Untreated chicken pox or shingles can result in life-threatening complications, including pneumonia, hepatitis, and encephalitis. Parents must make every effort to prevent exposure and watch for signs of these diseases while their child is on treatment.

Skin and Nail Problems

Minor skin problems often occur while on chemotherapy. The most common problems are rashes, redness, itching, peeling, dryness, and acne. Here are suggestions for preventing and treating skin problems:

- Avoid hot showers or baths, as these can dry the skin.
- Use moisturizing soap.
- Apply a water-based moisturizer after bathing, and once or twice daily, depending on the level of skin dryness.
- Rub cornstarch on itchy skin to help soothe it.
- Avoid scratchy materials such as wool. Your child may feel more comfortable in loose, cotton clothing.
- Have your child use sunscreen with a sun protection factor (SPF) of at least 30. This is especially important for areas that have been irradiated.
- Insist on head coverings or sunscreen every time your child goes outdoors if she is bald, especially if she had cranial radiation and/or is taking methotrexate.
- Buy your child lip balm with sunscreen.

    Matthew's lips would get very dry and eventually start to peel. It irritated him, and he developed a habit of biting on his lips. To minimize the problem, I learned that wiping a cool, wet cloth over his mouth many times a day worked well. I would then apply a light coating of Vaseline® to his lips to keep them moist.

If your child has chemotherapy drugs injected into the veins (rather than a central venous catheter), you may notice a darkening along the veins; this will fade after treatment ends. However, skin and underlying tissues can be damaged or destroyed by drugs that leak out of a vein. If your child feels a stinging or burning sensation, or if you notice swelling at the IV site, call a nurse immediately.

Call your child's doctor or nurse practitioner anytime your child gets a severe rash or is very itchy. Scratching rashes can cause infections, so you need to get medicine to control the itching.

Chemotherapy also affects the growing portion of nails located under the cuticle. After chemotherapy, you may notice a white band or ridge across the nail as it grows out. These brittle bands are sometimes raised and feel bumpy. As the white ridge grows out toward the end of the finger, the nail may break.

Steroid Problems

Most children with leukemia require therapy with steroid medications at intervals throughout treatment. Prednisone, dexamethasone, hydrocortisone, and others in this category can cause many unpleasant side effects, including fluid retention, high blood pressure, elevated blood sugar, sleep disturbances, muscle weakness, cataracts, and loss of bone mass. Most children and teens have profound mood swings and are very emotional when taking high-dose steroids. For more information about steroids, see Chapter 13, *Chemotherapy and Other Medications*.

Pets

Some oncologists recommend that parents rehome pets while their child is being treated for leukemia. Although it is very unlikely that your child will be harmed by living with a household pet, several common-sense precautions can help protect a child with a low ANC from disease, worms, or infection:

- Make sure your pet is vaccinated against all possible diseases.
- Have your pets checked for worms as soon as possible after your child is diagnosed, and then every year thereafter (more often for puppies). Give preventive treatments to your pets as directed by your veterinarian.
- Do not let pets eat off plates or lick your child's face.
- Keep children away from the cat litter box and any animal feces outdoors.
- Have all of your children wash their hands after playing with the pet.
- Make sure your pet has no ticks or fleas.
- If you have a pet that bites or scratches, consider finding another home for it. But if you have a gentle, well-loved pet, it may be a source of great comfort.

> *I think parents should know that you should not automatically get rid of your dog because your child has a low ANC. We went through a small crisis trying to decide whether to give away our large but beloved mongrel. The doctors wouldn't really give us a straight answer, but a parent in the support group said, "DO NOT get rid*

of your dog. Your son will need that dog's love and company in the years ahead." She was right. The dog was a tremendous comfort to our son.

If at all possible, try to delay getting a new pet until your child has finished treatment. If your child wants a pet while undergoing cancer treatment and the family is in a position to take care of it, follow these guidelines:

- Do not get a puppy. All puppies bite while teething, increasing the chance that your child may contract an infection.
- Do not get a parrot or parakeet, as these species can transmit an infection called psittacosis to humans.
- Do not get a turtle or other reptile (e.g., snake, iguana) as they sometimes carry salmonella.
- Get a calm animal that is unlikely to bite or scratch.

We bought Sarah a young adult dog. We were very selective about the breeder and the breed. The dog has given my little girl back to me. After she got the dog, she started to want to walk again. She started to laugh. She had reason to think beyond herself and how terrible this illness is. She had someone who needed her. Someone who was delighted to see her and made her feel special in a way no human can. It literally transformed my child.

The dog's name is Libbe, and after having Libbe for about a week, Sarah started asking when Libbe was going to die. She knew Libbe was young, but she really was asking about herself. We were able to tell her that Libbe will be around when she is a teenager and she can take Libbe with her on those big-girl sleepovers. Heck, she could take Libbe in the car for a ride, if she wanted. She beamed. It put the death and dying issue to rest.

If you have any concerns or questions about pets you already own or are thinking about purchasing, ask your oncologist and veterinarian for advice.

There were times during my son's treatment that I felt he suffered more from the side effects of treatment than from the disease. It was emotionally painful for me to watch him go through so much. I think one of the hardest moments for me was the day he lost all his hair. Up until that point I had been living in a semi-state of denial. His bald head was more proof of our reality—he really did have cancer. I had to learn how to accept our situation, because I needed to be strong for my child. To get through, I reminded myself every day that the treatments were necessary, and that without them he would die. It was a struggle, but the unpleasant side effects soon passed, and he was able to resume his normal activities. I was constantly amazed at his resilience.

Chapter 15

Radiation Therapy

"Nothing is so strong as gentleness,
and nothing is so gentle as true strength."

— St. Francis de Sales

RADIATION THERAPY is sometimes used to treat some children with very high-risk leukemia. Radiation to the brain, testes, or whole body can cause mild, short-term side effects, as well as permanent damage that may not be evident until months or years after treatment. The younger the child when treated, the greater the risk for side effects from radiation. For this reason, radiation treatment is avoided or postponed for very young children, and the benefits and risks of this treatment for any child or teen must be carefully weighed by both doctors and parents.

This chapter explains what radiation is, when and how it is used to treat children with leukemia, and its potential side effects. It explains what you and your child can expect from radiation treatment and shares stories from many families whose children were treated with radiation.

Overview

Radiation therapy, also called irradiation or radiotherapy, is the use of high-energy x-rays to kill cancer cells. A large machine called a linear accelerator directs x-rays to the precise portion of the body needing treatment. The radiation is given in doses measured in units called centigray (cGy) or gray (Gy).

Radiation is usually given every day for a specific number of days, excluding weekends. This process is called standard or conventional fractionation, and it is the most common way radiation is given to children and teens with leukemia. Radiation given more than once a day is called accelerated fractionation, or hyperfractionation. It uses smaller amounts of radiation for each treatment.

Children Who Need Radiation Therapy

Your child's oncologist may recommend radiation treatment, based on your child's type and risk level of leukemia. Because of the possibility of long-term damage, only a very small percentage of children with leukemia receive radiation treatment. Radiation may be prescribed for:

- Children who have a large number of leukemia blasts in their central nervous system (CNS) at diagnosis
- Children who are determined to be at extremely high risk for relapse
- Children who have relapsed in the CNS or testes
- Children who need stem cell transplants, although only some conditioning regimens include radiation

The types of radiation given to children with leukemia include cranial radiation (radiation to the entire brain), testicular radiation, and total body irradiation (TBI). Treatment for childhood leukemia is constantly evolving. Several ongoing clinical trials are evaluating other methods for preventing the spread of disease to the CNS and testes. Perhaps in the near future, no child with leukemia will need radiation. But for now, although side effects occur, radiation provides some children with their best chance to be cured.

> *After relapsing while on treatment, Stephan (7 years old) needed cranial radiation. They took him on a tour and explained in detail what would happen. All of his questions were answered. He would go in and hold perfectly still. We kept a bucket next to the bed, because he was on high-dose ARA-C, and after his radiation session, he would often need to lean over and vomit. He was so wonderful about it. He would go up to all of the older patients who were awaiting treatment and chat. He really reached out to them, and their eyes would just sparkle.*

Questions to Ask About Radiation Treatment

If radiation treatment has been recommended for your child, some questions you can ask the radiation oncologist include:

- Why does my child need radiation?
- What type of radiation does she need?
- What part of my child's body will be treated with radiation?
- What is the total dose of radiation that he will receive?
- How many treatments of radiation will she get?
- How much experience does this institution have in administering this type of radiation to children?

- How will he be positioned on the table?
- Will any restraints be used?
- Will anesthesia or sedation be needed?
- How long will each treatment take?
- What are the possible short-term and long-term side effects?
- Could this type and dosage of radiation cause cancer later?
- Are there any alternatives to radiation?
- Are any precautionary procedures needed prior to radiation therapy (e.g., sperm banking)?

Radiation Therapy Facilities

For optimal treatment, children should receive radiation therapy only at major medical centers with extensive experience treating children with cancer. Do not go to a local radiation center or the radiation department in your community hospital. State-of-the-art equipment, expert personnel, and vast experience with childhood cancer are what you should look for when choosing a center. Doctors who are experienced in pediatric radiation oncology should supervise all treatments. Pediatric anesthesiologists should administer sedation or general anesthesia to young children who require it during radiation.

> The radiation facility our children's hospital used was across town at another major hospital. So, we didn't need to travel for radiation (although we were already staying 120 miles from home because we needed to be there full time for the first eight months of treatment). We know another family from our small town whose teenaged son relapsed and needed cranial radiation. Rather than traveling the 120 miles to stay in the city for the two weeks of radiation, they chose to go to our small town's radiation facility. They ended up regretting that decision.

Radiation Oncologist

A radiation oncologist is a medical doctor with years of specialized training in using radiation to treat cancer. In partnership with the other members of the treatment team, the radiation oncologist will develop a treatment plan specifically tailored for your child.

The radiation oncologist will explain to you and your child what radiation is, how it will be given, and any possible side effects. She will also answer all your questions about the proposed treatment. You will be given a consent form to review prior to the first treatment. Take the consent form home if you need extra time to read it. Parents should not sign the consent form until they thoroughly understand the need for radiation and all benefits, risks, alternatives to, and possible short- and long-term side effects. The radiation oncologist will meet at least weekly with you and your child to discuss how the treatment is going and to address concerns or answer questions.

Radiation Therapist

Radiation therapists are specially trained technologists who operate the machine that delivers the dose of radiation prescribed by the radiation oncologist. This member of the medical team will give your child a tour of the radiation room, explain the equipment, and position your child for treatment. The technologist will operate the machine and monitor your child via closed-circuit television and a two-way intercom.

> When 3-year-old Katy was being given the tour of the radiation room by her technologist, Brian, he was just wonderful with her. He gave her a white stuffed bear, which he used to demonstrate the machine. He immobilized the bear on the table using Katy's mask (device to hold her head still during treatment), then moved the machine all around it so that she could hear the sounds made by the equipment. He then took a Polaroid® picture of the bear on the table, in the mask, for Katy to take home with her.

Radiation Simulation

Prior to receiving radiation therapy, measurements and a CT scan are performed to map the precise area to be treated. This preparation for therapy is called the "simulation" or "planning session." The simulation will take longer than any other appointment—from 30 minutes to two hours. Because simulation does not involve any high-energy radiation, parents may be allowed to remain in the simulation room to help and comfort their child. Young or active children require sedation for the simulation.

During simulation, the radiation oncologist and technologist use a specialized x-ray machine or a CT scanner to outline the treatment area. They will adjust the table the child lies on, the angle of the machine, and the width of the x-ray beam needed to give the exact dosage in the proper place. Ink marks are placed on the immobilization device to ensure treatment accuracy. After the simulation, you and your child can go home while the radiation oncologist carefully evaluates the imaging and measurements to design the treatment field.

Sedation

All infants, most preschoolers, and some school-aged children require sedation or a short-acting anesthesia (most commonly propofol is given intravenously) to ensure they remain perfectly still during radiation therapy. Parents will receive written instructions about pediatric anesthesia, including instructions about when to stop eating and drinking before sedation or anesthesia. Children can eat and drink after treatment, as soon as they are alert enough to swallow.

> *Joseph (age 5) had a good experience with the anesthesiologists who came to sedate him before each of his daily radiation treatments. They were kind and gentle, and explained each step of what would happen. They kept good records so once we figured out the medications and dosages that would allow him to go down and come back up quickly and cheerfully, they made sure to do that each day. It could have been a scary experience, but they smiled at him, encouraged him, and told him he was a champ. He was always happy to see them even when he felt pretty crummy.*

Anesthesia is given via gas or through the child's catheter or intravenous line (IV). Sometimes the parent can hold or comfort the child while anesthesia is given, but the parent must leave the room during radiation treatment. The entire procedure generally takes from 30 to 90 minutes. Nausea and vomiting are occasional side effects of anesthesia, but they are usually well controlled by anti-nausea drugs such as ondansetron (Zofran®).

> *Shawn was almost 3 years old when he needed his cranial radiation. He is an extremely active child, and we agreed with the medical team that he would have to be sedated. His appointment was always at 1 p.m., and we were told that he could have apple juice or Jell-O® at 6 a.m. but nothing to eat or drink after that. Every single morning he would drink the juice and then throw up. At the radiation room, I would hold him while he was anesthetized, then wait in the waiting room. They would bring him out to me in 30 to 45 minutes.*

During a course of radiation therapy, the dose, drugs, and methods used to sedate or anesthetize the child may need to change because some children develop a tolerance to certain drugs. Good communication between parents and members of the treatment team should prevent unnecessary anxiety about increased dosages or the use of a different drug. In some cases, less anesthesia is needed if the child is gently coached about ways to hold still.

> *Each time my young son came in for radiation, part of the routine was to place the hard plastic mesh mask over his face while he was awake, just for an instant, to get him used to the idea of trying to wear it for treatments without sedation. No pressure was ever put on him about it; it was just mentioned as a possibility of something he could try, something that would let him keep eating and drinking all through the day instead of having to fast for a few hours before each sedation, which was very hard for such a small boy.*
>
> *They left the mask on him for a tiny bit longer each time, until he was tolerating it for several seconds, and then close to a minute. His fifth birthday was at the exact middle*

of treatment, and he decided that since he was such a big boy now, he would try to do it without sedation. I know he was trying to please and impress all these kind people. He worked it out quietly with a favorite technician, asked the "sleepy medicine doctor" to wait outside the treatment room, let them screw the mask down to the table, and did the whole thing awake. I've never been more proud in my life. Everyone cheered and hugged him. He finished the rest of the treatments without sedation, sometimes eating and drinking on his way in the door just to show off that he could!

Cranial Radiation

Radiation to the whole brain is called cranial radiation. Because children who receive cranial radiation need to hold perfectly still during treatment, a mesh mask of the child's face is made and used to keep the head still the head during treatments.

Making the mask

Great care should be taken to ensure the mask-making procedure doesn't traumatize your child. It is helpful to use play therapy with young children to demonstrate the procedure beforehand. More time spent on preparation will mean less time spent on fitting the device. Also, if the fitting goes well, it creates trust and good feelings that will help the radiation treatments proceed smoothly.

The mask is made without sedation for well-prepared, calm children or it is done while young or active children are sedated. The following are parent suggestions for preparing a child for making the mask:

- Give the child a tour of the room where the fitting will take place
- Explain each step of the process in age-appropriate language
- Be honest in describing any sensations the child may experience
- For small children, put a mask on a mannequin or stuffed animal to demonstrate the process
- For older children or teenagers, show a video or read a booklet describing the procedure

Masks are made from a lightweight, porous, mesh material that your child can breathe through. First, the technologist should explain and demonstrate the entire mask-making process to your child. Some technologists make a mask of a child's hand to show how it looks and feels. Then, the child lies down on a table, and the technologist puts a sheet of the mask material in warm water to soften it. This warm mesh sheet is then placed over the child's face and quickly molded to her features. The child can breathe through the mesh material the entire time but must hold still for several minutes as the mask hardens. At some institutions, the mask is lifted off the child's face, and the technologist cuts holes in the mask for the eyes, nostrils, and mouth. At others, the mask is left in place while a CT scan is done and holes are not cut into the mask. You and your child should understand your institution's practices before the mask making starts so you will be prepared.

> *The cancer center staff had scheduled two hours for mask-making for my 3-year-old daughter. I asked them to explain very quietly every step in the process. I told her I would be holding her hand, and I promised that it would not hurt, but it would feel warm. I asked her to choose a story for me to recite as they molded the warm material to her face, to make the time go faster. She picked* Curious George Goes to the Hospital. *She held perfectly still; I recited the story; the staff were gentle and quick; and the entire procedure took less than 20 minutes.*

Very young children, or those who have difficulty holding still, are sedated while the mask is being made.

> *Shawn (2 years old) needed to be sedated for his 10 doses of cranial radiation. They also made his mask while he was anesthetized.*

Radiation treatment

To receive cranial radiation, children are given appointments to visit the radiation clinic for a specific number of days, most often at the same time each day. Cranial radiation is usually given five days a week for two weeks (weekends off). If your child will be sedated, the sessions are usually scheduled early in the morning, because he will not be able to eat or drink before coming in for treatments.

When you arrive each day, you'll check in at the front desk. The technologist or nurse then comes out to take your child into the treatment room. Often, parents accompany young children into the room. If your child requires anesthesia, it may be given in the treatment room or in a nearby anesthesia induction room.

> *I wanted my 4 year old to be able to receive the radiation without anesthesia. I asked the center staff what I could do to make her comfortable. They said, "Anything, as long as you leave the room during the treatment." So I explained to my daughter that we had to find ways for her to hold very still for a short time. I said, "It's such a short time, that if I played your Snow White tape, the treatment would be over before Snow White met the dwarves." Katy agreed that was a short time, and asked that I bring the tape for her to listen to. She also wanted a sticker (a different one every day) stuck on the machine for her to look at. I brought her pink blanket to wrap her in because the table was hard and the room cold. Each day, she chose a different comfort animal or doll to hold during treatment. So we'd arrive every day with tapes, blanket, stickers, and animals. She felt safe, and all treatments went extremely well.*

During the cranial radiation treatment, your child will lie on her back, the mask will be placed over his face, and the mask will be clamped to the table to keep your child's head perfectly still. Measurements are taken to verify that the child's body is perfectly positioned. Frequently, the technologist will shine a light on the area to be irradiated to ensure the machine is properly aligned. The technologist and parents leave the room, closing the door behind them.

At some institutions, parents are allowed to stay and watch the television monitor and talk to their child via the speaker system. If this is the case, the parent should be careful not to distract the technologist as he administers the radiation. At other institutions, parents are asked to wait in the waiting room. It's important that parents understand the department's policies; they should ask the radiation therapist if anything is unclear.

> Matthew had his own calendar outside the radiation treatment room. For every treatment he received, he picked a sticker to place on his calendar. It was a wonderful way to show him how far he had come and how much farther he had to go before he would be finished. Matthew loved rummaging through the sticker box for the perfect addition to his calendar. When the last treatment had been given, he was allowed to remove the calendar from the wall and bring it home as a keepsake. We still have Matthew's calendar.

The treatment takes only a few minutes and can be stopped at any time if the child has any difficulty. When the treatment is done, the technologist turns off the machine, removes the immobilization device, and parents and child can go home. If your child received anesthesia, he will need to recover from the anesthesia before he can go home. There is no pain at all when receiving radiation treatment, but some children report seeing flashing lights or noticing a burning smell. Both of these are normal experiences, but it is important to let the radiation oncologist know if your child mentions either of them.

> There was something about the radiation or the anesthesia that frightened 3-year-old Shawn terribly. He would scream in the car all the way to the hospital. It was a scream as if he was in pain. He had nightmares while he was undergoing radiation and every night after it was over. We decided a month after radiation ended to bring a box of candy to the staff who had been so nice. Shawn asked, "Do I have to go in that room?" When I explained that it was over and he didn't need to go in the room anymore, he asked if he could go in to look at it once more. He stood for a long time and just looked and looked at the equipment. Somehow he made his peace with it, because he never had any more nightmares.

Because radiation therapy is usually given at short, daily appointments, families that do not live within an hour or so of their treatment center often have to stay near the hospital. Your social worker can help you arrange to stay at a Ronald McDonald House or similar facility, at a hotel, or at a short-stay apartment near the hospital.

Testicular Radiation

For male children or teens with leukemic blasts in their testes, radiation may be part of the treatment plan; however, current clinical trials are evaluating the effectiveness of using more intensive chemotherapy rather than testicular radiation. Testicular radiation treatment is usually only given Monday through Friday, with weekends off. Treatment plans and the amount of radiation used vary among protocols and institutions. One example from a current Children's Oncology Group clinical trial for T-Cell ALL requires that boys or teens with testicular disease at the end of induction be given testicular radiation of 2,400 cGy (12 once-daily fractions of 200 cGy each) during the first two weeks of consolidation.

Different institutions use a variety of devices to immobilize children to ensure the radiation beam is directed with precision. Some of the products used are custom-made plaster of Paris casts, thermoplastic devices, vacuum-molded "bean-bag"-like molds, and polyurethane foam forms. Custom fitting the forms on a child who has already undergone numerous painful procedures requires skill and patience. The process that will be used to make the mold should be described clearly to your child or teen and all questions should be answered before mold-making begins. Prior to your son's first radiation treatment, the technologist should give him a tour of the facility, describe the machines, and explain exactly how the radiation sessions will be done.

> We told our 5-year-old son that he needed to have some special photos done, like x-rays, and he needed to lie very still to have them taken. A special mold was made of his bottom to hold him in the correct position. This was like a beanbag, and when he was in it at the radiation planning appointment, the air was sucked out of the cushion, leaving a firm cast of his bottom and legs, which he sat in for the radiation sessions. We had a dry run to be sure he didn't need sedation (which was a possibility and a team was on call for the first session). He had to lie on the cushion, and his penis was taped up and out of the way to enable the machine to be focused on the testes. Each session was very short, about 15 minutes from setup to finish.

> There were already stickers on the machine for him to look at, and he liked those. He took his favorite "pilly" into the room with him and that was nestled around his neck for the session. He also was covered up with a blanket until the very last second, as I think a little person's dignity is just as important as an adult's. We took a book along with us so I could read to him through the microphone while the radiation was happening. He had a reward after each session, which we supplied and the nurses gave him a chart to stick them to. We displayed this proudly in his room and I still have it!

To receive the radiation treatment, your child or teen will lie on the table, the technologist will place the child on the customized mold, and the penis will be taped up to keep it out of the radiation field. Each treatment will last less than five minutes, during which time your son must hold perfectly still. The technologist will watch your son by closed-circuit television and will be in verbal contact through a two-way intercom system.

Radiation therapy to the testes most often results in permanent sterility (survivors can have a normal sex life, but ejaculate will not contain sperm). For this reason, all boys who have gone through puberty should be offered sperm banking before any treatment begins. Frozen sperm can be kept viable for many years, and this allows male survivors the opportunity to become fathers later in life.

Total Body Radiation

Total body radiation (also known as total body irradiation, or TBI) is sometimes given prior to stem cell transplantation. There are numerous protocols, each with a different treatment schedule. Two examples are:

- 200 cGy given twice a day for three days
- 120 cGy given three times a day for four days

Prior to treatment, the child will be weighed and measured by the radiation therapist. The therapist will give the family a tour and show them the two machines that will be on either side of the stretcher in the middle of the room. Different institutions use different techniques to deliver TBI, so during the tour, the position of the child and how long each session will last will be explained.

On the first day of treatment, the child will be brought to the room (at some institutions, small children ride a tricycle or are pulled in a wagon) and may choose to watch TV or a movie, or listen to music. The therapist will remove all metal from the child's body and clothing—watches, rings, zippers, clamps. Anything with tight elastic, such as diapers or tight socks, will also be loosened or removed. The child or teen will lie on the stretcher, and the therapist will position her. Anti-nausea drugs are given to prevent vomiting, and these often make children drowsy enough to doze through the treatment. Some young or very active children will need to be sedated.

> The radiation was easy. When I wasn't sleeping, I watched TV or listened to the radio. I threw up once, but they gave me Benadryl® and I never was sick again from the radiation. The room was neat; it was painted lots of bright colors and had two big blue machines, one on each side of me.

Possible Short-term Side Effects

Generally, radiation treatments given to children with leukemia are completed in two weeks. Many children have no short-term side effects. If side effects do occur, it is often hard to differentiate those caused by radiation and those caused by the high-dose chemotherapy that is usually given at the same time. The radiation oncologist is familiar with all possible side effects and is responsible for managing them. Possible short-term side effects include the following:

- Loss of appetite
- Nausea and vomiting
- Fatigue
- Slightly reddened or itchy skin
- Temporary hair loss
- Low blood counts
- Changes in taste and smell (sometimes during the treatment)
- Increased or decreased saliva or dry mouth (ask your doctor about saliva substitutes such as Moi-Stir® or Salivant®)
- Sleepiness (somnolence syndrome)—from cranial radiation
- Swollen parotid (salivary) glands—from TBI

> Calories are most important; nutrition can come after treatment. We use whole milk, and put butter on everything: Ethan would eat any time, anything. When Ethan completely lost his appetite during radiation, we used Megace®, a prescription appetite stimulant. It has fairly few side effects and did seem to work for him.

One side effect uniquely associated with cranial radiation is somnolence syndrome. This is characterized by drowsiness, prolonged periods of sleep (up to 20 hours a day), low-grade fever, headaches, poor appetite, nausea, vomiting, and irritability. It may occur during radiation or as late as 12 weeks after radiation treatment ends; it can last from a few days to several weeks. Sometimes steroids are given to help the child recover from somnolence syndrome.

> Nine weeks after ending her cranial radiation, my daughter started having severe headaches. She would hold her head and just sob with pain. She also vomited several times. Then she became very sleepy, and dozed on the couch most of the day. She developed a low fever and choked when she tried to swallow liquids or solid food. This lasted for about a week.

Stephan (8 years old) had no side effects from the cranial radiation other than sleepiness, but he was very affected by it. First, he just started taking naps and generally slowing down. Then the naps got longer, and he was awake less. Finally, he only woke up to eat. Luckily, that part coincided with Christmas vacation, so he didn't miss much school. Altogether, it lasted about six weeks.

Possible Long-term Side Effects

Although short-term side effects appear and subside, long-term side effects may not become apparent for months or years after treatment ends. Specific late effects depend on the age of the child, the dose of radiation, the part of the body treated with radiation, and the vulnerability of each child. Children at greatest risk for cognitive problems are those treated with cranial radiation when younger than age five; those younger than age two are at highest risk. Chapter 20, *School*, discusses in detail the types of educational challenges some children face and ways to deal with them.

The effects of radiation on cognitive functioning, bone growth, soft tissue growth, teeth, sinuses, endocrine glands, puberty, and fertility range from no late effects to life-long impacts. Second tumors in the radiation field are also a possible long-term side effect. Detailed information about possible late effects are described in *Childhood Cancer Survivors: A Practical Guide to Your Future, 3rd edition* by Nancy Keene, Wendy Hobbie, and Kathy Ruccione.

When radiation treatment is complete, you should be given a summary of your child's care, including type of radiation, location, and dose. You also should be given a clear plan for any needed follow-up care. More information is available in Chapter 24, *End of Treatment and Beyond*.

My daughter had AML and had a bone marrow transplant when she was eight. She had total body irradiation and does have some late effects including ongoing endocrine problems, menstrual difficulties, and cataracts. She also has a reduced ejection fraction of the heart from the anthracyclines and had to deal with a second cancer in her thyroid gland. That said, you'd never pick her out of a crowd. She graduated from high school with a perfect 4.0 GPA and wants to specialize in biology with the intent to go into medicine (pediatric oncology) or molecular genetics with a focus on cancer genetics. There is hope.

Chapter 16

Stem Cell
Transplantation

*"Courage is being scared to death
and saddling up anyway."*
— John Wayne

STEM CELL TRANSPLANTATION (SCT) is a complicated procedure used to treat some children with leukemia. For this treatment, stem cells are collected from a donor's bone marrow, blood stream, or from umbilical cord blood. The child with leukemia is then given high-dose chemotherapy and sometimes radiation to kill as many cancer cells as possible. After these treatments, stem cells collected from the donor are infused into the child's central venous catheter (e.g., Hickman® or PICC). The stem cells migrate to the cavities inside the bones where new, healthy blood cells are then produced.

SCTs are expensive, technically complex, and potentially life-threatening. Understanding the procedure and its ramifications at a time of crisis can be very difficult, so this chapter offer parents information to help them make an informed decision. This chapter explains the types of SCT currently used to treat some children with leukemia, and it shares the experiences of several families.

When Are Transplants Necessary?

In some children, leukemia cannot be cured with conventional doses of chemotherapy, radiation, or targeted therapy. SCT allows the delivery of high-dose therapy to kill the cancer cells, followed by an infusion of donated stem cells to help the bone marrow begin to make healthy red blood cells, white blood cells, and platelets again. The donor's stem cells also play an important role in killing any leukemia cells not destroyed by the chemotherapy/radiation, a phenomenon known as the graft vs. leukemia (GVL) effect.

The use of SCT has declined as conventional chemotherapy and use of targeted drugs has improved cure rates of children and teens with leukemia. As a result, SCTs are currently recommended for some children who have:

- Juvenile myelomonocytic leukemia
- Early relapse of an acute leukemia
- A slow response to therapy
- Unfavorable cancer cell characteristics (cytogenetics)

Guidelines about which children need transplants change over time as new information becomes available, and practices vary among institutions.

> They said he would start chemo the next day, but that plan came to a grinding halt when they found out it was T-cell ALL with some AML characteristics. His blood work and test results were sent off to a bigger children's hospital for more tests. We signed up for a COG clinical trial for T-cell ALL. William was inpatient for all of induction and nothing seemed to go smoothly for him and there were many issues. I was so emotionally stressed that I literally felt like I might die. I asked loads of questions because I needed to understand what we were facing. Induction is all a blur. On day 29, his MRD [minimal residual disease] was 0.14 (supposed to be <0.01). After consolidation and three extra intensification blocks, he was still MRD positive. So, after seven months of being mostly inpatient for intensive chemotherapy treatment, he came off the trial and we were told he needed a transplant.

If an SCT has been recommended for your child or teenager, you may want to get a second opinion before proceeding. You also may want to ask the oncologist and transplant physician some or all of the following questions:

- What are all the treatment options for my child's type of leukemia?
- For my child's type of leukemia, history, and physical condition, what is the chance for survival with a transplant? What are my child's chances with other treatments?
- What are the risks and the benefits of this type of transplant?
- What will be my child's likely short-term and long-term quality of life after the transplant?
- Where would my child receive this type of transplant?
- What portion of the procedure will be outpatient versus inpatient?
- What is the average length of stay in the hospital for children undergoing this procedure?
- What are the anticipated and the rare complications of this type of transplant?
- Will my child have to take medicines after the transplant? For how long?
- What are the side effects of these medicines?

- Is this transplant considered to be experimental, or is it the current standard of care?
- Do insurance companies usually pay for this type of transplant?

> *My daughter was 6 years old when she was diagnosed with AML. When she relapsed four months into treatment, a transplant was her only hope.*

$$\bullet \quad \bullet \quad \bullet \quad \bullet \quad \bullet$$

> *After my son's second relapse from ALL, the doctors told us that a transplant was his last option for a cure.*

What Is a Match?

Everyone has proteins, called human leukocyte antigens (HLA), on the surface of their cells. These proteins allow a person's immune system to distinguish the body's own cells from those of another person. Half of a child's HLA genes are inherited from each parent. A child has one chance in four (a 25% chance) of being matched with a sibling who has the same biological parents. This pattern of inheritance explains why parents only rarely (1% of the time) match with their children. More distant relatives are even less likely to match, because they are more likely to have different HLA genes. When it is determined that an SCT might be needed, each full sibling and biological parent is HLA-typed. HLA genes come in many varieties (called alleles). Two people are considered to be a match if 8 to 12 of their alleles are identical.

> *We felt it was an omen that Jody's older sister and younger brother were perfect matches. They chose Marieke because she was older; but after all of the workup and tests, they discovered that she was CMV [cytomegalovirus] positive, so they used 2-year-old Christoph's marrow. Marieke was very disappointed.*

If a match is not found in the family, the search widens to the donor registries and umbilical cord blood banks. This search will identify any potential donors with the same HLA type as your child. The registry then contacts the potential donor to ask whether he or she will donate more blood samples for additional tests.

The odds of obtaining a match from an unrelated person were once slim. However, due to the increased number of people typed and listed on various national and international marrow registries, and the development of more accurate tissue typing methods, a complete or partial match can now be found for almost 70% of children. Registries currently contain more than 10 million potential donors. Because there is a strong association of some HLA types with a person's ethnic background, it is harder to find matches for children from certain ethnic backgrounds.

> *Christie had a rare HLA type, and we could not find a match in all the registries worldwide. We decided that we had to do it on our own and began a donor drive in*

our town, which is predominantly Italian. The Red Cross discouraged us, saying that we probably wouldn't get a good response, that they could not process the blood without the money ($45 per person) in hand, and that it would be better to spend quality time with Christie. But when the community of Rochester found out, it just snowballed. Dave and I went on TV and advocated for Christie, stressing the importance of Christie's bone marrow drive, and told people that this might help their own child one day. The first day of the drive, people lined up outside and stood for hours in the freezing rain and cold. The response was so overwhelming that late in the day they ran out of supplies. Large corporations became involved; one did a telethon that raised over $50,000. We typed over 4,000 people from Rochester and received letters from all over the country. It was just a beautiful thing. Christie was such a powerful little person, and she came to represent so much to our community.

Types of Transplant

The two types of transplants used for children with leukemia are syngeneic transplants (from an identical twin) and allogeneic transplants (from a person who is not an identical twin).

Syngeneic transplant

Syngeneic transplants are those in which the stem cell donor is the identical twin of the child with leukemia. These are the least complicated transplants because there is no risk of rejection or graft-versus-host disease (GVHD). Recovery is usually rapid after a syngeneic transplant. However, this type of transplant is often not favored because there is minimal GVL effect and a higher risk of relapse after transplant.

> *Jeremy had a syngeneic transplant from his identical twin brother as his donor to treat the AML that developed after treatment for Ewing's sarcoma. He received cyclophosphamide and radiation in his conditioning regimen. One of the worst side effects he experienced was the nausea and vomiting. He was released from the hospital on Day 9, readmitted on Day 11 because of an infection, and discharged again on Day 12. We stayed near the hospital, and then we were allowed to go home on Day 30. He has done very well.*

Allogeneic transplant

Allogeneic transplants are those in which the stem cells come from a person who is not the child's identical twin. Thus, the donor could be a sibling, parent, close relative, or an unrelated individual. The risk of complications increases if the donor is not a full match.

Allogeneic transplants can be further categorized based on the source of donor stem cells. Potential stem cell sources include:

- HLA-matched bone marrow or peripheral blood from a sibling
- HLA-matched bone marrow or peripheral blood from an unrelated adult
- Umbilical cord blood from a relative (e.g., sibling) or unrelated child
- Haploidentical (half-matched) bone marrow or peripheral blood from a relative

> *Adele was 5½ years old at the time of her transplant. Donor marrow was harvested from her brother Ben, 2½ at the time. Harvesting took approximately one hour, and after the marrow was prepared for infusion, Adele received it (about 45 minutes later). The actual infusion was very simple—just hanging an IV bag. The doctor and nurses were, understandably, extremely careful with it, and it was very dramatic!*
>
> *One hour after completion, Adele could get up, and she and Ben immediately went running to the playroom! She had not crashed yet from the preparative chemotherapy, which had been completed two days before. Just like her response to most of the treatment, however, this was not the norm. The nursing staff said they'd never seen a kid who felt well enough to do that following a transplant. Adele first showed something above a zero ANC [absolute neutrophil count] on Day 15. From then on, she improved quickly and steadily. She was released about six weeks after transplant, and met her goal of being at home and better (at least not sick!) for her sixth birthday. Because Adele showed basically no signs of graft-versus-host disease, she was taken off almost all meds early.*

HLA-matched sibling. The first step in identifying a suitable stem cell donor is to perform HLA typing on all siblings who have the same mother and father as the child with leukemia (called full biologic siblings). If a match is found, then that brother or sister will likely be used as the stem cell donor.

> *Jody's 2-year-old brother, Christoph, was a perfect match. I stayed with him when he donated marrow, and my husband stayed with Jody. Christoph seemed to handle the marrow donation easily. Although he had some nausea in the recovery room, he was up and running around late that afternoon saying, "I the donor." He felt very proud. I knew he was somewhat sore because he said, "My diaper hurts."*

Umbilical cord blood. Placental blood/umbilical cord blood is a rich source of stem cells. Some institutions perform transplants using the umbilical cord blood obtained during the birth of a sibling (and frozen for future use) or from preserved unrelated donor cord blood. The advantage of cord blood transplant is that the cord does not have to be a perfect match. The number of stem cells in cord blood is usually sufficient for most children, but it may not be adequate for larger children or teens.

> *Our 15-month-old son, Garrett, was diagnosed with AML and central nervous system involvement. He relapsed on treatment, and the doctors recommended a cord blood transplant. There was one perfect match in Barcelona, Spain. I wanted to fly to Barcelona and hug everyone I could see. He was so sick during treatment, which included a trip to the ICU [intensive care unit] and several periods of extended hospitalization for complications, that the transplant was almost anticlimactic. He had TBI [total body irradiation], then chemotherapy. He engrafted on Day 12 and was out on Day 21. He did wonderfully—he only got one fever, no GVHD, no other problems. He has not been inpatient since, and he's now in college.*

When transplanted stem cells enter the bloodstream, make their way to the bone marrow, and start making new blood cells, it is called engraftment. This usually occurs 10 to 30 days after a stem cell transplant. Engraftment after an umbilical cord blood transplant may take longer than with SCTs from other sources, but cord blood transplants may cause less GVHD than allogeneic transplants. In addition, cord blood is rarely contaminated by viruses such as cytomegalovirus (CMV) or Epstein Barr virus (EBV) that can cause life-threatening complications after a SCT. Cord blood SCT is one of many promising new directions in the research efforts to improve SCT. For information about public, private, and family cord blood banks, visit the Parent's Guide to Cord Blood Foundation at *www.parentsguidecordblood.org.*

> *Christopher received his cord blood unit after three days of TBI, testicular radiation, and other conditioning with chemotherapy. He had a feeding tube inserted during his final TBI, so we didn't have to worry about eating. He engrafted on Day 10 and had a little GVHD, which was treated with prednisone. After he was discharged from the hospital, he was readmitted a few times for fevers. Overall it went very well. Our biggest problems now are fixing his cataracts, waiting for results of his endocrine tests and bone tests, and getting educational support.*

Unrelated adult volunteer. Large registries of adult volunteer donors have been created in the United States and other countries. An HLA-matched or very nearly matched donor can often be identified through a computer-based search of those registries. More HLA proteins are evaluated with this type of donor, so you may hear the transplant team talk about an "8/8" or "10/10" match.

Haploidentical transplant. Haploidentical transplants are a newer form of treatment for children who do not have a matched donor. This type of transplant uses stem cells from a parent or sibling who is only half-matched with the child needing a transplant. The procedure is similar to an allogeneic transplant except that because the donor and recipient (child) are not fully matched, something must be done to remove T cells from the stem cell "graft" to prevent GVHD. This can be done by processing the graft to remove T cells before it is given to the child, or by administering a drug called cyclophosphamide after the transplant to kill T cells in the bloodstream.

Finding a Donor

Finding a donor can be a stressful and time-consuming task. The search may begin in first remission for children with acute myeloid leukemia (AML), during the chronic phase for children with chronic myelogenous leukemia (CML), and soon after diagnosis for children with JMML. Searches of the registries are expensive and usually take six to eight weeks. In some families, tests show that a sibling or parent is a partial or identical match. Other children, especially those from minority groups not well represented in the donor files, can wait months or years for a match, or a match may not be found. Appendix B, *Resource Organizations,* lists registries, foundations, and programs that can help you find a donor and obtain financial assistance, if necessary.

> My advice to parents just beginning the process is do not rely on anyone else to make all the arrangements for a donor search and financial arrangements with the transplant center. We were focused on my son's treatment and thought a donor search was ongoing. We then found out that over two precious months had been lost in a delay for financial approval. I foolishly relied on my doctor and his staff to make arrangements and follow through, and it just slipped through the cracks. I should have been on the phone several times a week making sure the search had begun and that the transplant center was happy with the financial arrangements. I have a lot of guilt over whether those months made a difference in my son's outcome. I'll never know.

If a sibling or other relative is identified as the best donor, that person needs to have the risks of donation fully explained. The medical team should explain that although the transplant is the best treatment, results of the transplant cannot be predicted and the success or failure of the transplant is not the donor's fault. The American Academy of Pediatrics has issued guidance for when the donor is a child, which can be found at *http://pediatrics.aappublications.org/content/125/2/392.*

> My son was 5 when he donated marrow to his younger brother who had refractory T-cell ALL. We didn't want to make too big a deal of it in case it didn't work. So, we told him that he had something his brother needed and we would be going to the hospital. He asked if it would hurt and we described the process in terms a preschooler could understand. They took cells from both hips, and he said three things as soon as he woke up: "It didn't hurt." "Did William get my bone marrow?" "When do I get a toy?" He needed pain meds for a few days, but a year later, he doesn't remember that there was any pain related to the donation.

If an unrelated donor is identified in the database searches, the potential donor is given an extensive explanation of the entire donation procedure and a complete medical exam. Because the amount of marrow that is removed contains less than 5% of the donor's developing blood cells, it only takes a few days for the body to replace the marrow. The donor is usually sore for a day or two and may feel a bit tired for several days.

The procedure often results in a mild anemia that resolves after several weeks. An iron supplement may be prescribed to hasten this process. The main risk of donating marrow is from the use of anesthesia. However, in an otherwise healthy donor, the risk of a severe complication is very small. After a discussion of these possible risks, the donor must then make a final commitment to provide stem cells for the child in need.

> While they were trying to find a match for JaNette, the church started a fundraiser and donor sign-up drive. They signed up over 600 people in two days, and United Blood Service had matching funds available to offset some of the costs. Meanwhile, we found an unrelated donor who lived in Milwaukee. She donated the marrow there, and a nurse from our transplant center flew out to pick it up.

Choosing a Transplant Center

If the institution where your child is treated is also an accredited transplant center, you may not need to travel for this part of your child's treatment. However, if you need to choose a transplant center, it is an important and often difficult decision. Institutions may just be starting an SCT program, or they may have vast experience. Some centers may be excellent for adults, but have limited pediatric experience. Some may allow you to stay overnight with your child; others may restrict access.

> We were lucky that my son was able to get his transplant at our local children's hospital, where he had been treated after diagnosis and after relapse. So, we knew everyone in ped onc and felt very comfortable. I'm a transplant nurse for adults—do stem cell collections and also do outpatient infusions. I don't know whether that was a blessing or a curse. I know a lot about adults who get transplants, but I learned that kids are really different. When our 4-year-old son relapsed six months into maintenance and we knew he needed a transplant, I was terrified. Our transplant doctor had to keep reminding me that kids are different. Later, it was good to have the medical knowledge because I could ask reasonable questions and manage a lot of his care at home.

The center closest to your home may not provide the best medical care available for your child or allow the necessary quality of life (social workers, child life services) that you need. In addition, your insurance plan may require your child to have the SCT at a specific center. To see a list of transplant centers, visit *www.bmtinfonet.org/before/choosingtransplantcenter.* Asking the following questions can help you learn about the policies of different transplant centers:

- Is your center accredited by the Foundation for Accreditation of Cellular Therapy (*www.factwebsite.org/AboutFACT*)? This agency inspects transplant programs and certifies programs that provide high-quality care.

- What are your program's 1-, 2-, and 5-year survival rates for different types of childhood leukemia? (Remember that some institutions accept very-high-risk patients, and their statistics will not compare to a center that performs less-risky transplants.)

- What is the nurse-to-patient ratio? Do all staff members have pediatric training and experience?

- What support staff is available (e.g., educators, social workers, child life specialists, clergy, support groups, volunteers)?

- Will my child be on a pediatric or combined adult–pediatric unit?

- What are the institution's rules about parents staying in the child's hospital room?

- Are children allowed to visit?

- What kinds of temporary and long-term housing are available near the center? What are the costs for this housing?

- What infection control measures does this center use for transplant patients? Isolation? Gown and gloves? Washing hands?

- What kinds of activities are available for children during their hospital stay?

- What is the average length of time before a child leaves the hospital? How long before he can leave the area to go home (if you live far from the center)?

- What long-term follow-up is available? Does the center have a post-transplant clinic that focuses on late effects?

- How does the center stay in contact with the child's primary doctor?

- Explain the waiting list requirements, if any.

- How much will this procedure cost? How much will my insurance cover?

Most transplant centers have videos and booklets for children and their families that explain services and describe what to expect before, during, and after transplant. You can call any transplant center that you are considering and ask that all available materials be sent to you.

> The head of oncology from a major transplant center comes to our city every two months to follow up with the kids who have been treated there. It was a big draw for us to have post-transplant follow-up at home, rather than having to travel a great distance to get back to the center. Family members weren't required to cap and gown, only scrub their hands. Since I'm allergic to those hospital gloves, this allowed me to stay with my daughter throughout. We did, however, call around to several centers to compare facilities, costs, and insurance coverage.

Making an informed consent is a serious decision when considering a life-threatening procedure such as an SCT. It is very important to work closely with your child's oncologist and treatment team when making this decision. Do not hesitate to keep asking questions until you fully understand what is being proposed. Record the conversation to review later, or take along a family member or friend to take notes. You do not need to sign the consent form until you feel comfortable that you understand the procedure and have had every question answered. Even after the consent is signed, you can change your mind up until the point that your child is admitted to the transplant unit and treatment begins.

> We were fortunate because our transplant facility keeps the kids in isolation but our son Austin could go out in the hallway. Only one kid was allowed in the hallway at a time, so they had a sign-up sheet. We didn't have to wear gowns, masks, and gloves, but we didn't let anyone in who was wearing shoes. In the room, we played, we did puzzles, and we watched TV. Each room had a little anteroom, so that's where my husband and I ate because we weren't allowed to eat in his room. I was obsessed with wiping down everything in the room (and everyone's cell phones) with Lysol® and made sure every person who walked in had to thoroughly wash his or her hands. I flipped out when someone blew his nose in the room—we asked him to leave.

Stem Cell Harvest and Storage

Stem cells are harvested from umbilical cord blood, bone marrow, or peripheral blood. Frozen umbilical cord blood is obtained from a registry, and stem cells come directly from donor bone marrow or peripheral blood.

Bone marrow

Collecting bone marrow stem cells from a family member or unrelated donor is a straightforward process that usually takes less than an hour. While the donor is under general anesthesia, doctors insert large needles into the bones of the hip and withdraw bone marrow. This procedure is repeated 50 to 150 times to collect enough stem cells. After marrow donation, some hospitals keep the donor overnight, while others discharge the same day if the donor is not in significant pain.

> After no match was found for Christie in the 4,000 donors that we signed up and typed, I became her donor. We were just a partial match. Being her donor was just wonderful. It was Mother's Day weekend, and I was just full of faith and love. I thought this is it; God has given me a second chance to give life to this child. I had a very powerful feeling that it was so special that I could do this for my daughter. I really felt that this was it, it was going to work. It was uncomfortable for a couple of days, and I was a little bruised. But the people there were wonderful, and they really followed me closely. I'm still on the registry; if someone called me tomorrow, I'd be on a plane.

The bone marrow that is collected is usually used immediately, but it can be frozen for later use.

Apheresis

To collect stem cells from a donor's blood, the donor self-administers granulocyte-colony stimulating factor (GCSF) injections for several days prior to collection day. GCSF stimulates the bone marrow to produce more stem cells. Those stems cells are released by the bone marrow into the peripheral blood. Peripheral blood is collected from an IV line and the cells are processed through a machine that separates stem cells from other blood cells. The stem cells are then collected and processed for donation. Other cells, such as red blood cells, are then infused back into the donor.

The Transplant

Prior to the SCT, the child's bone marrow is suppressed using high-dose chemotherapy and sometimes total body irradiation (TBI). This portion of treatment, called conditioning, kills cancer cells and makes room in the bone marrow for the new stem cells.

> Tanner was 17 months old when he had his transplant. My husband and I split time with him at the hospital. I was there the first part of the week, and he took off Fridays and came to the hospital so I could go home. When you have a little one and he's connected to all those IVs, it's so hard. I learned to block off a space in the hospital room so he had an area he could move around in, but keep the IV safe. Because we were worried about germs, neither of his brothers could visit. Video chat made a big difference. People from child life would come and play with him so I could get out, walk to a nearby park, and clear my head. Child life was awesome. Tanner came home on Day 23, but he was still on TPN [total parenteral nutrition] and oral pain meds. He was on the TPN for about three weeks after he came home. He is doing very well now and is an energetic and happy little boy!

Conditioning regimens vary according to institution and protocol; they also depend on the medical condition and history of the child. Sometimes all or part of the therapy is given in an outpatient setting. If your child receives conditioning chemotherapy as an outpatient, he will need to go to the transplant unit no later than the evening before the transplant for hydration.

> Conditioning was four days of chemotherapy and three days of TBI delivered twice a day in fractions. Our 4-year-old son was sedated each time for the TBI. The transplant took six hours because they got so many stem cells from the donor's bone marrow. Even though it was his new birthday, it wasn't so joyous because the IV Benadryl® they gave him upset him so he screamed most of the six hours it took to transfuse the liter of cells. The mucositis started after four days, so he couldn't eat or drink. He got continuous intravenous pain meds, and I was stringent about the oral care. He was on TPN through the PICC line. He needed lots of platelets, but never needed a red blood cell transfusion because the donated marrow had such a high red

cell count. He had no complications or infections and we were home four weeks after the transplant (close to the record for that facility).

The transplant itself consists of infusing the stem cells through a central venous catheter into the child, just like a blood transfusion. The stem cells travel through the blood vessels, eventually settling in the bone marrow.

I cannot say enough good things about the transplant center. They were very family-oriented, allowed us in the room 24 hours a day. I was allowed to sleep in bed with her (I just told the nurses to make sure to poke her and not me). The nurses were wonderful, and I still think of them as family.

A transplant doctor will monitor your child during the stem cell infusion. The infusion of donor stem cells is typically uneventful. However, a variety of minor to major complications might occur, especially if the stem cells have previously been frozen, including:

- Abdominal cramps
- Difficulty breathing
- Slow heartbeat
- Tightness in the chest
- Chills
- Cough
- Diarrhea
- Skin rash
- Fever
- Flushing
- Headache
- Changes in blood pressure
- Nausea and vomiting
- Unpleasant taste in the mouth
- Kidney failure

Some of the complications that occur are caused by the substance (dimethyl sulfoxide) used to keep the stem cells alive while frozen. Washing the stem cells prior to infusion minimizes the risk of these complications, but is not standard practice at all transplant centers. However, most stem cells used in allogeneic transplants are fresh, not frozen.

Emotional Responses

SCT can take a heavy emotional toll on the child, the siblings, and the parents. It can be a physically and mentally grueling procedure, with the possibility of late effects. Most transplant team members are extensively trained to meet the needs of the child and family during the transplant itself and throughout the recovery period that follows. The team usually includes doctors, nurses, social workers, educators, nutritionists, child life specialists, and physical, occupational, and speech therapists.

Levi's transplant experience was like watching someone wake up from a deep sleep. For two weeks he was flat on his back, suffering greatly from mucositis and a tummy bug that caused diarrhea for days straight. It was a real horror. Then one evening he sat up and said, "What's all that stuff?" He was referring to all the gifts that had piled up in the corner of his room. He opened every toy, got down on the floor, and drew pictures of all the foods he was craving, and he never looked back. It was like an instant transformation. I think my own recovery was longer. I believe part of me froze in order to survive the transplant, and it took a long time to thaw.

• • • • •

My teen-aged daughter struggled with anxiety throughout treatment. The things that helped us were a structured day (lights on at 8 a.m., wash, dress, eat, go for a walk or a wheelchair ride when she couldn't walk), daily visits from the child life specialist, and help from nurses. The child life specialist stayed with us the entire first day of diagnosis, explaining things and helping us to stay calm. During my daughter's hospitalizations and the transplant, the child life folks came every day to do crafts, art therapy, music therapy, walks, and visits to the teen room. We didn't worry about school that year, just focused on staying calm and getting through it.

• • • • •

What helped me the most were the decorations and having a positive attitude. My mom decorated the area outside the transplant room with balloons, cards, and posters. It was hard to take the medicine, so my mom made a huge poster to mark off how well I did. Every time I took my medicine, I got a sticker. When I got one hundred stickers, I got some roller blades.

• • • • •

My son had standard risk B-cell ALL, diagnosed at age 8, and relapsed in his testicles, marrow, and CNS [central nervous system] after front-line treatment ended. He relapsed again in the CNS soon after he had completed his relapse therapy, at age 14. So, we were five years post diagnosis when he had a transplant using cells from his triplet sister who was a perfect match. He was in a new transplant wing at a big children's hospital. Everyone who came in the room had to thoroughly wash

their hands, and non-family members had to wear gowns and masks. The continu-
ous pressure vent was right over where I slept, and it made enough noise that it
drowned out the hospital noises. He was an angry teenager by then, so he basically
slept, refused to eat, and yelled at the physical therapists every time they came in the
room. He did, however, bond with the music therapist who taught him to play the
ukulele.

Sometimes, unrelated donors wish to meet the child or teen who received their donated stem cells. This is usually allowed a year after transplant, and both parties must provide written consent before any information is exchanged. These reunions can be very emotional and in some cases life-long friendships are formed.

Austin's bone marrow donor wanted to meet us after the year of waiting, and we
wanted to meet him too. So, when we were in Philadelphia for a follow-up visit, he
drove up. Austin hugged him and hugged him. Those two have become very close—
two peas in a pod. Every time we come east now, Doug and his girlfriend drive to
Philadelphia and spend a weekend with us doing fun things. We feel very fortunate
and very blessed that things turned out the way they did.

Paying for the Transplant

SCTs are expensive. Some transplants are considered standard of care, so insurers cover the procedure without problems. However, you will need to work with the transplant center coordinator to find out whether your insurance company considers the type of transplant proposed for your child to be experimental, and possibly not covered. All transplant centers have coordinators who will help obtain insurance approval for your child's transplant. Most insurance plans have a lifetime cap on benefits, and many only pay 80% of the costs of the transplant up to the cap. Often, transplant centers will not perform the procedure without all of the money guaranteed. With time being of the essence, this can cause great anguish for families who struggle to raise funds or need to take out a second mortgage to pay for an SCT.

Our first quote from the transplant center was $350,000, but we were able to negoti-
ate a lower price.

Most insurance companies will assign your child's care to a case manager who is responsible for making arrangements with the transplant center and helping with financial issues. Case managers can be valuable resources during this stressful time, especially if you get to know them and share you needs and concerns. If the insurance company does not assign a case manager, you can request to have one assigned or you can speak with a benefits manager about coverage and costs.

Right at the beginning, our doctor explained the different treatment options, including a stem cell transplant. The insurance company denied coverage for the transplant because they considered it experimental, even though our oncologist wrote several appeals. Social workers and the doctor dealt with the insurance company but we felt the stress of it. You shouldn't have to stress over that when your kid is so sick!

At the time this book was written healthcare policy was in flux. So if you don't have insurance, you may be able to go to *www.healthcare.gov* to see whether your family is eligible for government-sponsored insurance plans. Another option is the National Cancer Institute (*https://ccr.cancer.gov*), which offers transplants free of charge to children who qualify for one of its research studies.

We were one of the fortunate families because I had excellent insurance from the hospital where I worked (the coverage isn't as good now). We did not pay anything out of pocket for the transplant, and the hospital was in our town so we didn't have to travel. The insurance company assigned a case worker who called every week to check that the billing was correct and that things were okay. Most families we know are not so lucky. Community members held two fundraisers for us, and we didn't need to touch that money. So, we donated it to nonprofits that help kids with cancer.

In Canada, each province and territory has a provincial health plan that usually covers the medical costs of transplantation. However, many other expenses will need to be covered by the family. Children often have to travel long distances to facilities that can perform an SCT. Travel, accommodations, and related costs are paid by parents.

Complications after Transplant

Some children have a smooth journey through the transplant process, but others bounce from one complication to another. There is no way to predict which children or teens will develop problems, nor is there any way to anticipate whether the new development will be a mere inconvenience or a major health crisis.

The transplant center was very clear about all of the potential problems. That was good because it prepared me. My attitude is watch for them, hope they don't happen, if they do, then live with them. My daughter had an easy time with the transplant. She's a happy third grader, she's alive, and we feel so, so very lucky.

The biggest risk of transplant is that your child's leukemia may return despite having undergone the transplant procedure. If this happens, your transplant physician and your child's oncologist will talk with you about further treatment options.

Short-term side effects

The transplant itself can result in a number of immediate and late complications. One concern after transplant is rejection of the donor cells by the child's body. The new stem cells must relocate and grow in their new body. If the immune system of the child with leukemia was not suppressed adequately, the new stem cells may be rejected. Rejection is uncommon with HLA-matched sibling or unrelated volunteer adult donor transplants (<5%). This risk is somewhat higher with partially matched and umbilical cord blood transplants. If rejection does occur, a second transplant may be required, often using stem cells from a different donor. The rest of this section presents (in alphabetical order) some of the major complications that can develop post-transplant and the experiences of several families who coped with these problems.

Eating difficulties. Almost all children undergoing SCT require nutrition support during their recovery. Some centers feed children using tubes inserted through the nose to the stomach or small intestine. This is a good choice if your child is not experiencing nausea and vomiting. Other children require intravenous (IV) nutrition (see Chapter 22, *Nutrition*). Most transplant centers start IV or tube feeding promptly after transplant and continue until the child's appetite and ability to take in adequate calories by mouth have returned. This usually occurs a few months after the transplant.

GVHD. GVHD is a reaction of the donor stem cells (graft) against the patient (host). It may be triggered by HLA antigen differences, by the chemotherapy and radiation used to prepare the child for transplantation, or by infections. It affects approximately 30 to 50% of children who have undergone an allogeneic transplant and 10 to 12% of children who have a cord blood transplant. It affects a higher percentage of children whose transplants used mismatched marrow or marrow from an unrelated donor. Although GVHD is a serious complication, it may decrease the likelihood that the child will relapse after transplant.

Hemorrhagic cystitis. Hemorrhagic cystitis (bleeding from the bladder) may result from certain chemotherapy drugs (e.g., cyclophosphamide) used in your child's conditioning regimen. To prevent this, during conditioning your child will receive IV hydration and the drug mesna to help coat the bladder lining to prevent damage. Occasionally, hemorrhagic cystitis is caused by a bacterial or viral bladder infection. Signs of infection include blood or blood clots in the urine, pain when urinating, and bladder discomfort.

Infection and fever. Virtually all children will develop a fever soon after the transplant. A cause of the fever, such as an infection, may or may not be identified. Although the immune system of healthy children quickly destroys any foreign invaders, this is not the case for children who have undergone a transplant. Until the new stem cells begin to produce a functioning immune system, children are at risk of developing serious infections. Although the probability of infection decreases after engraftment, the immune system does not function normally until 6 to 12 months after the transplant.

> *After Hunter's stem cell transplant, we had to follow many precautions. We had to be careful when we took him out, avoiding large crowds or public places (especially those indoors). He needed to wear a mask when we took him to his doctor's visits. We took him to plenty of outdoor places for fun.*

To help prevent bacterial infections, children receive prophylactic antibiotics during the first weeks after transplant when their white blood cell count is low. IV antibiotics are started if the child has a fever. Fungal infections can also occur after transplant. The risk of fungal infections can be reduced by use of prophylactic medications such as fluconazole.

After transplant, children are also susceptible to serious viral infections; the most common are herpes simplex virus, influenza, RSV parainfluenza virus (the virus that causes croup), varicella zoster virus (which causes chickenpox and shingles), and cytomegalovirus (CMV). Viral infections are often very hard to treat, so many centers use prophylactic medications, such as acyclovir, to prevent them.

> *Our daughter (age 9) had a stem cell transplant. It's been several months and her white blood cell count is still low, but we have come to the conclusion that we can't make her live in a bubble anymore. We are careful to avoid potential risks, though, such as being around large crowds of people.*

Following are suggestions to minimize exposure to bacteria, fungi, and viruses:

- Have medical staff members and all family members thoroughly wash their hands before touching your child.
- Keep your child away from crowds and people with infections.
- Do not let your child receive live virus inoculations until the immune system has fully recovered; your child's oncologist will determine the appropriate date for getting immunizations.
- Keep your child away from anyone who has recently been given a live virus such as chicken pox, polio, MMR (measles, mumps, and rubella), or FluMist®.
- Keep your child away from zoos, barnyard animals, and all animal feces.
- Avoid remodeling your home while your child is recovering.
- Avoid areas of active construction where ground digging is occurring.
- Shampoo all home carpets and rugs before your child returns home from transplant.
- Bathe and shampoo all family pets prior to your child's return home from transplant.

- Thoroughly wash fruits and vegetables prior to eating and completely cook all meat, poultry, and fish.
- Do not allow your child to share utensils, dishware, or drinks with other people.
- Call the doctor at the first sign of a fever or infection.

During recovery, children must redevelop immunity to common organisms, which may require redoing the usual childhood immunizations. You should discuss the plan for reimmunization with the transplant physician.

Mucositis. Mucositis (inflammation of the mucous membranes lining the mouth and intestines) and stomatitis (mouth sores) are common complications following an SCT. Symptoms include reddened, discolored, or ulcerated membranes of the mouth; pain; difficulty swallowing; taste alterations; and difficulty speaking. The majority of children undergoing transplant experience this problem. Your child will require frequent mouth care, changes in diet, and pain medications. To make daily mouth care less painful, try to ensure that it happens after pain medicine has been given. Likewise, it helps to make sure your child receives pain medication before eating. When the bone marrow starts making white blood cells again, your child's mouth will heal.

> *High-dose chemo kills your taste buds, and I wanted to only eat sweet or spicy food, anything else tasted like cardboard. I'd eat ribs with BBQ sauce. KFC® mashed pota- toes and gravy was great. Drinking was hard. I used to suck on ice cubes. It's gross when the lining of your mouth comes out. It just pulls out, it's white, but it doesn't hurt. It comes out during bowel movements, too. You can't swallow because of the sores, so you have to spit a lot.*

Veno-occlusive disease (also known as sinusoidal obstruction syndrome or SOS). Veno-occlusive disease (VOD) causes the flow of blood through the liver to become obstructed. Children who have had more than one transplant, previous liver problems, or past exposure to intensive chemotherapy are more at risk of developing VOD. It can occur gradually or very quickly. Symptoms of VOD include jaundice (yellowing of the eyes and skin), enlarged liver, pain in the upper right abdomen, fluid in the abdomen, unexplained weight gain, and poor response to platelet transfusions.

> *Our 15-month-old son had JMML and was treated with two allogeneic transplants from a matched unrelated donor [MUD]. He had several side effects including a reaction to cyclosporine (they switched to tacrolimus) and two bouts of VOD. One of the hardest things for him to cope with was the restrictions on liquids when he had VOD. He cried because he was so thirsty and it was hard for me to watch. His potassium went way up once from tube feedings and they were worried about his heart, but the level came back down and everything was fine. His ANC is beginning to stabilize after receiving monthly IVIG infusions.*

Long-term side effects

Increasing numbers of children are being cured of their disease and surviving years after an SCT. The intensity of the treatment prior to, during, and after transplant can cause major effects that are not apparent for months or even years. This section describes a few of the possible long-term side effects that sometimes develop after transplant. Your child should have life-long follow-up from experts to identify and treat any long-term effects that develop after an SCT.

Dental development. Certain chemotherapy drugs, given in high doses prior to transplant, may result in improper tooth development and short or absent tooth roots in children who had a transplant when they were younger than age 5. Your child should have a comprehensive dental exam prior to the transplant and a dental follow-up every six to twelve months after recovery from the SCT.

Thyroid function. Children who receive only chemotherapy before transplant do not usually develop thyroid deficiency. If, however, your child receives radiation therapy to the head or neck (e.g., cranial radiation or TBI), she should have life-long monitoring for thyroid deficiency. Tablets containing thyroid hormone are effective in treating the problem, if it develops.

Puberty, fertility, and growth. Depending on prior treatment and the conditioning regime used, problems with puberty or fertility can develop. For this reason, boys who have gone through puberty should bank sperm, if possible, before treatment begins. You may also consider methods to preserve fertility in girls (e.g., freezing eggs before treatment). Any child or teen who had a transplant should be followed closely by a pediatric endocrinologist who can prescribe hormones, if necessary (testosterone for boys, estrogen and progesterone for girls), to assist in normal pubertal development and who can assess fertility in older survivors. Your child's growth may also be affected by the agents used for pre-transplant conditioning, especially TBI. Growth should be monitored for years after transplant and consultation with an endocrinologist obtained if your child is not growing normally.

Second cancers. Children who receive an SCT have a small risk of developing a second cancer. The risk depends on the chemotherapy drugs given, whether any radiation treatment was given, and genetic factors.

Summary. Overall impact and long-term effects of an SCT on individual children and teens are not known. Your child's oncologist can explain known risks given your child's disease and treatment. You can also read about late effects in *Childhood Cancer Survivors: A Practical Guide to Your Future*, 3rd ed. by Nancy Keene, Wendy Hobbie, and Kathy Ruccione. It is very important that any child who had a transplant be followed for life by an expert in the late effects of treatment for childhood cancer. Many of these late effects, if found early, are treatable.

The road of chemotherapy treatment was long and harsh, but transplant was a test of faith and patience. Knowing that Mia's immune system would be zapped to the point of no return was scary. However, it felt like the last step in killing off any sign of cancer in my little girl's body and a step closer to the end of this nightmare. Isolation was tough on both of us but once again the staff, the programs, the volunteers, and everyone in the hospital were amazing. Mia's room was personalized and decorated just for her. She only asked to leave the room the day before we left for good, day 38! The nurses and doctors did everything in their power to make the whole transplant process go as smoothly as possible for all of us. They kept us informed, called us on their days off, helped me clean Mia up when she was sick, and even played dress up to help get her out of bed and to the shower. We survived, and Mia was discharged on Day 39. She walked out dressed like a princess.

Chapter 17
Siblings

"Why was his hair falling out?
Why was he going to the hospital all the time?
Why was he getting so many presents?"

— Chet Stevens
Straight from the Siblings:
Another Look at the Rainbow

CHILDHOOD CANCER TOUCHES all members of the family, with especially long-lasting effects on siblings. The diagnosis creates an array of conflicting emotions in siblings. Not only are they concerned about their ill brother or sister, but they usually resent the turmoil the family has been thrown into. They may feel jealous of the gifts and attention showered on the sick child, yet feel guilty for having these emotions. The days, months, and years after diagnosis can be extremely difficult for the sibling of a child with cancer.

Ways to explain the diagnosis to siblings are discussed in Chapter 7, *Telling Your Child and Others*. This chapter focuses on common emotions and behaviors of siblings and provides insight into how to cope from parents and siblings who have been through this experience.

Emotional Responses of the Siblings

Brothers and sisters are shaken to the very core by cancer in the family. Parents, the leaders of the family clan, sometimes have no time, and little energy, to focus on the siblings. During this major crisis, siblings sometimes feel they have no one to turn to for help. They may feel concerned, worried, fearful, guilty, angry, sad, abandoned, or other powerful emotions. If you understand that these ever-changing emotions are normal, you will be better able to help your children talk about and cope with their strong feelings.

Although the months or years of treatment are emotionally potent for every member of the family, research has shown that most siblings have good psychological outcomes, particularly if they have been assured they are valuable, contributing members of the family whose thoughts and feelings matter. In the years afterwards, siblings frequently report the experience as life-changing in many positive ways. Following are descriptions and stories about the emotions felt by siblings.

Concern for sick brother or sister

Children really worry about their sick brother or sister. It is difficult for them to watch someone they love be hurt by needles and sickened by medicines. It is scary to see a brother or sister lose weight and go bald. It is hard to feel so healthy and energetic when the brother or sister has to stay indoors because of weakness or low blood counts. The siblings may be old enough to know that death is a possibility. There are plenty of reasons for concern.

> *Christine's younger sister has really developed the nurturing side of her personality as a result of the leukemia. She frequently puts her arm around her sister, comforts her with soothing words or touches, and seems to feel her pain.*

• • • • •

> *I'm the mother of three children. Logan was 19 months old when diagnosed. It was very hard on all of us. Kathryn (5 ½ at the time of diagnosis) felt that she had to take so much on herself. She was there with us the entire time Logan was in the hospital. She had a cot right next to Logan's bed, and only she and I were the ones who could take care of "our Logan."*

> *She used to love to visit the other kids on the hospital floor and entertain them. She hated to go home. She would get so involved with the other kids and didn't want to leave them. She actually got very close to two little girls who lost the battle, so here she was at 6, dealing with the loss of two friends.*

Fear and worry

It is extremely common for young siblings of children with cancer to think the disease is contagious—that they can "catch it." Many also worry that one or both parents may get cancer. The diagnosis of cancer changes children's view that the world is a safe place. They may feel vulnerable and afraid. Many siblings worry that their brother or sister may get sicker or may die.

> *When my infant daughter was diagnosed, I had two older daughters—5 and 3 years old. They are having a hard time because my husband and I have been gone most of the last three months staying in the hospital. Our oldest is very worried. She's been talking to her counselor at school once a week, and she's expressed that that she was worried that her sister is going to die. We think she understands our explanations that her sister needs to stay in the hospital to get medicine to make the cancer go away. It's been hard.*

Fears of things other than cancer may emerge: fear of being hit by a car, fear of dogs, fear of strangers. Many fears can be quieted by accurate and age-appropriate explanations from parents or medical staff.

> My 3-year-old daughter vacillated between fear of catching cancer ("I don't ever want those pokes") to wishing she was ill so that she would get the gifts and attention ("I want to get sick and go to the hospital with Mommy"). She developed many fears and had frequent nightmares. We did lots of medical play, which seemed to help her. I let her direct the action, using puppets or dolls, and I discovered that she thought there was lots of violence during her sister's treatments. She continues to ask questions, and we are still explaining things to her, four years later.

Jealousy

Despite feeling concern for the ill brother or sister, almost all siblings also feel jealous. Presents and cards flood in for the sick child. Mom and Dad stay at the hospital with the ill sibling, and most conversations revolve around that child. When the siblings go out to play, the neighbors ask about the sick child. Even at school, the teachers are concerned about their ill sibling. Is it any wonder brothers and sisters feel jealous?

The siblings' lives are in turmoil and they sometimes feel a need to blame someone. It's natural for them to feel it's the sick sibling's fault that family life has changed, or to feel upset with the sibling for taking all the adults' attention, or to feel angry and blame the parents for daily life being disrupted. Some siblings even develop symptoms of illness in an attempt to regain attention from the parents.

> Our 9-year-old son seemed to be dealing with things so well until one evening as I was tucking him in, he confided that he had tried to break his leg at school by jumping out of the swing. He began to cry and told me he doesn't want his brother to be sick anymore; that he needs some attention, too. As parents, we were always so concerned with our sick child that we didn't realize how much our healthy child was suffering.

Guilt

Young children are egocentric; they are not yet able to see the world from any viewpoint but their own. Some children believe they caused their brother or sister to get cancer. They may have said in anger, "I hope you get sick and die," and then their sibling got sick. Any such fears should be dispelled right after diagnosis. Children need to be told, many times, that cancer just happens and no one in the family caused it. They need to understand that no one can make something happen just by thinking or talking about it.

Many siblings feel guilt about their normal responses to cancer, such as anger and jealousy. They think, "How can I feel this way about my brother when he's so sick?" Assure them that the many conflicting feelings they are having are normal and expected.

It is also common for some children (and parents) to feel guilt about being healthy. It is important for parents to frequently remind their healthy children that there is no connection between their health and their sibling's illness and that no one, including the sick brother or sister, wants them to feel bad about being healthy.

Abandonment

If parental attention revolves around the sick child, siblings may feel isolated and resentful. Even when parents make a conscious effort not to be so preoccupied with the ill child, siblings sometimes still feel they aren't getting their fair share of attention and may feel rejected or abandoned.

> Months after his 4-year-old sister's treatment ended, my 6-year-old son confided to his grandmother that his parents loved her more than him. He still has never told his father or me, but he does sometimes ask if his sister is going to die. When I say no, he looks sort of disappointed.

Sometimes it's necessary to have the siblings stay with relatives, friends, or babysitters. Parents may have to miss activities they would otherwise have attended, such as soccer games or school events. Vacation plans may be scrapped. The reasons may seem obvious to parents, but the siblings may interpret these changes as evidence that they are not as well-loved as the sick child. Parents should explain in detail the reasons for any alterations in routines and try to find solutions that work for everyone in the family.

> When Jeremy was very sick and hospitalized, we sent his older brother Jason to his grandparents for long periods of time. We thought that he understood the reasons, but a year after Jeremy finished treatment, Jason (9 years old) said, "Of course, I know that you love Jeremy more than me anyway. You were always sending me away so that you could spend time with him." It just broke my heart that every time he made that long drive over the mountains with his grandparents, he was thinking that he was being sent away.

Sadness

Siblings have many very good reasons to be sad. They miss their parents and the time they used to spend with them. They miss the life they used to have—the one they were comfortable with. They miss their sick sibling. They worry that he or she may die. Some children show their sadness by crying often; others withdraw and become depressed. Sometimes children confide in relatives or friends that they think their parents don't love them anymore.

We always, always explained everything that was happening to Brian's older brother Zack (8 years old). He never asked questions, but always listened intently. He would say, "Okay. I understand. Everything's all right." We tried to get him to talk about it, but through all these years, he just never has. So we just kept explaining things at a level that he could understand, and he has done very well through the whole ordeal. The times that he seemed sad, we would take him out of school and let him stay at the Ronald McDonald House for a few days, and that seemed to help him.

Anger

Children's lives are disrupted by the diagnosis of a sister or brother with cancer, and siblings often feel very angry. Questions such as "Why did this happen to us?" or "Why can't things be the way they used to be?" are common. Children's anger may be directed at their sick sibling, their parents, relatives, friends, or doctors.

Children's anger may have a variety of causes. They may resent being left with babysitters so often or having extra responsibilities at home, or they may notice that the sick child is not always held to the same standards of behavior as the other children. Because each member of the family may have frayed nerves, explosions of temper can occur.

As we were driving home from school one day, Annie was talking, and I was only half listening. All of a sudden I realized that she was yelling at me. She screamed, "See, this is what I mean. You never listen, your mind is always on Preston." I pulled the car over, stopped, and said, "You're right. I was thinking about Preston." I told her that from now on I would try to give her my full attention. I realized that I would really have to make an effort to focus on what she was saying and not be so distracted. This conversation helped to clear the air for a while. I tried to take her out frequently for coffee or ice cream to just sit, listen, and concentrate on what she was saying.

Worry about what happens at the hospital

Children have vivid imaginations, and when they are fueled by disrupted households and whispered conversations between teary parents, children can imagine truly horrible things. Seeing how their ill sibling looks upon returning from a hospital stay can reinforce their fears that awful things happen at the clinic or hospital. Or the siblings may think they are missing some grand parties when they see their sister or brother and parent come home from the hospital with presents and balloons.

My son is only in kindergarten. He has separation anxiety worse than a 6 month old. He doesn't want to go to bed alone. The last time Karissa had the flu, I thought he was going to die from worrying so much. He cried himself to sleep every night and woke up crying. He was so worried. He hasn't gotten much better since she has started feeling better, either. He doesn't even want to go near the hospital with his sister.

Age-appropriate explanations can help children be more realistic about what they think happens at the hospital, but nothing is as powerful as a visit. Of course the effectiveness of a visit depends on your child's age and temperament, but many parents say that bringing the siblings along helps everyone. The sibling gains an accurate understanding of hospital procedures, the sick child is comforted by the presence of the sibling(s), and the parents get to spend more time with all the children.

> *Alissa's older brother Nicholas is her best friend. We are at the hospital for appointments and therapy three nights a week, every week. Nicholas helps Alissa with "hospital homework" and he also helps with her therapy. Nicholas is doing great at school. We include him in everything.*

Another way to help a worried sibling is to read age-appropriate books together. Many children's hospitals have coloring books for preschoolers that explain hospital procedures with pictures and clear language. School-age children may benefit from reading more detailed books with a parent (see Appendix C, *Books, Websites, and Support Groups*). Adolescents might be helped by watching videos, reading books, or joining a sibling support group.

Several parents suggested that another way to reduce siblings' worries is to allow even the youngest children to help the family in some way. When children have clear explanations about the situation and concrete jobs to do that will benefit the family, they tend to rise to the occasion. Make them feel they are a necessary and integral part of the family's effort to face cancer together.

Concern about parents

Exhausted parents are sometimes not aware of the strong feelings their healthy children are experiencing. They may assume children understand they are loved and that they would be getting the same attention if they were the one who had cancer. Siblings frequently do not share their powerful feelings of anger, jealousy, or worry because they love their parents and do not want to place more burdens on them. It is all too common to hear siblings say, "I have to be the strong one. I don't want to cause my parents any more pain." But burdens are lighter if shared. Parents can help themselves and the siblings by talking about their own feelings and encouraging children to share their feelings, especially the difficult ones. Try to listen without becoming defensive, and use those moments as a chance to grow together and strengthen each other.

> *Ethan had been sharing a room with his eldest brother, Jake, prior to his diagnosis, but after the first surgery either my spouse or I slept in the room with Ethan. Ethan gradually improved over the first couple of months to the point where he was more independently mobile and Jake said he wanted to sleep in Ethan's room again so that my spouse and I could go back to sleeping together. Jake has always been calm,*

thoughtful, and responsible, and he really seemed to handle Ethan's illness the best of the boys. When he and I participated in a survey to evaluate Post Traumatic Stress Disorder (PTSD) in siblings, I found out that he was much more distressed than I had imagined. We took some time to talk about how the stress affected each of us, and I was really grateful that we had agreed to do the research project.

Sibling Experiences

Simply understanding the pain and fears of your healthy children eases their journey. Being available to listen and say, "I hear how painful this is for you," or "You sound scared. I am, too," reminds siblings they are still valued members of the family. They need to understand that even though their brother or sister is absorbing the lion's share of their parents' time and care, they are still cherished. Siblings need to hear that what they feel matters, especially if parents don't have a lot of time to spend with them. If parents understand that overwhelming emotions are normal, expected, and healthy, they can provide solace to all their children.

Brothers and sisters of children with cancer shared the following stories about some of the difficulties they faced.

Silent hurting heart

Dayna E. wrote the following poem when she was 13 years old. Two of Dayna's brothers had cancer—one lived and one died. This poem was published in *Bereavement* magazine and is reprinted with permission.

"Oh, nothing's wrong," she smiled,
grinning from ear to ear.
The frown that just was on her face
just seemed to disappear.

But deep down where secrets are kept,
the pain began to swell.
All the hurt inside of her
just seemed to stay and dwell.

All the pain in her heart
was too much for her to take.
Pretending everything's OK
is much too hard to fake.

She'd duck into the bathrooms
and hide inside the stalls.
Because no one could see her tears,
behind those dirty walls.

She was sick and tired of losing
and things never turning out right.
She had no hope left in her.
She was ready to give up the fight.

But she wiped away the teardrops,
put a smile back on her face,
pulled herself together, and
walked out of that place.

Life went on and things got better.
She thought that was a start.
But still, no one could see inside
her silent hurting heart.

Alana's story

Alana F. (11 years old) remembers how family life changed when her sister, Laura, had cancer.

My sister was in fifth grade and had been sick for the last week or so. Laura always seemed to be my hero. Although we got into arguments, all siblings get into fights, so I didn't worry. I didn't know what was about to happen, but neither did anyone else.

I don't quite remember how my parents told me she had cancer, but I do remember a lot of tears.

As time progressed, my life changed. I lived with my best friend and her parents, Catherine and Bill, but that changed too. Kelsie (my friend) and I got into a lot of arguments, but we still do. I don't know if that is why my grandmother and grandfather moved up to live in our house so that they could take care of me. Living with them was different. My grandmother had different expectations of me than my mother did.

My parents would each take turns staying at the hospital. Some nights I would live with my mom, grammy, and grandpy; and the next it would be with my dad and them.

Of course going through this dilemma I felt left out. Here I was living with my grandparents, and my sister got to live with our parents. She got lots of flowers, cards, and gifts, and all I got was the feeling of love from my relatives. I know that love is better than material things, but when you are 6 years old, you don't think so.

Things stayed the same for a long time. Then my sister went into remission and started living at home. I had to get used to my parents again and missed my grandparents.

My sister was spoiled at home, too. They bought her a waterbed, so she wouldn't get cold. What did I get? A heating blanket; a used heating blanket.

Having a sister with cancer

Alison L. (6 years old) describes the experience of having a sister with cancer.

I think having a sister with cancer is not fun. My mom paid more attention to my sister. I had to stay with Daddy. Mommy picked Kathryn up and not me. My mommy wanted to stay with me, she did not want to leave my sister alone. Sometimes I felt like I was going to throw up.

For brothers and sisters

Ellen Z. discusses the impact that her cancer had on her siblings. (Reprinted with permission from *Candlelighters Youth Newsletter.*)

I am the first of four children and the only girl. When I was diagnosed with ALL at the age of 14, it affected all our lives. My brother Wes was 13, Matthew was 4, and Erik was 2. They and my parents were my support system.

When I was first diagnosed and in the hospital, Dr. Plunkett asked if I wanted anyone besides my parents present when he gave us the diagnosis. I told him I wanted Wes with me. Wes is only 14 months younger than I am, and we have always been very close. He took it all in, and we all decided that we would face this thing, and beat it, as a family. Then he and I sent our parents off so we could have some private time together.

Wes was my support at school and at home. He stuck up for me and kept an eye on me. I lost some of my "friends" after I was diagnosed because of my illness and their fear of it. Wes was always there for me. That's not to say we didn't have our fights. Poor Wes—I could hit him, but he couldn't hurt me physically because of my low blood counts. Sometimes I took advantage of that.

Matt and Erik were also a great source of comfort and support. They would accompany my mom and me to treatments and hold my hand when I got stuck. If one of them wasn't with me when I went in, the nurses would ask me where they were. These little boys made it easier for me to be brave.

I hope my brothers know how much I appreciate, too, the extra time they gave me with our parents during my illness. My parents were very good about splitting time between me and my brothers. If one was with me at treatment or the hospital, then the other was spending time with the boys. Family and friends were also a big help.

I've been out of treatment for 10 years now. I teach second grade and spend a week of my summer as a counselor at a camp for kids with cancer. I am the proud sister of three Eagle Scouts. Wes is married now and lives in another state. I realize how much he meant to me during that trying time and how much he means to me now.

If you are a sibling to someone with cancer and wonder if you make a difference to your sick brother or sister, I would like to tell you that you make a very big difference.

My sister had cancer

Eleven-year-old Jeff P. explains what happened when "My Sister Had Cancer." (Reprinted with permission from Candlelighters Childhood Cancer Foundation Canada's *CONTACT* newsletter.)

My sister Jamie got cancer when she was 23 months old. I was 8, and my two other sisters were 6 and 4. My sisters and I were scared that Jamie was going to die. We weren't able to go to public places and also weren't allowed to have friends in our house. We missed a lot of school when there was chicken pox in our school. I got teased in school sometimes because my sister had no hair. Once an older kid called my sister a freak. My mom was sad most of the time. It was very hard. We are all pleased that Jamie is doing well, and our lives are getting back to normal. It was an experience I'll never forget, and I hope it has made me a stronger person.

From a sibling

Fifteen-year-old Sara M. won first prize in a Candlelighters Creative Arts Contest with her essay, "From a Sibling." Her work is reprinted with permission.

Childhood cancer—a topic most teens don't think much about. I know I didn't until it invaded our home.

Childhood cancer totally disrupts lives, not only of the patient, but also of those closest to him/her, including the siblings. First, I was numbed with unbelieving shock. "This can't be happening to me and my family." Along with this came a whole dictionary full of incomprehensible words and a total restructuring of our (up to that time) fairly normal lifestyle.

One day I was waiting for my parents to pick me up from summer camp and anticipating the start of our family vacation to Canada. When they arrived, they informed me that my older brother Danny was very sick, and we wouldn't be taking that trip after all. The following day, the call came that confirmed the diagnosis. Instead of packing for vacation, we packed our bags and headed for Children's Hospital in Denver, 200 miles away, where Danny was scheduled for surgery and chemotherapy.

I developed my own disease (perhaps from fear I would "catch" what Danny had) with symptoms similar to my brother's:

Sympathy pains. I asked, "Why him?" when he came home from the hospital, exhausted from throwing up a life-saving drug for three days.

Fear. How much sicker is Danny going to get before he gets well? He is going to get well, isn't he?

Resentment. My parents seemed so worried about him all the time. They didn't seem to have time for me anymore.

Confusion. Why couldn't Danny and I wrestle around like we used to? Why couldn't I slug him when he made me mad?

Jealousy. I felt insignificant when I was holding down the fort at home.

The parts I hated the most were: not understanding what was being done to him, answering endless worried phone calls, and hearing the answers to my own questions when my parents talked to other people.

I was helped to sort out these feelings and identify with other siblings when I attended a program held just for teens who had siblings with cancer. We got together, tried to learn how to cross-country ski, and talked about our siblings and ourselves.

Perhaps you remember this story: US speed skating star Dan Jansen, 22, carrying a winning time into the back straightaway of the 1,000 meter race, inexplicably fell. Two days earlier, after receiving word that his older sister, Jane, had died of leukemia, Dan crashed in the 500 meter race. Having a sibling with cancer can immobilize even an Olympic athlete. Dan was expected to bring home two gold medals, but cancer in a sibling intervened. He became, instead, the most famous cancer sibling of all time. He shared his grief before a television audience of two billion people. Dan later went on to win the World Cup in Norway and Germany, and capture the gold at the Olympics. He is the first to tell you the real champions can be found in the oncology wards of children's hospitals across our nation, and the siblings who are fighting the battle right along beside them.

Helping Siblings Cope

The following are suggestions from several families about ways to help brothers and sisters cope.

- Make sure you explain leukemia and its treatment to the siblings in terms they understand. Create a climate of openness so they can ask questions and know they will get answers. If you don't know the answer to a question, write it on your list to ask the doctor at the next appointment, or ask your child if he would like to go to the appointment with you and ask the question himself.

    We drew a lot of pictures of red cells, white cells, and platelets. We showed each doing its job: red cells carrying oxygen around, white cells gobbling up cold germs as well as leukemia blasts, and platelets clumping up to form scabs. Drawing opened the floodgates of questions, and I was always amazed at how each child understood some things so clearly, and was confused and frightened by other things.

- Make sure all the children clearly understand that cancer is not contagious. They cannot catch it, nor can their ill brother or sister give it to anyone else. Impress upon them that nothing the parents or brothers and sisters did caused the cancer.

- Bring home a picture of the brother or sister in the hospital, and encourage the children to talk on the phone or send emails or text messages when their sibling is hospitalized.

  My daughter was 18 months old when her 3-year-old sister was diagnosed. Each member of the family flew in to stay at the house for 2-week shifts, so she had a lot of caregivers. A friend of mine gave her a big key chain that held eight pictures. We put a picture of each member of the family (including pets) on her key chain, and she carried it around whenever we were away. It seemed to comfort her.

- Try to spend time individually with each sibling.

  We began a tradition during chemotherapy that really helped each member of our family. Every Saturday each parent would take one child for a 2-hour special time. We scheduled it ahead of time to allow excitement and anticipation to grow. Each child picked what to do on their special day—such as going to the park, eating lunch at a restaurant, riding bikes. We tried to put aside our worries, have fun, and really listen.

- If people only comment about the sick child, try to bring the conversation back to include the sibling. For example, if someone exclaims, "Oh look how good Lisa looks," you could say, "Yes, and Martha has a new haircut, too. Don't you think she looks great?"

- Share your feelings about the illness and its impact on the family. Say, "I'm sad that I have to bring your sister to the hospital a lot. I miss you when I'm gone." This gives the sibling a chance to tell you how she feels. Try to make the illness a family project by expressing how the family will stick together to beat it.

  I never kept my feelings secret from Shawn's two older brothers (5 and 7 years old). If I was scared, I talked about it. Once when we thought he was relapsing, my stomach was so knotted up that I could barely walk. Kevin said, "Mom, I'm really worried about Shawn." I told him that I was, too, and then we both just hugged and cried together. They really opened up when we didn't hide our feelings.

- Include siblings in decision-making, such as giving them choices about how extra chores will be divided up or devising a schedule for parent time with the healthy children.

> We always gave the boys choices about where they would stay when Shawn had to be in the hospital. I felt like it gave them a sense of control to choose babysitters. They usually stayed at a close neighbor's house where there were younger children. It allowed them to ride the same bus to school and play with their neighborhood friends. Their lives were not too disrupted. They also really pitched in and helped with the younger kids. I think it helped them to help others.

- Allow siblings to be involved in the medical aspects of their brother or sister's illness, if they want to be. Often the reality of clinic visits and overnight stays is easier than what siblings imagine. Many siblings are a true comfort when they hold their brother or sister's hand during procedures.

> Just yesterday, Spencer out of the blue said "Mom, I wish I could have donated my marrow to Travis." And he's 5! He also donated money to plant a tree in Israel today at Sunday school and asked us to write that it was "In honor of God and my brother, Travis." Oh man, we can never forget how this experience is seared in the memory of our children who don't have cancer. I am convinced that for Spencer, too, we will be seeing effects of this entire experience in many ways, long into the future.

- Give lots of hugs and kisses.

> We assumed everything was fine with Erin because she had her grandma, who adored her, staying with her. We made a conscious decision to spend lots of time with her and include her in everything. But we realized later that she felt very left out. My advice is to give triple the affection that you think they need, including lots of physical affection such as hugs and kisses. For years, Erin felt jealous. She thought her brother got more of everything: material things, time with parents, opportunities to do things she was not allowed to do. She finally worked it out while she was in college.

- Be sure to alert teachers of siblings about the tremendous stress at home. Many children respond to the worries about cancer by developing behavior or academic problems at school. Teachers should be vigilant for the warning signals and provide extra support or tutoring for the stressed child or teen. Continue to communicate frequently with the siblings' teachers to make sure you are aware of any developing problems.

- Expect your other children to have some behavior problems as part of living with cancer in the family. This is a normal response.

When my 4-year-old healthy child screams and sobs over a minor skinned knee, she gets as much sympathy as my child with cancer does when having her port accessed. I put a bandage on the knee, rock her, sing a song, and get her an ice pack. The injuries are not equal, but the needs of each child are. They both need to be loved and cared for; they both need to know that mom will help, regardless of the severity of the problem. I even let her use EMLA® for routine shots. The pediatrician laughs at me, but I just tell him, "Sibs need perks, too."

- The child with cancer receives many toys and gifts, which can result in hurt feelings or jealousy in the siblings. Provide gifts and tokens of appreciation to the siblings for helping out during hard times, and encourage your sick child to share.

My daughter Jacqueline is 7 years old. We have three other children, ages 14, 8½, and 3. We found (through trial and error) that letting them know as much as they were able to handle, and making sure they felt comfortable asking any questions they might have, helped a great deal. We also made sure we called them two or three times a day from the hospital, and talked to them about how THEIR day was. We let them come to the hospital any time they wanted, after checking that it was okay with the docs. The second time around, we made sure that anyone coming to visit, or sending her something through the mail, either brought something small for the other three kids, or didn't bring anything at all. We also kept a small stock of wrapped presents for those who didn't remember our rule.

- Encourage a close relationship between an adult relative or neighbor and your healthy children. Having a "someone special" when the parents are frequently absent can help your child feel cared for and loved.

We tried very hard to attend to the feelings of Ethan's siblings ourselves, but we realized early on that we were going to need help. We have a friend who is a children's librarian. She and her husband took the boys out every week and spent the evening with them. The kids picked out books at the library with her help and input, talked about the things they were doing at school, what was going on in their lives, got an ice cream, and were made to feel wanted and special. When Ethan had to go to the hospital for chemotherapy, the children's music teacher would have a sleepover for the boys at her house. She made them a favorite meal, rented a movie, made popcorn, and had a pajama party at her house so that they felt there was something special for them.

You can also take advantage of any workshops, support groups, or camps for siblings. These can be of tremendous value for siblings, providing fun and friendships with others who truly understand their feelings.

Positive Outcomes for the Siblings

After reading about all the difficult emotions your children might experience, it is important to note that many siblings exhibit great warmth and active caretaking while their brother or sister is being treated for cancer. Their empathy and compassion seem to grow with the crisis.

Some brothers and sisters of children with cancer feel they have benefited from the stressful experience in many ways, such as increased knowledge about disease, increased empathy for the sick or disabled, increased sense of responsibility, enhanced self-esteem, greater maturity and coping ability, and increased family closeness. Many of these siblings mature into adults interested in the caring professions, such as medicine, social work, or teaching. Character can grow from confronting a personal crisis, and many parents speak of their healthy children with admiration and pride.

Brothers and sisters of those with cancer go through much adversity, as we parents do. At times, much is overlooked, unintentionally of course, because of the many changes in our lives that we experience at such a difficult time. Well, today, I want to pay a small tribute to Tommy's 15-year-old brother, Matt. From the time Tommy was diagnosed, Matt has been by his side. The first night Matt wouldn't go to bed, just so he could stand by Tommy's bedside and be close to him. When we got back home, Matt took over and made sure Tommy would get his "daily laugh." Every evening, even when Tommy felt too sick to sit up, Matt would be there and always made us smile and laugh. As we all know, the siblings sacrifice much of their own lives during this time. Whether it be their social activities or school work, much of their "normal" lifestyle is changed. They even show their courage through the wide range of emotions, including much sorrow, that they experience. It is said, "Angels shine their light on us that we may see more clearly." So as our angel on earth, thank you Matt for shining your light on your brother Tommy, and may you also be blessed with the light of angels.

Chapter 18

Family and Friends

"Shared joy is double joy,
shared sorrow is half sorrow."
— Swedish proverb

THE INTERACTIONS BETWEEN the parents of a child with cancer and their family members and friends are complex. Potential exists for loving support and generous help, as well as for bitter disappointment and disputes. The diagnosis of childhood cancer creates a ripple effect, first touching the immediate family, then reaching extended family, friends, coworkers, neighbors, schoolmates, members of religious groups, and, sometimes, the entire community.

This chapter begins with how family life can be restructured to cope with treatment. It then provides many practical ideas about helpful things that extended family members and friends can do to support the family of a child with cancer. To prevent possible misunderstandings, parents of children with cancer also share their thoughts about things that are not helpful.

Restructuring Family Life

Every family of a child with leukemia needs assistance. Many people have a hard time asking for, and accepting, help from others. However, learning to ask for help when it's needed and accepting it gracefully will help you get the support your family needs. Many family members, friends, and neighbors will want to assist, but they need direction from you about what is helpful, but not intrusive.

> My advice to newly diagnosed families is to say yes to help. It's very humbling to accept help. Our friends, moms' group, and church ran a meal train for months after diagnosis. They also dropped off hundreds of dollars' worth of restaurant cards, so my husband could pick up dinner at a restaurant and not have to shop or cook when our daughter and I were in the hospital (133 days inpatient!). People babysat our young son when I was in the hospital with our daughter and my husband was at work. Learn to say yes and it will change your world.

Jobs

In two-parent families in which both parents are employed, decisions must be made about their jobs. Single parents who are employed full-time also need to make tough decisions about whether to take a leave of absence from work or cut back on hours to care for their child. It is better, if possible, to use all available sick leave and vacation days before deciding whether a parent needs to leave his or her job. Parents need to be able to evaluate their financial situation and insurance availability; this requires time and clarity of thought—both of which are in short supply in the weeks after diagnosis.

> When Garrett got sick, I used up all of my vacation. At that time, our head of human resources called me in and informed me that I now had to take unpaid leave if I wanted to stay out of the office any longer. He then added that in order to continue my benefits, I had to pay "my share" of all benefits costs during this leave. This included insurance, retirement, and other contributions. The weekly outlay was not insignificant. I was dismayed to say the least.

> Fortunately, our senior management and common sense prevailed. We came to an informal arrangement where I "made up" lost time by working weekends and extended days when Garrett was home and doing okay. When he was inpatient (most of the first year and the first three months of the second), I would stay with him in the hospital on the weekends (Friday night through Sunday evening) and on Tuesday night and all day Wednesday. This would give my wife a break from the hospital and let me spend time with my son. It worked very well. Pam later calculated that I worked more hours in make-up than I missed for Garrett. The company came out ahead. Every situation is different and every solution will be different in these circumstances. There is only one constant: You will never ever regret the precious time you spent with your child.

You may have some legal protections for your job. The Family and Medical Leave Act (FMLA) protects the job security of employees of large companies who:

- Take a leave of absence to care for a seriously ill child or other family member
- Take medical leave because the employee is unable to work because of his or her own medical condition
- Take leave after the birth or adoption of a child

The FMLA:

- Applies to all public employers (federal, state, county and local, including schools) and private employers with 50 or more employees within a 75-mile radius.
- Applies to employees who have worked at a qualified place of employment for at least 12 months, and who have worked at least 1,250 hours during those 12 months.
- Provides 12 weeks of unpaid leave during any 12-month period.

- Requires employers to continue providing benefits, including health insurance, during the leave period.

- Requires employers to return employees to the same or equivalent positions upon return from the leave. Some benefits, such as seniority, need not accrue during periods of unpaid FMLA leave.

- Requires employees to give 30-day notice of the need to take FMLA leave, when the need is foreseeable.

- Is enforced by the Wage and Hour Division, U.S. Department of Labor, or by private lawsuit. You can locate the nearest office of the Wage and Hour Division by visiting *www.dol.gov/whd*.

Your state government may provide family leave benefits broader than what are mandated by the federal government. For example, California, New Jersey, and Rhode Island have a paid family leave benefit as part of their state disability insurance programs. Other states do not provide paid leave, but do require certain employers to allow more unpaid family leave than the federal minimum. Visit the website of your state's employment department to find out what rights and benefits you may be legally entitled to.

In Canada, a parent may be entitled to benefits under the Employment Insurance Act. Consideration is provided in the act for a parent having to leave work to care for an ill child. Entitlement to benefits is made on a case-by-case basis. Should a parent qualify, benefits are determined by the number of hours the parent has worked prior to making the claim. For more information, parents should contact the nearest Employment and Social Development Canada office.

Marriage and partnerships

Diagnosis and treatment place enormous pressure on marriages and partnerships. Couples may be separated for long periods of time, emotions run high, and coping styles and skills may differ. Initially, family life is disrupted; couples then must work together to figure out how to proceed. Following are parents' suggestions and stories about how they managed.

- Share medical decisions

> *My husband and I shared decision-making by keeping a joint medical journal. The days that my husband stayed at the hospital, he would write down all medicines given, side effects, fever, vital signs, food consumed, sleep patterns, and any questions that needed to be asked at the next rounds. This way, I knew exactly what had been happening. Decisions were made as we traded shifts at our son's bedside.*

I made most of the medical decisions. My husband did not know what a protocol was, nor did he ever learn the names of the medicines. He came with me to medical conferences, however, and his presence gave me strength.

. . . . .

I was in a new relationship when my toddler daughter was diagnosed with JMML. My boyfriend had just met her a few months before. He bought her an Easter basket and just stole my heart. Soon after Easter, she was diagnosed. He has been with us for bone marrow biopsies, hospitalizations, and numerous appointments. He changed his work schedule to be at her bedside when I couldn't be. He has been a rock and we are so blessed. It's now two years later, and we are getting married in three weeks.

- Take turns staying in the hospital with your child

  We took turns going in with our son for painful procedures. The doctors loved to see my husband come in because he's a friendly, easygoing person who never asked them any medical questions. We shared hospital duty, also. I would be there during any crisis because I was the person better able to be a strong advocate, but he went when our son was feeling better and needed entertaining company. It worked out well.

  . . . . .

  My husband fell apart emotionally when our daughter was diagnosed, and he never really recovered. He stayed with her once in the hospital and cried almost the whole time. She never wanted him there again, so I did all of the hospital duty.

  . . . . .

  My wife took care of most of the medical information gathering because she had a scientific background. But my work schedule was more flexible, so I took my son for almost all of his treatments and hospitalizations. I cherish my memories of those long hours in the car and waiting room.

- Share household duties

  We both worked full-time, so we staggered our shifts. He worked 7 to 3 during the day; I worked 3 to 11 at night. He did every single dressing change for the Hickman® catheter—584 changes, we counted them up. Wherever I left off during the day, he took over. He was great, and it really worked out well for us. We shared it all.

  . . . . .

  My husband really didn't help at all. I couldn't even go out because he wouldn't give the pills. He kept saying that he was afraid he would make a mistake.

- Accept differences in coping styles

    We both coped differently, but we learned to work around it. I didn't want to deal with "what if" questions, but he was a pessimist and constantly asked the fellow questions about things that might happen. I felt that it was a waste of energy to worry about things that might never happen. I didn't want to hear it and felt that it just added to my burden. It was all I could do to survive every day. We worked it out by going to conferences together, but I would ask my questions and then leave. He stayed behind to ask all of his questions.

    · · · · ·

    My husband didn't have the desire to read as much as I did. However, whenever I read something that I felt he should read, he always took the time to do so and then we discussed it.

    · · · · ·

    My husband and I have always been a team. We complement the strengths and weaknesses of each other and I think that was the reason we managed to hold everything together. When I was down, he would bring me up. When he was down, I would do the same for him. With the exception of the initial trauma when our son was diagnosed, we handled things in that manner throughout treatment.

- Seek counseling

    I went for counseling because I couldn't sleep. At night, I got stuck thinking the same things over and over and worrying. I ended up spending two years on antidepressants, which I think really saved my life. They helped me sleep and kept me on an even keel. I'm off them now, my son is off treatment, and everything is looking up.

    · · · · ·

    My husband and I went to counseling to try to work out a way to split up the child rearing and household duties because I was overwhelmed and resenting it. I guess it helped a little bit, but the best thing that came out of it was that I kept seeing the counselor by myself. My son wanted to go to a "feelings doctor," too. I received a lot of very helpful, practical advice on the many behavior problems my son developed. And my son had an objective, safe person to talk things over with.

Most marriages and partnerships survive, but some do not. Those that deteriorate often have serious pre-existing problems that are further strained by cancer treatment.

My husband had a lot of problems that really brought my daughter and me down. The cancer really opened my eyes to what was important in life. We stayed together through treatment, but we divorced after the transplant. I just realized that life is too short to spend it in a bad relationship.

My husband went to work rather than go with us to the hospital when our son was diagnosed. It went downhill from there. He started using drugs and mistreating us, so we divorced.

Blended families

Many children diagnosed with cancer live in blended families. Parents may be separated or divorced, remarried, or living as single parents. There may be foster parents, biological parents, step parents, or legal guardians. Communication between involved adults may be open and amiable or it may be strained. It is best for the child when all parents/ guardians put their differences aside and work together to provide an environment focused on caring for and supporting the ill child. Counseling is often very helpful.

> *My son's dad and I are divorced and we are both remarried with kids. We found it to be helpful and important to have all four parents at all of the meetings that discussed treatments and options, as well as any follow-up meeting where decisions needed to be made. While the forms that needed to be signed for treatments and protocols only needed to be signed by my ex-husband and me, we found it to be especially important that all four of us signed the paperwork. On one hand, it provided a way for step parents to take part in and feel included in something that was so important to a child who they, too, loved, but it also alleviated the potential of someone casting blame later on if treatment didn't work out in our favor. The doctors gladly added two more signature lines underneath the two signatures that were required.*

If the child with cancer has two homes due to a blended family, it often helps to have a journal that goes with the child to each family. It keeps everyone involved up to date. It can contain information about medications given, dose changes, blood test results, and upcoming procedures.

Unfortunately, the diagnosis of cancer in a child can make strained family relations even worse. It is important that all parents/guardians with a legal right to information about all aspects of the illness receive that information and are able to participate in the decision-making process. In some situations, a social worker or psychologist will work with all parties to set up family meetings to make this possible.

> *We have a blended family (although my husband and I have been married for 20 years now) and have two teenagers in the house. My recommendation is counseling. Both of my teenagers and I see a therapist individually. My husband and I also had to go to marriage counseling at various times during our marriage. Serious illness will put a strain on any marriage. If you have issues before cancer strikes, they will become exacerbated. We have good insurance and it pays for most of our sessions. I paid about 20% out of pocket. It is so worth it. Raising a family is hard work. Add*

cancer on top of it and, quite frankly, it can become overwhelming. Counseling helps each member of the family have an outlet to express their concerns and worries.

Single parents

Some parents are single and do not share parenting with an former spouse or partner (e.g., widows, widowers, single parents who adopted children, parents whose former partner is no longer involved). Going through a crisis of this magnitude with no one to talk to or help with daily tasks can leave a single parent feeling isolated, helpless, lonely, and overwhelmed. Also, many single parents are both the sole breadwinner for the family and the sole caretaker of the child with cancer and any siblings. Single parents shared the following suggestions on ways to cope:

- Involve a best friend in making the medical decisions and providing care
- Ask a family member to stay with you at the hospital for support
- Have a friend bring you changes of clothes, bring meals and snacks you can keep in the room or put in a fridge (if one is available), or relieve you for an hour while you take a walk
- Talk with a therapist or other single parent about medical choices and your feelings

> *It's really difficult being a single parent when your child is in the hospital, as there is no other parent to take turns sitting with your child, running errands, helping make medical decisions, or supporting you emotionally as you are watching your child suffer. It can feel incredibly lonely! That is when friends become your lifeline. One day we rushed to the ER for what I thought would be a quick visit, and my daughter ended up being admitted for a week's stay. I had no extra clothes, no laptop, no cell phone charger, none of her comfort items, nothing! And my dog was home alone with no food or way to get outside. Before my phone died, I sent out some texts and a Facebook post to friends, coworkers, and church members. Then I dissolved into tears, feeling totally sad and overwhelmed.*
>
> *Next thing I knew, church members had arranged to pick up our dog; my best friend went to my home and brought me a change of clothes, my laptop and chargers, my daughter's favorite CDs and movies, and warm food. Then a food delivery guy showed up at the door of the hospital room with a bunch of Italian food that my coworkers had ordered for me. And by day's end I had more than 100 Facebook comments from friends, sending their love, prayers, and hopes. At that moment, I realized that though I did not have a partner to share my burdens, I was not alone and never would be. Through my daughter's entire illness, I was supported by friends and church members. It taught me that it is okay to ask for help; it doesn't mean you are weak or incapable of parenting alone. Quite simply, being a single parent, full-time worker, and full-time caregiver is really hard, and you cannot do it alone. Don't be afraid to ask for help! People can be incredibly compassionate and generous when you give them a chance.*

The Extended Family

Extended family—grandparents, aunts, uncles, cousins—can cushion the shock of diagnosis and treatment with loving words and actions. Extended family members sometimes cancel their plans to rush to the side of the newly diagnosed child, and often remain steadfast throughout the months or years of treatment. Regrettably, some family members are not helpful, either out of ignorance about what your family needs or simply because they are frightened by the diagnosis or overwhelmed by events in their own lives.

Some extended families, and even entire communities, rally around the family; for other families, support never appears. Several factors affect the strength of support that is offered, including well-established community ties, good communication within the extended family, physical proximity to the extended family, and clear exchange of information about the needs of the affected family. If any of these elements are missing, support may dissolve or never appear.

> We had just moved 3,000 miles away from family and friends for my husband to accept a new job. We had no family close by, no friends. Each family member and some close friends used their vacations to fly out and take 2-week shifts at our new house to help out. Thankfully, they got us through the first eight months, but the rest of treatment was lonely.

Families with strong community ties often receive support throughout treatment.

> Shortly after Jesse relapsed, I was praying with my Bible study group. With four children ages 1 to 9, I just didn't know how we would manage with one parent 100 miles away at the hospital and one parent working. The group decided to collect enough money to allow my sister to quit her job and move in to take care of our other three children while I was at the hospital with Jesse. She stayed for eight months. It was such a wonderful thing. They didn't even ask us; they just said they would support her financially so she could care for my children and keep the household running.

Grandparents

Grandparents grieve deeply when a grandchild has cancer. They are concerned not only for their grandchild, but also for their own child (the parent). Cancer wreaks havoc with grandparents' expectations, reversing the natural order of life and death. Grandparents frequently say, "Why not me? I'm the one who is old." A cancer diagnosis in a grandchild is a major shock to bear. Many parents reported that the grandparents responded to the crisis with tremendous emotional, physical, and financial support.

My mother was a rock. She lived far away, but she put her busy life on hold to come help. She took care of the baby and kept the household running when I was living at the hospital with my very ill child. She was strong, and it gave me strength.

Some parents express tremendous gratitude for the role played by the grandparents in providing much-needed stability to the family rocked by cancer. When grandparents are able to care for the siblings or help with meals and other home chores, the parents can focus on the most urgent needs, such as caring for the sick child or putting in necessary time at work.

Judd was in isolation at Children's for a month. I stayed with him full time, and my husband took a month off work to be there. Luckily, my mother had moved to our town just the year before and was able to immediately move to our house to take care of Erin, my 10-year-old daughter. Grandma was great because she cooked special meals for Erin and helped with cleaning and transportation.

Other families are not as fortunate. Many grandparents are too old, too ill, or simply unable to cope with a crisis of this magnitude. Some simply fall apart.

My mother-in-law became hysterical when my daughter was diagnosed. She called every day, sobbing. Luckily, she lived far away, and this minimized the disruption. We had to ask her not to come, because we just couldn't handle the catastrophe at home and her neediness too. It hurt her feelings, but we just couldn't cope with it.

• • • • •

We've been in treatment for eight years—three relapses. I tell families you never know where support will come from, so it helps to stay open to everyone. I've met a wonderful group of people through our cancer journey. Some people surprise you with their support, and others disappoint. My mother only came to the hospital once; she said it was just too hard. But other people we hardly knew, or didn't know at all, stepped up and really helped out.

Some grandparents allow pre-existing problems with their adult child to color their perceptions of what the family needs or what role they should take on during the crisis. For example, sometimes cancer allows grandparents to renew criticism of the way grandchildren are being raised.

While we stayed at the hospital, the grandparents moved into our house to care for our 8-year-old daughter. They decided that this was their chance to "whip her into shape, teach her some manners, and get her room cleaned up." Our daughter was in tears, and we ended up saying, "We appreciate your help, but we will take over."

It is hard to predict how anyone will react to the diagnosis of childhood cancer; grandparents are no exception. Some respond with the wisdom gleaned from decades of living, others become needy or overbearing, and some withdraw. It is natural in a time of grave crisis to look to your parents for support and help, but it is important to remember that grandparents' ability to respond also depends on events in their own lives. If problems between family members develop, help can be obtained from hospital social workers or through individual counseling.

Helpful things for extended family members to do

Families differ in what is truly helpful for them. The suggestions in this chapter are snapshots of what some families appreciated. Connections can be made in many different and personally meaningful ways. Extended family members should try to support the family of the child with cancer in ways that respect their wishes, while also honoring their privacy. Parents of ill children shared the following suggestions for helpful actions by family members.

- Be sensitive to the emotional state of both the sick child and the parents. Sometimes parents want to talk about the illness; sometimes they just need a hand to hold. The same is true for the child or teen with cancer. Some will want to share their feelings, but others will prefer to be distracted and do "normal" fun things with you to whatever extent they can. Ask them what feels right.

- Encourage all members of the extended family to keep in touch through visits, calls, video chats, mail, email, text messages, and social media. When visits are welcome, make them brief and cheerful. Not only do long visits sometimes distress sick children and teens, but they can also overtax a tired parent.

    Our relatives who lived close to the hospital had teenagers. One was a candy striper at Children's on Saturdays. The aunts, uncles, and cousins came to visit several times a week any time he was in the hospital during his years of treatment. They were all very supportive, very positive, and fun to be around.

- Be understanding if the parents do not want phone calls while in the hospital. Remember that parents often have to stay very close to their sick child, and the child can hear what is being said in phone conversations, so text or voicemail messages are sometimes better.

- A cheerful hospital room really boosts a child's spirits. Send balloon bouquets, funny cards, posters, signs with messages on them, toys, or humorous books. Most hospitals do not allow latex balloons, so only send mylar balloons. Flowers are rarely allowed in children's rooms.

    We plastered the walls with pictures of family and friends, and so many people sent balloons that the ceiling was covered. It was a lovely sight.

- Laughter helps heal the mind and body, so stage a fun event, send funny videos, or arrive with a good joke if you think it is appropriate.

My brother and sister-in-law created an exciting "trip" for my 4-year-old daughter. She was bald, big-bellied from prednisone, and her counts were too low to leave the house, but her interest in fashion was as sharp as ever. Bill and Cathleen bought 10 outfits, rigged up a dressing room, and with Cathleen as saleswoman, turned Katy's bedroom into a fashion salon. She tried on outfits, discussed all of their merits and shortcomings, and had a fabulous time. It was a real high point for her.

- Distraction is the name of the game. Puzzles, card games, picture books, coloring books, age-appropriate video games, new movies, and craft kits are welcome. For a child who cannot get out of bed, a remote control car or a foam dart launcher can be a fun way to extend their reach and have more active play while they are stuck in one spot.

  A friend who was a nurse came to my son's room shortly before Christmas and brought an entire gingerbread house kit, including confectioner's sugar for the icing. We had a very good time putting it together.

- Offer to give the parent(s) a break from the hospital room. A walk outside, shopping trip, haircut, dinner out, or just a long shower can be very refreshing.

- Bring a fresh, home-cooked meal to the hospital for the parents. This can be a wonderful respite from hospital food for parents who are staying with their child.

  My coworkers had Italian food from a nice restaurant delivered to me while my daughter was in the hospital and it made my week!

- Donate frequent flyer miles to distant family members who have the time but not the money to help.

  A close friend (who lived 3,000 miles away) had just lost her job and wished she could be there for us. My parents gave her their frequent flyer miles. She flew in for three weeks during a hard part of treatment and helped enormously.

- Donate blood. Your blood may not be used specifically for the child you know, but it will replenish the general supply, which is depleted by children with cancer.

  Our family friend John is terrified of needles. John always avoided giving blood. John doesn't like going to the doctor. But John showed up to donate platelets once, early on, and we found that he was a great platelet match for Deli. So, he kept returning to that awful two-needle machine that you stay hooked onto for three hours at a time, probably a couple dozen times, because we needed him. Then we had Beth, who was one of my professional acquaintances. Beth was always pretty nice to us, but she found out that she too was a good "sticky" platelet donor. Probably at least a dozen times she took hours out of her work day and donated platelets whenever Deli needed some. We concentrated on the few "star" friends and relatives, the one or two people whose attitude, abilities, and circumstances allowed them to be the most helpful.

Friends

Like family, friends can cushion the shock of diagnosis and ease the difficulties of treatment with their words and actions. It is very helpful if a friend creates an online task calendar. These free programs allow the family to list tasks they need help with (e.g., meals, pet care) on certain dates, such as scheduled hospitalizations or clinic days. This way, helpers can sign up to take care of chores or be on call for tasks such as snow shoveling or lawn mowing. You can find a list of online calendars in Appendix C, *Books, Websites, and Support Groups.*

Mother Theresa once said, "We can do no great things—only small things with great love." The family of a child being treated for cancer is overwhelmed. The list of helpful things to do is endless, and following are suggestions from parents who have traveled this hard road.

Household

- Provide meals. It is helpful to find out whether anyone in the family has food allergies or whether there are types of food the family prefers to eat—or prefers to avoid. It is best to be thoughtful when delivering meals, as the family may feel too tired or the child too ill to welcome friends in for an extended chat.

   One of the biggest ways our extended family helped us was by setting up a Care Calendar online. Then they would provide meals based on the specific need. For example, if we were inpatient, it would be gift cards and hospital-delivered meals. Big chemo weeks would be several meals delivered to our home the next couple of days. Full-day infusions meant someone would bring a meal that evening. They worked to anticipate what our needs would be. I was also able to add photos and updates on how she was doing for the volunteers.

- Take care of pets or livestock.
- Mow grass, shovel snow, rake leaves, water plants, and weed gardens.

   We came home from the hospital one evening right before Christmas, and found a freshly cut, fragrant Christmas tree leaning next to our door. I'll never forget that kindness.

- Clean the house or hire a cleaning service.

   My husband's cousin sent her cleaning lady over to our house. It was so neat and such a luxury to come home to find the stove and windows sparkling clean.

- Grocery shop (especially when the family is due home from the hospital).
- Do laundry or drop off and pick up dry cleaning.

Siblings

An entire chapter of this book is devoted to the complex feelings that siblings experience when their brother or sister has cancer. Chapter 17, *Siblings*, provides an in-depth examination of the issues from the perspective of both siblings and parents. Below is a list of suggestions about how family and friends can help the siblings.

• Babysit younger siblings whenever parents go to the clinic or emergency room, or need to be with their child for a prolonged hospital stay.

• When parents are home with a sick child, take siblings somewhere fun to get their minds off of the stresses at home. Find out what they would enjoy, and spend special time with them going to the park, a sports event, miniature golfing, bowling, the zoo, or a movie.

• Invite siblings over for meals.

• If you bring a gift for the sick child, bring something for the siblings, too.

> *Friends from home sent boxes of art supplies to us when the whole family spent those first 10 weeks at a Ronald McDonald house far from our home. They sent scissors, paints, paper, and colored pens. It was a great help for Carrie Beth and her two sisters. One friend even sent an Easter package with straw hats for each girl, and flowers, ribbons, and glue to decorate them with.*

• Offer to help siblings with homework.

• Drive siblings to lessons, games, or school.

• Listen to how they are feeling and coping. Siblings' lives have been disrupted; they have limited time with their parents, and they need support, attention, and care.

Psychological support

There is much that can be done to help the family maintain an even emotional keel.

• Call frequently, and be open to listening if the parents want to talk about their feelings. Also, talk about non-cancer related topics (e.g., neighborhood or school news) to help them feel less isolated.

> *What I wished for most was that friends and family had been able to call more often to see how we were doing; that someone could have handled my confidence on the good days and my tears on the bad days. It somehow took too much emotional energy to make a call myself, but I valued any phone call I received.*

• Visit the hospital and bring fun stuff such as bubbles, Silly String®, water pistols, joke books, funny movies, rub-on tattoos, and board games.

I've had two children diagnosed with cancer. The first time, I felt like it was a burden to ask anyone for help. Really, about 90% of the time I went without rather than ask. After my second child was diagnosed, a friend who was a massage therapist asked if she could come by to chat and give me a massage, and I said yes. Another friend was a therapist who mostly worked with couples. He would visit, let me vent, and really helped me come up with ways to cope with difficult situations. My best friend, who has multiple sclerosis so travel is difficult for her, showed up at the hospital (a 2-hour drive) and splurged for me to have a pedicure. She took me out to lunch and stayed with my daughter so I could go for a walk outside. She brought albums of pictures of our family before cancer entered our lives. It was lovely.

- Drive the parent and child to clinic visits.
- Send email, cards, and letters.

  Word got around my parents' hometown, and I received cards from many high school acquaintances who still cared enough to call or write and say we're praying for you, please let us know how things are going. It was so neat to get so many cards out of the blue that said, "I'm thinking about you."

- Babysit the sick child, and any siblings, so the parents can go out to eat, exercise, take a walk, or just get out of the hospital or house.

  Joseph's kindergarten teacher would come to play with him so we could get out of the hospital and eat and take a break for an hour or so. She just seemed to understand how much we needed that and how hard it would be for us to do it otherwise.

- Ask what needs to be done, and then do it.

  A close friend called to ask what I needed the day after Michelle was diagnosed. I asked if she could drive our second car the 100 miles to the hospital so my husband could return in it to work. She came with her family to the Ronald McDonald House with two big bags containing snack foods, a large box of stationery, envelopes, stamps, books to read, a book handmade by her 3-year-old daughter containing dozens of cut-out pictures of children's clothing pasted on construction paper (which my daughter adored looking at), and a beautiful, new, handmade, lace-trimmed dress for my daughter. It was full-length and baggy enough to cover all bandages and tubing. She wore it almost every day for a year. It was a wonderful thing for my friend to do.

- Give lots of hugs.

Financial support

Helping families avoid financial difficulties can be a very important form of support. In the United States, medical bills are the top cause of personal bankruptcy. It is estimated that even fully insured families spend 25% or more of their income on deductibles, co-payments, travel, motels, car maintenance, meals, childcare for siblings, and other expenses that aren't covered by insurance. Uninsured or underinsured families may struggle to pay even the most basic household bills while trying to keep up with medical bills, and some lose their car or home when they cannot keep up with payments.

At the same time, families can face a substantial loss of income while caring for their critically ill child. Caring for a child or teen with cancer is complex and intensive, and one parent often needs to leave work for the entire duration of treatment. A single parent usually has no other source of employment income, but may need to reduce hours or take FMLA to care for the child—often causing financial distress. Most families need financial assistance, and there are many ways to help.

- **Start a support fund:** There are many ways to start a support fund, but certain guidelines should be followed to protect everyone involved. Always check with the parents first. It is important to respect any privacy concerns they may have, and to allow them to have a say over anything organized in their child's name. Some people are embarrassed to have their personal financial situation or sensitive medical information shared with others in the community, while others are comfortable freely sharing that with anyone. Also, the parents may need to work with the hospital social worker to ensure that any bank account created to assist the family is set up in such a way that it does not endanger any state or federal benefits the child is receiving. Volunteers should not have access to the account, though the parents can designate someone to pay bills for them directly out of the fund,

  > A friend of mine called and asked very tentatively if we would mind if she started a support fund. We felt awkward, but we needed help, so we said okay. She did everything herself, and the money she raised was very, very helpful. We did ask her to stop the fund when volunteers started calling us to ask if they could use giving to the fund as an advertisement for their business.

In a smaller community, a fundraising drive can be as simple as leaving jars at local stores for contributions or sending an email to family, friends, and the local newspaper that includes the address of a bank account where contributions can be dropped off or mailed. A newer method of collecting donations for a family in need is to use an online resource such as *www.youcaring.com* or *www.gofundme.com*. You can create a fundraising site with photos and stories from the family and share a link to the site on social media to reach family and friends all over the world. These companies charge fees to host your fundraising page and process the donations, so it is important to carefully read the fine print. Find out more about online fundraising sites in Appendix C, *Books, Websites, and Support Groups.*

• **Share leave with a coworker:** Governments and some companies have leave banks that permit people who are ill, or taking care of someone who is ill, to use coworkers' leave so they will not have their pay docked for taking time off work.

> *My husband's coworkers didn't collect money, they did something even more valuable. They donated sick leave hours so he was able to be at the hospital frequently during those first few months without losing a paycheck.*

• **Job share:** Some companies allow job-share arrangements in which a coworker donates time to perform part of the parent's job so the parent can spend extra time at the hospital. Job sharing allows the job to get done, keeps peace at the job site, and prevents financial losses for the family. Another possibility is for one or more friends with similar skills (e.g., word processing, filing, sales) to rotate through the job on a volunteer basis to cover for the parent of the ill child.

> *After my son's diagnosis, the Board of Directors requested that the balance of my school year contract be paid—even though I was unable to fulfill my obligations. It was handled by using my sick days (I had only been on the job a little over six months) and then maternity/ disability. I was expecting a baby eight weeks after Matt's diagnosis, so I went right into the maternity/disability benefit. How they figured it on paper to carry the rest of my contract, I don't know. I did not return to my job until the second school year into Matt's illness. I then began to work on a job-share basis, which I still do. To this day, I have not used any family medical leave time. My agency has been absolutely the exception, and it has been one of our blessings to be working for such a compassionate agency.*

• **Collect money by organizing a bake sale, dance, spaghetti supper, silent auction, or raffle:**

> *Coworkers of my husband held a Halloween party and charged admission, which they donated to us. We were very uncomfortable with the idea at first, but they were looking for an excuse to have a party, and it helped us out.*

• **Offer to help keep track of medical bills:** Keeping track of bills is time-consuming, frustrating, and exhausting for the parents. If you are a close relative or friend, you could offer to review, organize, and file (either on paper or into a computer spreadsheet) all the stacks of paperwork. Making the calls and writing the letters over contested claims or errors in billing can also be very helpful.

Religious support

Following are a few suggestions for families who have religious affiliations:

• Arrange for church/synagogue/mosque members and clergy to visit the hospital, if that is what the family wants.

• Arrange prayer services for the sick child.

> *The day our son was diagnosed, we raced next door to ask our wonderful neighbors to take care of our dog. The news of our son's diagnosis quickly spread, and we found out later that five neighborhood families gathered that very night to pray for Brent.*

• Have your child's religious education class send pictures, posters, letters, balloons, or audio or videotapes.

Accepting help (for parents)

As a parent of a child with cancer, one of the kindest things you can do for your friends is to let them help you. Let them channel their time and worry into things that will make your life easier. Think of the many times you have visited a sick friend, made a meal for a new mom, babysat someone else's child in an emergency, or just pitched in to do what needed to be done. These actions probably made you feel great and provided a good example for your children. When your child is diagnosed with cancer, both you and your friends will benefit immensely if you let them help you and if you give them guidance about what you need.

> *Asking for help is tricky because no one magically knows what you need. Yet it's hard to ask for someone to pick up the sibs from school, mow the lawn, or bring dinner. That said, most people have really good intentions. Lots of families I know set up one of those online calendars such as Lotsa Helping Hands that folks can fill in. We had a women's club in our town (I wasn't even a member) that decided to adopt our family and they brought meals for months. Adorable little old ladies would drop off meals every day. It was such a lovely thing for them to do.*

· · · · ·

> *My best advice is to keep lines of communication open with family and friends. We parents tend to bottle things up, especially when things are at their worst. We often put ourselves on the back burner to keep the focus on our child. When we don't release that stress and express those emotions, the damage is done and we need to deal with it later. If our child survives, we beat ourselves up for not letting people in more. If our child dies, we beat ourselves up for things we did or did not do. I've had two children with cancer—one lived and one died. So, I suggest you let people in, let them help, and be gentle with yourself. You're doing the best you can.*

What to say (for friends)

Following are some suggestions for friends about what to say and how to offer help. Of course, much depends on the type of relationship that already exists between you and the family you want to help; but a specific offer can always be accepted or graciously declined.

- "Our family would like do your yardwork. It will make us feel as if we are helping in a small way."
- "Would it help if we took care of your dog (or cat, or bird)? We would love to do it."
- "I walk my dog twice times a day. May I walk yours, too?"
- "The church is setting up a system to deliver meals to your house. When is the best time to drop them off?"
- "I will take care of Jimmy whenever you need to take John to the hospital. Call us anytime, day or night, and we will come pick Jimmy up."

Things that do not help

Sometimes people say things to parents of children with cancer that are not helpful and can even be hurtful. If you are a family member or friend of a parent in this situation, please do not say any of the following:

- "God only gives people what they can handle." (Some people cannot handle the stress of childhood cancer, and it is painful to be told that your child was singled out to have cancer because you are strong.)
- "I know just how you feel." (Unless you have a child with cancer, you simply don't know.)
- "You are so brave," or "so strong." (Parents are not heroes; they are normal people struggling with extraordinary stress.)
- "They are doing such wonderful things to save children with cancer these days." (The prognosis might be good, but what parents and children are going through is not wonderful.)
- "Chemo killed my aunt/grandma/sister. That stuff is terrible. Those doctors can't really cure cancer." (Cancer is not a death sentence. Many people don't understand that cancer treatments for both adults and children have improved a great deal over the years.)
- "All those chemicals are unnatural! I learned about a guy whose cousin's daughter used kale juice/essential oils/shark cartilage/ground apricot pits/exotic spices instead." (Most people are well-meaning, but undermining a family's decision to seek evidence-based medical care for a child with a life-threatening illness is not supportive.)
- "It's God's will" or "Everything happens for a reason." (These are just not helpful things to hear.)

- "At least you have other kids," or "Thank goodness you are still young enough to have other children." (A child cannot be replaced.)

> *A woman whom I worked with, but did not know well, came up to me one day and out of the blue said, "When Erica gets to heaven to be with Jesus, He will love her." All I could think to say was, "Well, I'm sorry, but Jesus can't have her right now."*

Parents also suggest the following things:

- Rather than say, "Let us know if there is anything we can do," make a specific suggestion.

> *Many well-wishing friends always said, "Let me know what I can do." I wish they had just "done," instead of asking for direction. It took too much energy to decide, call them, make arrangements, etc. I wish someone would have said, "When is your clinic day? I'll bring dinner," or "I'll baby-sit Sunday afternoon so you two can go out to lunch."*

- Do not make personal comments about sick children in front of them, such as, "When will his hair grow back in?" "He's lost so much weight." or "She's so pale."

- Do not do things that require the parents to support you, such as repeatedly calling them up and crying.

Losing friends

It is an unfortunate reality that most parents of children with cancer lose some of their friends. For a variety of reasons, some friends just cannot cope and either suddenly disappear or gradually fade away.

> *We had friends and family we thought would be the greatest sources of support in the world. Yet, they pulled away from us and provided nothing in the way of help, emotional or otherwise. We also had friends that we never expected to understand step up in surprising ways. My wife's friend, Leslie, a busy single woman, actually negotiated time off with a new employer so she could fly from her home in Tampa and help out after Garrett's transplant. She stayed with us for over a week, then came back a few months later to do it again. A couple of my SCUBA diving buddies who we liked, but didn't know well, have since become our best friends. They would visit us in the hospital, bringing gifts for both of our kids, and giving us a much-needed break. They were the only folks who regularly came by when Garrett was home after the transplant and who always followed our strict rules without complaint. Of course, the best support we had was from other parents of kids with serious illnesses or problems.*

Telling your friends about cancer is difficult, but it's not as hard as keeping it a secret would be. Fighting this cancer has been a family effort and, frequently, an effort involving our larger circle of friends. The more people we've been able to call on for support, the better. We've had to keep in mind that we've had an opportunity to adjust. But, the news is brand new to our friends, and it can be a shock. People often don't know what to do or say when they've been told that someone they care about has cancer. After we've given them some time, and when they ask what they can do, we tell them something constructive: mow the lawn, take back the recyclables, go to the store, bring over a pizza on Friday night, whatever would help.

Before my son was diagnosed, I had no idea what this experience was like, and I try to remember that my friends don't really know either, unless I tell them. They can't know the sleepless nights, the anxiety over tests, the fear when your child says he doesn't feel well, or the terror that we might lose our precious child. Some of us have found great support and others none. I hope your family and friends come to your side.

I want to say that I hope that cancer does not become your life. For us, it used to be an "elephant in the living room," and now it's maybe a "zebra in the kitchen." There are times when it demands everything you can give, no doubt, but there will be moments when there is time for the rest of your life.

Chapter 19

Communication and Behavior

"When I approach a child, he inspires in me two sentiments:
tenderness for what he is, and respect for what he may become."

— Louis Pasteur

UNDER THE BEST OF CIRCUMSTANCES, child rearing is a daunting task. When parenting is complicated by a tremendous crisis such as childhood cancer, normal family life is disrupted, and all sorts of confusing and distressing feelings and behaviors may appear. When people are under great stress, they often behave in ways they would not under normal circumstances. In response, parenting styles may need to adjust to the frequently shifting needs and behaviors of the ill child and affected siblings.

This chapter discusses feelings that many children have about their disease and some emotional and behavioral changes that may arise in both children and parents. It also offers suggestions for maintaining effective communication and appropriate behavior within the family. Parents share stories about what they experienced and how they coped with their and their ill child's powerful, and sometimes overwhelming, emotions. For more stories about the emotions of siblings, please see Chapter 17, *Siblings*.

Communication

Chapter 1, *Diagnosis*, lists many of the feelings parents may have after their child's diagnosis of leukemia. It is helpful to remember that children, both the ill child and siblings, are also overwhelmed by strong feelings, and most often have fewer coping skills than adults. At different times and to varying degrees, children and teens may feel fearful, angry, resentful, powerless, violated, lonely, weird, inferior, incompetent, or betrayed. Children have to learn ways to deal with these strong feelings to prevent "acting out" behaviors (aggression, risk taking) or "acting in" behaviors (depression, withdrawal).

Good communication is the first step toward helping your family identify how cancer is affecting behavior and family functioning, and how family members can work with each other, and with professionals, to maintain a nurturing climate. Clear and loving communication with your children or teens is the foundation for trust. Children need to know from the very beginning that you will answer questions truthfully and take the time to talk about feelings.

Honesty

Children can face almost anything if they know their parents will be at their side. For your ill child and other children to feel secure, they must always know that they can depend on you to tell them the truth, be it good news or bad. This trust you build with your children reduces feelings of isolation and disconnection within the family.

> We were always very honest. We felt that if she couldn't trust us to tell her the truth, how scary that would be. I've seen a few incidents in the clinic of people with totally different styles who don't tell their kids the truth. I ran into the bathroom at the clinic crying after overhearing a mother who had deceived her child into coming to the clinic. Then he found out he needed a back poke and completely lost it. It makes me cringe. Children just have to be prepared. If they can't trust their parents, who can they trust?

Listening

Just trying to get through each day consumes most of a parent's time, attention, and energy. Thus, one of the greatest gifts parents can give their children is time—time when they are fully present in the moment and really focus on what their children are saying and the feelings that generate the words. This can be difficult when you are physically and emotionally exhausted. But children notice when you aren't really paying attention and are distracted by other thoughts and worries.

> After my relapse at age 13, the chemotherapy was much more difficult to tolerate. My appearance changed dramatically due to hair loss and rapid weight gain from prednisone. The L-asparaginase made my legs stiff and sore, so that it was difficult to walk. After a 2-month absence, when I returned to school, the treatment I received from the other students was unbearable. I finally refused to go to school. I felt so strongly about not going to school that once, on the way there, I jumped out of the car at an intersection. This helped mom and dad listen to me and make the decision to send me to a private school. The kids and staff at the new school knew my situation and were very compassionate. The decision to change schools was one of the best things my parents ever did for me.

Talking

If you are not in the habit of sharing your feelings with your children, it is hard to start doing so during a crisis. But now, more than ever, it is important to try. Parents can create an opening for discussion by simply stating how they are feeling, for example, "I have lots of different feelings at the same time. Sometimes I really get mad at the cancer because it is making your life so tough, but I am also happy that the medicine is working."

Telling your healthy children what you are feeling can strengthen your connection and reassure them of your love: "I really miss you when I have to take your sister to the hospital. I'll call you every night just so I can hear your voice," or "I wish the family didn't have to be separated so much, and I feel sad that you have to go through this." Such statements reassure children of your continued love for them and distress about being separated from them; they also create a chance for children to share with you how they feel about what is happening to the family.

> My daughter, diagnosed at 1 year old and now entering fifth grade, has three older siblings, so we have been through many developmental stages as far as communication goes. I try to answer their questions honestly, but I only tell them what I think they can understand without overwhelming them with information. I remember one of my boys, soon after my daughter's diagnosis, asked me if she was going to die, and I said "no" emphatically. I regretted it immediately, and realized that I would have to deal with my fears about the possibility of her dying, then go back and tell him the truth. So, later, I told him that I hadn't given an accurate answer because I was scared and that we didn't know if she was going to die. We hoped not, but we would have to wait and see. I have found that as their understanding deepens, they come back with more questions, needing more detailed answers. So, my motto is, be honest, but don't scare them. If you say everything is okay, but you are crying, they know something is wrong, and that they can't trust you for the truth.

Common Behavioral Changes in Children

Parenting is challenging, even when family life is going well. But when a child has cancer, parents are stressed, siblings may be angry or worried, and the ill child is scared and upset. Parents may find themselves reaching their emotional breaking points, and children may begin behaving in negative ways, making the situation very difficult.

The first step to improving family life is to decide whether the ill child is going to be treated as if she only has a few months to live, or as if she will survive and needs to learn strategies for how to manage difficult emotions. Step two is to examine your own behavior to see whether you are modeling the conduct you expect from your children.

If your child becomes angry or destructive, step three is to develop a consistent, healthy response to the behaviors to help him learn ways to deal with his strong emotions. In the following sections, parents share how they handled their children's range of emotions and behaviors.

Anger

Parents sometimes respond to the diagnosis of childhood cancer with anger, and so do children. Not only is the child angry at the disease, but also at the parents for bringing her in to be hurt, at having to take medicine that makes her feel terrible, at losing her hair, at losing her friends, and on and on. Children with cancer and their siblings have good reasons to be angry. The parents' task is to help the child learn to channel the anger appropriately.

We have a case of the halo or the horns. Our son is either very defiant or an absolute angel. He argues about every single thing. I really think that it is because he has had so little control in his life. I have very clear rules, am very firm, and put my foot down. But I also try to choose my battles wisely so we can have good times, too. My husband reminds me when I get aggravated that if he weren't this type of tough kid, he wouldn't have made it through so many setbacks. Then I am just glad to still have him with us.

· · · · ·

I was initially excited when my son finished treatment. I really expected to have a normal life again. In reality, the whole family had a hard time adjusting. He has a twin brother, and both boys had a very rough transition to junior high school. They were frequently in trouble and began failing most of their subjects. It added a lot of stress to our home life to have the principal calling us two to five times a week. Although we started counseling, we still had major blow-ups at home.

Tantrums

Healthy children have tantrums when they are overwhelmed by strong feelings, and so do children with cancer. In some cases, tantrums can be predicted by parents paying close attention to what triggers the outburst (for example, a missed nap or anxiety about an upcoming procedure). This knowledge can help parents prevent tantrums by avoiding situations that create emotional overload for their child; but sometimes there is no warning of the impending tantrum. It also helps to know that many tantrums and behavioral changes are due to medication side effects and are out of the child's control.

We never knew what would set off 3-year-old Rachel, and to tell the truth, she didn't know what the problem was herself. She was very verbal and aware in many ways, but she had no idea what was bothering her and causing the anger. I would just hold

her with her blanket, hug her, and rock until she calmed down. Later she would say,
"I was out of control," but she still didn't know why.

Of course, if your child is destructive, she needs help learning safer ways to vent her anger. A chapter in Larry Silver's book *The Misunderstood Child* (see Appendix C, *Books, Websites, and Support Groups*) explains in detail how parents can initiate a behavior modification program at home. For a child who is frequently destructive, professional counseling is needed.

When my son needed to get out a good old temper tantrum just to unload, I'd let him. Then he'd fall into my reassuring arms and soak up some good ole momma lovin' and just whimper till he slept...my hand stroking his hair, and I'm whispering things like, "I know, honey, I know. It's just so wrong. I'm here, baby. I love you. I know. I know. Just sleep for now. I'll be here when you wake. I'm not moving. I'm not going anywhere. I love you. There now."

Withdrawal

Some children deal with their feelings by withdrawing rather than blowing up in anger. Like denial, withdrawal can temporarily be helpful as a way to come to grips with strong feelings. However, too much withdrawal is not good for children, and it can be a sign of depression. Parents or counselors need to find gentle ways to allow withdrawn children to express how they feel.

My daughter became very depressed and withdrawn as treatment continued. She started to talk only about a fantasy world that she created in her imagination. She seemed to be less and less in the real world. She didn't ever talk to her therapist about her feelings, but they did lots of art work together. At the beginning, she only drew pictures of herself with her body filling the whole page. With time, she began to draw her body more normal sized. As she got better, she began to draw the family again. When she drew a beautiful sun shining on the family, I cried. She just couldn't talk about it, but she worked so much out through her art.

The emotional impact of cancer is very strong during the teenage years, a time when appearance is particularly important. When adolescents look different from their peers, they may feel sad, angry, embarrassed, bewildered, helpless, and scared. Teens may go through a period of withdrawal and/or grieving; it is crucial that they receive support and counseling during these times.

I had cancer when I was 15. I tried so hard as a freshman in college to put it all behind me and get on with my life. It just didn't work. Next to treatment, that was the worst year of my life. It showed me that if I didn't deal with it consciously, I was going to deal with it subconsciously. I had nightmares every night. I'd wake up feeling that I had needles in my arms. I decided to start taking better care of myself in a different kind of way. I do something fun every day. I try to see the positive side of situations. I read more and write a lot. I unplug from the cancer community whenever I feel overwhelmed. I try to explore my feelings with my counselor rather than shove them in the back corner. It's like garbage; if you don't take it out, it starts to stink. Once I started dealing with these feelings, things really improved.

Comfort objects

Some parents worry when, after diagnosis, children regress to using a special comfort object. Many young children ask to return to using a bottle, or cling to a favorite toy or blanket. It is reasonable to allow your child to use whatever he can to find comfort against the difficult realities of treatment. The behaviors usually stop either when the child starts feeling better or when treatment ends.

> *Matthew had a special teddy bear that a friend had bought for him in Germany. Mr. Bear, as he was called, went through everything Matthew went through. When he received cranial radiation, Mr. Bear had his skull irradiated, too. If Matthew needed oxygen, they both got a mask. That little teddy bear even had surgery a few times. Each time my son was admitted to the hospital, Mr. Bear went along and got his own hospital identification bracelet. They went through a lot together. It's amazing how much comfort he received from a stuffed toy.*

Talking about death

Part of effective parenting is allowing children to talk about topics that may cause feelings of discomfort in parents and children. No parent wants to talk, or even think, about the possibility of a child's death. In some cultures, the subject of death is taboo. But a diagnosis of cancer forces both parents and children to acknowledge that death is a very real possibility. Even children as young as age 3 may think about death and what it means. They need to be able to talk about their feelings, fears, or questions without their parents shutting down the conversation.

> *Eighteen months into treatment, 5-year-old Katy said, "Mommy, sometimes I think about my spirit leaving my body. I think my spirit is here (gesturing to the back of her head) and my body is here (pointing to her belly button). I just wanted you to know that I think about it sometimes."*

Trusting your child

Sometimes children will tell you what they need to do to persevere through this trial. Their coping choices may not be what the parents would choose—the decisions may even make the parents nervous. But it is the child or teen's way to make peace with the day-to-day reality of diagnosis and treatment.

More than half of my son's life has been hijacked by cancer (8 years) and he has had so little control. So, when he could be in control he was. He often chose not to communicate or make eye contact. Or he'd say, "I will do that but not right now." In the beginning, I was embarrassed and talked to him about cooperation. Then I decided it was my hang-up and his right. His life has really sucked for a long, long time. So, I let him decide how he wanted to communicate and participate, and I'm glad that I did.

• • • • •

Early one summer morning, 12-year-old Preston and I left the hospital after a week-long stay for chemotherapy. He had been heavily sedated and was groggy and shaky on his feet. My husband and daughter were getting ready to go on a boat trip, and I felt Preston was too sick to go. We sadly saw them off, then returned to the car. Preston said, "Mom, I really need to go fishing. I know you don't understand, but I really need to do this."

It made me very uncomfortable, but we went home to get his equipment. We then drove up to the mountains to a very deserted spot on the river, and Preston said that he needed to be out of my sight. So I watched him put on his waders, walk into the swift river, and disappear around a bend upstream. I went out into the river and sat on a rock. I waited for two hours before Preston came back. He said, "That's what I needed; I feel much better now."

There is a fine line between providing adequate protection for our children or teens and becoming overly controlling because of worry about the disease. You might ask yourself, "If she didn't have cancer, would I let her do this?"

Coping

Some children, because of both temperament and the environments in which they have lived, are blessed with good coping abilities. They understand what is required, and they do it. Many parents express great admiration for their child's strength and grace in the face of adversity. However, most children and parents have a hard time coping during parts of treatment, or throughout treatment. Help is available (e.g., private therapy, hospital social worker, or psychologist) if this is your situation.

My daughter, Lilly, did not have many coping skills due to preexisting mental issues and PTSD, and this was one of the biggest challenges during hospital visits. We were helped by a home therapist who came twice a week to the house and spent time teaching Lilly how to recognize emotions and healthy ways of dealing with them, as well as healthy ways to express anger, sadness, hurt, etc., rather than hurting herself or me.

. . . . .

Stephan has not had any behavior problems while being treated for his initial diag-
nosis (age 5) or his relapse (age 7). He has never complained about going to the hos-
pital and views the medical staff as his friends. He has never argued or fought about
painful treatments. Unlike many of the parents in the support group, we've never
had to deal with any emotional issues. We are fortunate that he has that confident
personality. He just says, "We've got to do it, so let's just get it done."

Common Behavioral Changes in Parents

It is impossible to talk about children's behavior without discussing parental behavior.
A child's development does not occur in a vacuum; it occurs within the context of the
family, and parents set the tone for their home's atmosphere. At different times during
their child's treatment, parents may be under enormous physical, emotional, financial,
and existential stress. The crisis can cause parents to act in ways that reflect their own
fear and lack of control—ways they would not behave under normal circumstances.
Some of the common problem behaviors mentioned by parents follow.

Dishonesty

As stated earlier, children feel safe when their parents are honest with them. If parents
start to keep secrets from a child to protect her from distressing news, she may feel
isolated and fearful. She might think, "If Mom and Dad won't tell me, it must be really
bad," or, "Mom won't talk about it. I guess there's nobody I can talk with about how
scared I am."

Denial is a type of unconscious dishonesty. This occurs when parents say things to
children such as, "Everything will be just fine," or, "It won't hurt a bit." This type of
pretending just increases the distance between child and parent, leaving the child with
no support. However horrible the truth, it seldom is as terrifying to a child as what he
imagines if he doesn't know the truth.

I try so hard to be honest with my 5-year-old son, but blood draws, which he thinks
of as "shots," are just so hard for him. Every doctor's visit, that's his first question,
"Am I going to get a shot?" and I just want to say no. My husband's the one who
started saying, "It'll be fine," but the anxiety that came up later at the appointment
was so much worse that I put an end to that pretty quickly. Now I say, "Yes, but just
once," because if I say, "I don't know," it just makes him worry.

Depression and anxiety

Parents of children with cancer often feel sad, depressed, or overwhelmingly anxious.
Responses to stress can include changes in sleeping patterns, appetite, and sex drive as

well as racing thoughts, poor concentration, suicidal thoughts, or drug/alcohol abuse. If you are consistently experiencing any of those symptoms, it may help to speak with a counselor or psychologist.

> *Find a counselor you click with. Stick with that person until you truly feel some peace about your experiences and strength for dealing with the ongoing stress of treatment or whatever else might come up. I regret that I toughed it out and didn't recognize the depression I was experiencing for such a long time. I think finding sources of support in a variety of ways at the earliest moment possible can greatly mitigate long-term difficulties in coping.*

If you have an underlying tendency toward anxiety or depression, having a child diagnosed with cancer can cause more symptoms. Depression and anxiety are extremely common and very treatable, and they should be dealt with early on.

> *It was two years after my son finished treatment that my depression became severe enough that I recognized it. I actually had a lot of suicidal thoughts and my husband urged me to see a doctor. He started me on Zoloft® and it has helped me tremendously.*

Losing your temper excessively

All parents lose their tempers sometimes. They lose their tempers with spouses, healthy children, pets, and even strangers. When you are living with the chronic stress of having a child with cancer, you may find that you lose your temper much quicker than in the past and over situations that normally wouldn't upset you. In part, this is because chronic stress leads to prolonged, higher cortisol levels—a hormone that is released as part of our "flight or fight" response.

There are many ways to naturally lower your cortisol levels, such as exercise, yoga, meditation, eating a healthy diet, watching a funny movie, and listening to music. Also, if you start to notice when you are close to losing your temper, get away from the situation until you can respond more calmly—take a walk, listen to music, do breathing exercises, find a private place to cry or yell, pet the family dog or cat, or ask another adult to step in and give you a break. Self-care is vital to preserving healthy relationships and avoiding saying or doing things you will later regret.

> *I had my share of temper tantrums. The worst was when my son was having his radiation. I tried to make him eat because it would be so many hours before he could have any more food. He always threw up all over himself and me, several times, every morning. It seemed like we changed clothing at least three times before we even got out of the house each day. I remember one day just screaming at him, "Can't you even learn how to throw up? Can't you just bend over to barf?" I really flunked*

mother of the year that day. I can't believe that I was screaming at this sick little kid, who I love so much.

Emotional and/or physical abuse of children and spouses may begin, or increase, when either or both spouses feel incompetent and powerless, and when there is chronic stress in their lives. If you find yourself unable to manage your temper, seek professional counseling immediately. Counseling can help you prevent or repair any damage your outbursts may have caused to your family relationships. It takes courage and strength to seek help. But asking for help is a sign that you care deeply about your family and want your home atmosphere to be healthier and happier.

I had always taught my children that feeling anger was okay, but we had to make good choices about what to do with it. Hitting other people or breaking things was a bad choice; running around outside, or punching pillows were good choices. But, as with everything else, they learned the most from watching how I handled my anger, and during the hard months of treatment my temper was short. When I found myself thinking of hitting them, I'd say, in a very loud voice, "I'm afraid I'm going to hurt somebody so I'm going in my room for a time-out." If my husband was home, I'd take a warm shower to calm down; if he wasn't, I'd just sit on the bed, cry, and take as many deep breaths as it took to calm down.

Unequal application of household rules

You will guarantee family problems if the ill child gets a pass while the siblings are asked to step up and do extra chores. Granted, it is hard to know the right time to insist that your ill child resume making his bed or setting the table, but it must be done. Siblings need to know from the beginning that any child in the family, if sick, will be excused from chores, but that she will have do them again as soon as she is physically able.

I spoiled my sick daughter and tried to enforce the rules for my son. That didn't work, so I gave up on him and spoiled them both. He was really acting out at school. What he needed was structure and more attention, but what he got was more and more things. They both ended up thinking the whole world revolved around them, and it was my fault.

Overindulgence of the ill child

Overindulgence is a very common behavior of parents of children with cancer. There are a variety of reasons for this: parents are trying to make up for the suffering their child is enduring or they are trying to make other parts of the child's life more enjoyable. In some cases, parents overindulge their sick child because it makes the parents feel better.

I bought my daughter everything I saw that was pretty and lovely. I kept thinking that if she died she would die happy because she'd be surrounded by all these beautiful things. Even when I couldn't really afford it, I kept buying. I realize now that I was doing it to make me feel better, not her. She needed cuddling and loving, not clothes and dolls.

· · · · ·

Four days into Selah's diagnosis, we were doing anything to keep her happy. Our sweet little 4 year old had turned into a demon child in that short time. Luckily, my very dear friend took me outside into the hallway, pushed me against the wall, and demanded to know exactly what I was doing. I just looked at her and said, "I have no idea." I just didn't want my daughter to die and that was my only focus. She then told me I was giving my daughter no boundaries, no behavior expectations, and she had no respect for anyone who walked into the room. Through my tears and our hugs, she assured me that the way we were going, if she didn't die from cancer, we were going to want to kill her because of the monster we were creating. I am still so grateful that she wasn't afraid to tell me what I needed to hear.

Not spending enough time with the sibling(s)

While acknowledging that there are only so many hours in a day, parents interviewed for this book felt the most guilt about the effect that diagnosis and treatment had on the siblings. They wished they had asked family and friends to stay with the sick child more often, allowing them to spend more of their precious time with the siblings. Many expressed pain that they didn't know how severely affected the siblings had been.

I try to find some time in each holiday, weekend, or whenever that is just for Christopher and me. No matter how ill Michael is, someone else can cope with it for an hour or two, and nothing is allowed to interfere with that. We still go out, even if it is only Christopher and me at McDonald's®. Bottom line is that all mothers have to accept that along with the baby is delivered a large package of guilt, and whatever we do for one we will wish we had done for the other. But I don't think you can put one child on hold for the duration of the other's illness, because the year that Christopher has lost while Michael has been ill won't ever come again. He'll only be 11 once, just as surely as Michael will only be 14 once (or possibly forever), and we owe it to our healthy kids to allow them to be just that.

Using substances to cope

Some parents find themselves turning to alcohol or drugs to help them cope. Some parents use illegal drugs for stress relief and escape, while others overuse over-the-counter and prescription drugs. If you find yourself drinking so much that your behavior is affected, or using drugs to get through the day or night, seek professional help.

Coping

Many parents find unexpected reserves of strength and are able to ask for help from friends and family when they need it. They realize that different needs arise when there is a great stress to the family, and they alter their expectations and parenting accordingly. Parents and families that had strong and effective communication prior to the illness most often pull together as a unit to deal with it. Most families, however, have periods of calm alternating with times when nerves are frayed and tempers are short. In the end, most families survive intact and are often strengthened by the years of dealing with cancer.

Improving Family Life

Parents suggest the following ways to keep the family more emotionally balanced.

- Make sure the family rules are clearly understood by all of the children. Stressed children feel safe in homes with regular, predictable routines.

    After yet another rage by my daughter with cancer, we held a family meeting to clarify the rules and consequences for breaking them. We asked the kids (both preschoolers) to dictate a list of what they thought the rules were. The following was the result, and we posted copies of the list all over the house (which created much merriment among our friends):

    1. No peeing on rug

    2. No jumping on bed

    3. No hitting or pinching

    4. No name calling

    5. No breaking things

    6. No writing on walls

    If they broke a rule, we would gently lead them to the list and remind them of the house rules. It really helped.

- Have all caretakers consistently enforce the family rules.

    We kept the same household rules. I was determined that we needed to start with the expectation that Rachel was going to survive. I never wanted her to be treated like a "poor little sick kid," because I was afraid she would become one. We had to be careful about babysitters, because we didn't want anyone to feel sorry for her or treat her differently. I do feel that we avoided many long-term behavior problems by adopting this attitude early.

- Give all the kids some power by offering choices and letting them completely control some aspects of their lives, as appropriate.

  For a few months we ignored Shawn's two brothers as we struggled to get a handle on the situation. We just shuttled them around with no consideration for their feelings. When we realized how unfair we were being, we made a list of places to stay, and let them choose each time we had to go off to the hospital. We worked it out together, and things went much smoother.

- Take control of the incoming gifts. Too many gifts may cause the ill child to worry ("If I'm getting all of these great presents, things must be really bad") and the siblings to feel jealous. Be specific if you prefer that people not bring or send gifts, or if you prefer gifts for each child, not just the sick one.

  Paige has a sister, Chelsea, who was 5 at diagnosis, and a brother, Dan, who was 4 months old. Chelsea had a very difficult time. She didn't like it that Paige was getting so many presents, and she often felt left out. When I would try to do something special for her, she would get mad—she just wanted normalcy.

- Recognize that some problems are caused solely by treatment. It helps to remember that children with cancer are not naturally defiant or destructive. They are feeling sick, powerless, and altered by surgery, radiation, and/or drugs, and parents need to try to help by sympathizing, yet setting limits. Remember, with time, their real personalities will return.

  In the beginning, my 2-year-old daughter was incredibly angry. She would have massive temper tantrums, and I would just hold her until she changed from angry to sad. When she was on certain chemotherapy drugs, she would either be hugging me or pinching, biting, or sucking my neck. It drove me crazy. Now she's not having as many fits, but she still pushes her sisters off swings or the trampoline. She has a general lack of control. Sometimes, when I can't stand it anymore, I swat her on the bottom, and then I feel really bad.

- If your child likes to draw, paint, knit, collage, or do other artwork or crafts, encourage it. Art is both soothing and therapeutic, and it gives children a positive outlet for feelings and creativity. This is true for kids with cancer and their siblings.

  Recently, when Cami was going through another "This-is-the-last-time-I'm-going-to-the-doctor" outburst, we spent the waiting time writing a list of all the horrible things we want to do to cancer (step on it; put needles in its eye; not let it have cake). I also draw cells—good and bad. We give lollipops to the good cells and scribble out the bad ones. It sounds simplistic, but it really helps.

- Allow your child to be totally in charge of her art. Listen carefully if your child offers an explanation about the art, but do not pry if he says it is private. Being supportive will allow your child to explore ways to soothe himself and clarify strong feelings.

    Jody was continually making projects. We kept him supplied with a fishing box full of materials, and he glued and taped and constructed all sorts of sculptures. He did beautiful drawings full of color, and every person he drew always had hands shaped like hearts. If we asked him what he was making, he always answered, "I'll show you when I'm done."

- If your child does artwork or likes to write, recognize that powerful emotions may surface for both child and parents.

    At my daughter's preschool, once a week each child would tell the teacher a story, which the teacher wrote down for the child to take home. Most of my daughter's prediagnosis stories were like this: "There was a rhinoceros. He lived in the jungle. Then he went in the pool. Then he decided to take a walk. And then he ate some strawberries. Then he visited his friend." But during treatment, she would dictate frightening stories (and this from a kid who wasn't allowed to watch TV and had never seen any violence). Two examples are: "Once there were some bees and they stung someone and this someone was allergic to them and then they got hurt by some monkeybars and the monkeybars had needles on them and the lightning came and hit the bees," and, "Once upon a time there were six stars and they twinkled at night and then the sun started to come up. And then they had a serious problem. They shot their heads and they had blood dripping down."

- Come up with acceptable ways for your child to physically release her anger. Some options are: ride a bike, run around the house, swing, play basketball or soccer, pound nails into wood, mold clay, punch pillows, yell, take a shower or bath, or draw angry pictures. In addition, teach your child to use words to express his anger, for example, "It makes me so angry when you do that," or "I am so mad I feel like hitting you." Releasing anger physically and expressing anger verbally in appropriate ways are both valuable life skills to master.

    Our kids go along okay for a while, dealing with stuff. Then suddenly (because they're tired, have reached a new point developmentally, or are not feeling well in a way they can't describe), they lose it. It seems that every kid needs something different at these times, but what works best for Cami is for us to help her find words for her frustration. We talk about how unfair cancer is, how terrible treatment is, how no one else really knows what she's going through. Sometimes she just bursts out crying with relief that someone understands!

· · · · ·

Shawn was very, very angry many times. We had clear rules that it was okay to be angry, but he couldn't hit people. We bought a punching bag, which he really pounded sometimes. Play-Doh® helped, too. We had a machine to make Play-Doh® shapes, which took a lot of effort. He would hit it, pound it, push it, roll it. Then he would press it through the machine and keep turning that handle. It seemed to really help him with his aggression.

• Get professional help whenever you are concerned or run out of ideas about how to handle emotional problems. Mental health professionals (see Chapter 21, *Sources of Support*) have spent years learning how to help resolve these kinds of problems, so let them help your family.

Every possible grouping of our family has been in therapy at one point or another. We have all done individual therapy, family therapy, and my husband and I did couples therapy. I feel that each of these sessions was a gift to our family. It helped us vent, cry, plan, and forge stronger bonds. We are all happy together many years after our daughter's cure, and every single penny we spent was worth it.

• Most emotional problems resulting from cancer treatment can be resolved through professional counseling. However, some children and parents also need medications to get them through particularly rough times.

My daughter was doing really well throughout treatment until a combination of events occurred that was more than she could handle. Her grandmother died from cancer during the summer, one of her friends with cancer died on December 27, then another friend relapsed for the second time. She was fine during the day, but at night she constantly woke up stressed and upset. She had dreams about trapdoors, witches brewing potions to give to little children, and saw people coming into her room to take her away. She would wake up smelling smoke. She was awake three or four hours in the middle of the night, every night. Her doctor put her on sleeping pills and anti-anxiety medications, and the social worker came out to the house twice a month.

• Have reasonable expectations. If you are expecting a sick 4 year old to act like a healthy 4 year old, or a teenager to act like an adult, you are setting your child up to fail.

It seemed like we spent most of the years of treatment waiting to see a doctor who was running hours behind schedule. Since my child had trouble sitting still and was always hungry, I came well prepared. I always carried a large bag containing an assortment of things to eat and drink, toys to play with, coloring books and markers, books to read aloud, and Play-Doh®. He stayed occupied and we avoided many problems. I saw too many parents in the waiting room expecting their bored children to sit still and be quiet for long periods of time.

- As often as possible, try to end the day on a positive note. If your child is being disruptive, or if you are having negative feelings about your child, here is an exercise you can use to end the day in a pleasant way. At bedtime, parent and child each tell one another something they did that day that made them proud of themselves, something they like about themselves, something they like about each other, and something they are looking forward to the next day. Then a hug and a sincere "I love you" bring the day to a calm and loving close.

Our children look to us to learn how to handle adversity. They learn how to cope from us. Although it is extremely difficult to live through your child's diagnosis and treatment, it must be done. So, we each need to reach deep into our hearts and minds to help our children have hope, endure, and grow.

I used a method with my son that I called, "Why are we here?" I used it for everything from IV pokes to taking meds. Anything we needed him to cooperate with got the "Why are we here" talk. He was 3 ½ when he was diagnosed and parenting him and guiding/coaching him through procedures is something I'm pretty proud of.

Before a blood test, for example, I would say, "Why are we here? We can't see what is going on inside your body, but your blood tells us a story. It can tell us how you're doing and how healthy your body is and how to help you feel better. But we need to take some blood out to be able to find all this out. How do you think we should get it?" This made my son feel empowered and he would offer suggestions and make some of the decisions. Once he has chosen to cooperate on his own terms, he could move on; we just need to give him the tools to do it. Many times, he still wouldn't want to, but now he understands why we have to.

There can always be choices. Do you want to use freezing cream so it hurts less? Do you want the nurse to take it from your hand or arm? Which arm, right or left? Do you want mom or dad to help you? Hold you? Do you want a treat for cooperating? (The treat box didn't work for long for us.) Do you want to watch?

Explain clearly what is expected of him. Acknowledge that it will hurt. Tell him that I'll be right there with him so he doesn't have to do it alone. Sometimes we would ask him how the nurse is supposed to do it to make sure she/he did things according to his preference. Kids watch everything so they know things like cleaning the arm takes 30 seconds of wiping, or you clean the port site with three cleaning sticks and let it dry before poking. Consistency with details like that can cut down on anxiety.

Chapter 20

School

*"Most of us had two feelings at the same time: wanting
to go back to school and being scared of going back."*

— Eleven children with cancer
There Is a Rainbow Behind Every Dark Cloud

CHILDREN AND TEENS WITH LEUKEMIA have disruptions in their education because of frequent hospitalizations and side effects from the disease or treatment. As their health improves and their treatment schedule allows, returning to school can be a relief or a challenge.

For many children, school is a refuge from the world of hospitals and procedures—a place for fun, friendship, and learning. School is the defining structure of children's daily lives and returning to school can signal hope for the future and a return to normalcy. Some children and teens, however, may dread returning to school because of temporary or permanent changes to their appearance or concerns that prolonged absences may have changed their social standing with friends.

In addition, physical limitations caused by cancer treatment may prevent children from participating in games, physical education class, athletics, or other activities. These physical impairments sometimes require time out from the regular classroom for physical or occupational therapy. School can also become a major source of frustration for children who learn differently because of treatment.

Although educating children who have or had cancer can be a complex process, many challenges can be successfully managed through careful planning and good communication. This chapter covers ways to work with the school during and after treatment. It also includes information about avoiding communicable illnesses at school and getting any help your child needs to learn.

Keeping the School Informed

A school-aged child diagnosed with leukemia is usually admitted to a children's hospital (sometimes far from home) and will not be able to return to school for weeks or months. To prevent your child from being dropped from school rolls due to nonattendance, you need to notify the school in writing about your child's medical situation. This notification allows planning to begin for your child to return to school or to receive hospital- or home-based schooling when able. Following is a sample letter, reprinted with permission from Sharon Grandinette, Exceptional Education Services.

Date

Dear [Name of Principal],

Our child, [name of your child], [date of birth], a student at [name of school], was diagnosed with leukemia in [month/year] and is hospitalized. He is unable to attend school at this time, and will undergo treatment with chemotherapy for [length of treatment].

We are requesting that a Student Study Team meeting be scheduled with the school nurse in attendance. The purpose of the meeting is to discuss [your child's name] current medical status and how it may affect [his/her] school attendance and functioning. [Your child's name] may require accommodations or special education services, and we would like to discuss those options at the meeting. Depending on [your child's name] medical status, we may be able to attend the meeting in person, but if not, we request that it take place by phone.

Please send us the appropriate release forms so that we can authorize an exchange of information between the school and the medical professionals treating [your child's name].

Sincerely,

[Parent/guardian name(s) and contact information]

Your child may want to send a letter to her class, which can help the teacher begin one of many discussions about why the classmate isn't in school. The letter below was sent by 7-year-old Madison to her classmates. It was handwritten and decorated with beautiful red hearts.

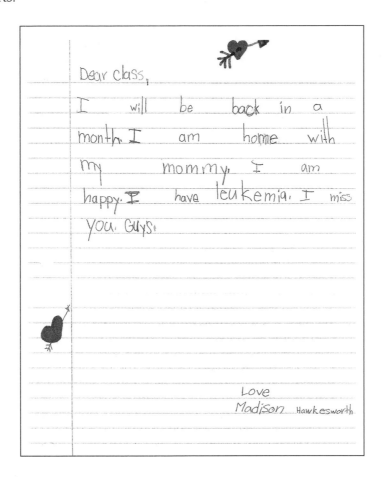

Dear class,

I will be back in a month. I am home with my mommy. I am happy. I have leukemia. I miss you. Guys.

Love
Madison Hawkesworth

Treatments for leukemia (e.g., chemotherapy, radiation, and stem cell transplantation) may cause changes in children's behavior and ability to function in school, both during and after treatment. Thus, the study team meeting can lay the foundation for any needed support or accommodations.

At the meeting, you may wish to distribute booklets about how to help children with cancer in the classroom, as well as age-appropriate information that can be shared with the classmates. You can create a communicable disease notification strategy, if needed, and do your best to build a rapport with the entire school staff. Take this chance to express appreciation for the school's help and your hopes for a close collaboration in the future to create a supportive climate for your child.

> *My daughter Julia was diagnosed with T-cell ALL when she was in second grade. We had her tutored at home by a district-sponsored, certified teacher and it was a great experience. She received the tutoring right through the end of the school year. (She started around mid-January with the tutoring, and it continued through June.) The teacher we had was fabulous, and Julia stayed caught up with (and even ahead of) her class. Our school district has everything in place for kids who, for medical reasons, need to be tutored at home. I think it was much less stressful than trying to get into school for a day or two at a time and not being able to keep track of homework. Plus, we didn't have to worry about all the germs floating around. When Julia went back to school last year, she had no adjustment problems and did very well.*

At the meeting, the school will assign a person (e.g., child's teacher, guidance counselor, special education expert) to communicate with a designated person at the hospital (e.g., school liaison).

> *I still feel unbelievable gratitude when I think of the school principal and my daughter's kindergarten teacher that first year. The principal's eyes filled with tears when I told her what was happening, and she said, "You tell us what you need and I'll move the earth to get it for you." She hand-picked a wonderful teacher for her, made sure that an illness notification plan was in place, and kept in touch with me for feedback. She recently retired, and I sent her a glowing letter, which I copied to the school superintendent and school board. Words can't express how wonderful they were.*

· · · · ·

> *We had a very difficult time with the school. They viewed my daughter as another problem they had to deal with. Her first grade teacher was impatient with her, at one point telling her she was too slow getting ready for the bus home, and closing her in the room by herself. The door was too heavy for her to open (she was weak from chemo and radiation), and another parent heard her crying, got her out, and put her on the bus. We withdrew her from that school and homeschooled her.*

The designated liaisons will work to keep information flowing between the hospital and school and will help pave the way for a successful school reentry for your child. The liaison from the hospital should encourage questions and address any concerns the school staff have about having a seriously ill child in the school. The hospital liaison may also help school staff understand how the child's illness might affect school attendance or performance. Privacy laws prohibit liaisons from communicating unless parents sign a release form authorizing the school and hospital to share information. These forms are available at schools and hospitals.

Robby was diagnosed in January of his kindergarten year. He returned to kindergarten the same day he got out of the hospital. His teacher was wonderful. She moved the desks around in the classroom so that if Robby got tired, she would go get his cot and put it in the center of the classroom so he could lay down and still listen. If a child had a cold, she would move him/her to the other side of the classroom. The kids washed their hands at least four times a day. The teacher's aide would sit in the rocking chair holding Robby if he was sad (prednisone days). Also on prednisone days, Robby was allowed to have his lunch box, which weighed at least 10 pounds a day, at his desk, and he could eat all day.

In the months and years after diagnosis, try to maintain an open and amicable relationship with the school in the hope that your child, who may be emotionally or physically fragile, continues to be welcomed and nurtured.

Keeping the Teacher and Classmates Involved

While your child is hospitalized, it helps to stay connected with the teacher and classmates. Parents can call the teacher periodically and send notes or audiotaped messages from their child to classmates. Following are some suggestions for keeping the teacher and classmates involved with your child's life:

- Have the hospital's school liaison give a presentation to your child's class about what is happening and how their classmate may look and feel when he returns to school. This talk should include a question and answer session to clear up misconceptions and alleviate fears. All children, especially teenagers, should be involved in deciding what information will be discussed with classmates and whether or not the child/teen wants to be present.

- Encourage your child's classmates to keep in touch. The class can make a card or banner or send a group photo. Individual students can call on the phone or send notes, emails, text messages, or pictures.

- If possible, use Skype®, FaceTime®, or a similar webcam software application to allow your child to interact "face-to-face" with classmates using a laptop, tablet, or smartphone. Use of this technology provides a chance for classmates to see changes in appearance as they gradually occur during treatment. This may lessen the surprise about changes in appearance when your child returns to school.

My daughter missed 13 months of school (all of kindergarten). Most of that time, she was in the hospital. The district sent a tutor two to three times a week. A foundation called Omar's Dream (http://omarsdream.org) provided an iPad® for home/hospital and one for the classroom. This allowed her to Skype® into class to participate, talk to classmates, and be part of the parties. Her classmates saw what she looked like and it made the transition back much easier. She was ahead academically at diagnosis, so she wasn't behind when she returned to school.

Keeping Up with Schoolwork

As treatment progresses, your child may return to school either part time or full time, but extended absences due to infections or complications from treatment are common. A child who is out of school longer than two weeks for any medical reason is entitled by law to instruction at home or in the hospital. It is a good idea to request offsite instruction as soon as you find out your child may be out of school for longer than two weeks. The school will require a letter from the doctor stating the reason and expected length of time offsite instruction will be needed. Four ways to continue education are:

1. Homebound or hospital education

2. Video teleconferencing of classes

3. Online classes

4. Homeschooling by parents

If your child is hospitalized far from home, the hospital will provide onsite teachers or make arrangements with teachers from the local community. If your child is hospitalized close to home or is at home but cannot attend school, your school district provides the teacher (called a homebound teacher). The hospital teacher or homebound teacher is responsible for gathering materials from the child's school.

> Communication was the key. I wrote weekly updates and made copies for each teacher, put their names on them, and delivered them to school. I learned that a single copy of a letter didn't get passed around to everyone. (Joel was in high school.) Some classes used a tape recorder; they all kept a record of what he'd missed. His math teacher got together with the librarian and arranged to videotape his math classes. They did so much on the board, on overheads, and with discussion in that class that an audiotape would not have helped. All teachers were willing to meet with him after or before school to essentially reteach the concepts that he had missed.
>
> I also told his teachers it was okay to discuss Joel, his leukemia, and his treatment with the other kids in his classes. They would never have done it without my okay. I knew that in the absence of information, there would be rumors flying. This might not work for everyone, but it served us well.

Technology provides many ways to keep up with schoolwork. For example, some school systems provide a computer so the student can keep up via teleconferencing and online classes. In some cases, parents choose to homeschool their child. Check with your local school district to find out the requirements for homeschooling.

We used Skype® and had a weekly time set up so that Patrik could see his class-mates, and they could see him. If an oral presentation was due, he heard a few of theirs, and presented his. If nothing shareable was due, they just traded jokes or did a show and tell of something that had happened that week. If he was not feeling well or was hospitalized, it was cancelled for that week. It sure helped make him still feel a part of his class, and the teacher said it really helped his classmates to see he was still okay, and still himself. He wasn't allowed to attend school at all for frontline treatment (almost 10 months). Patrik started the first day of 5th grade this year. He was able to walk in the building, feel welcome, and step right back into his friend-ships. No problems at all with that. I really thank his teacher last year for keeping him a part of his class despite not being in school.

• • • • •

One thing we did in the hospital was ABC Reading Eggs®—an online learn-to-read app (http://readingeggs.com). There were of course times where we wasted hours watching TV and DVDs, but we also encouraged Flynn academically—we didn't try hard, just provided alternative opportunities. By doing Reading Eggs® and by always having books on hand, he learned to read very young. I was always so proud of this because the chemo took away so much of my boy, but it was all only temporary. I think he was clever to realize that reading was an excellent form of distraction, and even now at 6.5 years old he will still go to his room to read when he's upset. By escaping into his world of books, he becomes calm and happy once again. I will be forever grateful for this positive that emerged from the darkness.

Helping Siblings

The diagnosis of cancer affects all members of the family. Siblings can be overlooked when the parents need to spend most of their time caring for the ill child. Many sib-lings feel frustrated, angry, frightened, neglected, or guilty, but they may try to keep their feelings bottled up to prevent placing extra burdens on their parents. Often, these complicated feelings emerge at school. Siblings may cry easily, fall behind in classwork, do poorly on tests, cut classes, challenge teachers, or withdraw from friends or school activities.

Lindsey was in kindergarten when Jesse was first diagnosed. Because we heard nothing from the kindergarten teacher, we assumed that things were going well. At the end of the year, the teacher told us that Lindsey frequently spent part of each day hiding under her desk. When I asked why we had never been told, the teacher said she thought that we already had enough to worry about dealing with Jesse's illness and treatment. She was wrong to make decisions for us, but I wish we had been more attentive. Lindsey needed help.

To help prevent problems from developing, you can send a letter to each sibling's school principal requesting that teachers, counselors, and nurses be informed of the cancer diagnosis in the family and asking for their help with, and support for, the siblings.

If possible, try to include the siblings' teachers in some of the school discussions concerning the ill child. Teachers of siblings need to be aware that the stressors facing the family may cause the siblings' feelings to bubble to the surface during class. Chapter 17, *Siblings*, deals exclusively with siblings and contains tips about how to help them cope.

Returning to School

Preparation is the key to a successful return to school. You and the hospital school liaison may want to prepare a package for the school staff that contains the following information:

- A doctor's statement that describes your child's health status; ability to safely return to the school environment; physical restrictions, including any limits to physical education or recess; and possible attendance disruptions.

    My son was diagnosed at age 14. He was starting ninth grade, the last year of junior high. He missed about a third of that year. He was able to keep up, thanks to some terrific teachers and a very cooperative administration, not to mention being a really motivated kid. He hated missing school and would go even when he didn't feel very good, just to say he'd been to school that day, even if only for two periods.

- Whether your child will attend full or half days.
- A description of any changes in physical appearance, such as weight changes or hair loss, and suggestions about how to help classmates handle them appropriately.

    Jeremy's kindergarten teacher was the pits. Jeremy was on chemotherapy, and she told Jeremy not to wash his hands, as it took too long. I was disappointed that even after the nurse came to class and gave a presentation, the kids still teased my son. They would say things like, "You've got Jeremy germs; you are going to catch cancer," and "You can't get rid of cancer; you always die." During his kindergarten year, Jeremy needed to have heart surgery. I called the teacher to let her know, but my son did not hear from anyone in his class, not one card or phone call, even from the teacher. She didn't even tell the class why Jeremy was absent.

- A request that your bald child be permitted to wear a wig, hat, or scarf to school.
- An explanation of possible effects medications may have on academic performance and a list of medications or other health services that will need to be provided at school (see section later in this chapter called "Individual healthcare plan").

- A list of signs and symptoms requiring parent notification (e.g., fever, nausea, vomiting, pain, swelling, bruising, or nosebleeds) and notification procedures to be followed.

- Concerns about exposure to communicable diseases, if needed (e.g., if you live in an area with low immunization rates, you will need to know whenever students in the school have chicken pox, whooping cough, measles, or mumps).

- Any accommodations needed, such as extra snacks, rest periods, extra time to get from class to class, use of the nearest restroom (even if it is the staff restroom), and the need for restroom breaks without permission. This list should also include any requests for academic accommodations such as extended time for tests, reduced workload, or access to online textbooks. (These services are discussed in greater detail later in this chapter.)

> *My 16-year-old son was allowed to leave each textbook in his various classrooms. This prevented him from having to carry a heavy backpack all day. They also let him out of class a few minutes early because he was slower moving from room to room.*

School reentry plans require peer education and teacher education, but the guiding principle should be meeting the individual needs of the returning student. Therefore, frequent communication among school personnel, parents, the student, and the hospital liaison is vital before, during, and after school reentry. The following are parent suggestions for preventing problems through preparation and communication:

- Keep the school informed and involved from the beginning to foster a "we're all in this together" spirit.

- Bring a pediatric oncology nurse or school liaison into the classroom to talk about childhood cancer, explain that it is not contagious, and answer questions. Make sure to ask whether your child wants to be part of the presentation. If treatment is lengthy, this should be done at the beginning of each school year to prepare new classmates. Because the sick child may be given accommodations that could cause other students to feel upset or jealous, the nurse or school liaison should explain that the student has some different rules because of the illness.

> *Elizabeth was in preschool at the time of her diagnosis. The manager did a wonderful job of integrating her back into the fold. All of the other children at the school were taught what was happening to Elizabeth and what would be happening (such as hair loss). They learned that they had to be gentle with her when playing. The manager was a former home health nurse, so I was very confident that she would be able to take care of my daughter in the event of an emergency. She was already familiar with central lines and side effects from chemotherapy. She was a gem!*

- Arrange places for your child to rest if she is too tired to participate in class.

- Have a mental health therapist talk with your child about his emotions and life both inside and outside of school.

My son Zachary has been out of school for over a year. Zachary received a stem cell transplant, and school was not an option for him in the months afterwards. He is taught by a teacher provided by our county for "homebound" students. She's great, and Zach is ahead of the regular second grade curriculum. Zach is so comfortable with his teacher that he doesn't want to return to school in the fall. He feels everyone will think he's weird and will tease him. I realize this is an important issue for him, so he is seeing a therapist in preparation for return to school.

- Realize that teachers and other school staff can be frightened, overwhelmed, or discouraged by having a child with a life-threatening illness in their classroom. Accurate information and words of appreciation can provide much-needed support.

It can be so helpful for the school staff to have periodic meetings to address concerns, fears, progress, or to learn about upcoming procedures. I don't think enough parents know they can request meetings (for an Individual Education Plan [IEP] or otherwise) as they feel the need, and so can school staff. When Matt started elementary school, I requested monthly inclusion meetings with his IEP team for the first semester and then every other month during the second semester. We wrote this in his IEP so it actually happened. I learned to do this from a parent much wiser than me!

A helpful and free handbook for school personnel is available at *www.lhsc.on.ca/Patients_ Families_Visitors/Childrens_Hospital/Programs_and_services/HelpingSchools.pdf.*

Avoiding Communicable Diseases

The dangers of communicable diseases to immunosuppressed children are discussed in Chapter 14, *Common Side Effects of Treatment.* Parents of children with low white blood cell counts need to work closely with the school to develop a plan for outbreaks of chicken pox, whooping cough, measles, mumps, or flu if the school does not already have a communicable disease notification plan in place. If you know that children at school have these illnesses, you can keep your child at home. If your child is exposed to an illness at school, the school should immediately notify you so you can tell the oncologist.

Several methods can be used to ensure rapid reporting of outbreaks. Some parents notify all the classmates' parents by letter to ask them for prompt reports of illness. If you have a good rapport with the teacher, ask that he or she immediately tell you about any cases of communicable disease.

My daughter's preschool was very concerned and organized about the disease reporting. They noted on each child's folder whether he or she was immunized against measles, whooping cough, and chicken pox. They told each parent individually about the dangers to Katy, and then frequently reminded everyone in the monthly newsletters. The parents were absolutely great, and we always had time to keep her out of school until there were no new cases.

Other parents enlist the help of the office staff who answer the phone calls from parents of absent children.

We asked the two ladies in the office to write down the illness of any child in Mrs. Williams' class. That way the teacher could check daily and call me if any of the kids in her class were ill.

After Treatment

State-of-the-art treatment for childhood cancer has resulted in greater numbers of long-term survivors, but not without cost. Radiation, chemotherapy, and stem cell transplant can cause changes in learning abilities, motor skills, and social skills. Parents and educators need to remain vigilant for these changes and intervene as early as possible. Teachers and other school personnel may not be aware of how long-term effects can influence learning potential and school performance. The hospital school liaison can provide materials to help school personnel understand these issues, and can attend school meetings to provide additional information. Regardless of where your child is on the treatment continuum, there are federal laws that will assist you in the process of obtaining appropriate educational services for your child.

Federal Laws

Two federal laws protect the education rights of children ages 0 to 22 who have disabilities that affect education—Section 504 of the Rehabilitation Act of 1973 and the Individuals with Disabilities Education Act (IDEA). These laws guarantee every public school student the right to education regardless of physical, mental, or health impairment. Every state has a department of education website that describes state guidelines about how these laws are implemented and ways to obtain more information.

Examples of impairments affecting school performance that may develop during or after treatment for childhood leukemia include the following:

- Problems with small motor and gross motor skills (temporary or permanent) due to vincristine neuropathy
- Learning disabilities
- Difficulties with attention
- Slow processing speed
- Post-traumatic stress, depression, and anxiety
- Hormonal issues (e.g., chronic fatigue)

No matter how good your relationship is with the school, any services needed by your child should be documented in a written and signed Individual Education Plan (IEP) or 504 Plan (see information about both below). A written plan will document your child's legal right to services and accommodations, and if your family moves, the new school will be legally required to follow the former school's plan until a new one is agreed upon and put into place.

Section 504 of the Rehabilitation Act of 1973

Some children are eligible for services under Section 504 of the Rehabilitation Act whether on or off treatment. Commonly referred to as Section 504, this civil rights law prohibits discrimination against any individual with a physical or mental impairment that substantially limits one or more major life activity. Section 504 comes into play when a student with a disability attending a public school—or any private school, college, or university that receives federal funds—needs accommodation to access the educational opportunities available to children who are not disabled. Children who do not need special education services can be eligible for an educational plan under Section 504.

The school's Section 504 team determines whether a child is eligible for a 504 Plan based on information from a variety of sources, including the findings and recommendations of the treatment team about how the illness and treatment affect school participation. For example, a child being treated for leukemia might need a Section 504 Plan that provides:

- Exemption from regular attendance/tardy policies
- A school-based health plan
- Reduced homework when ill or hospitalized
- Occupational and/or physical therapy

Section 504 can also be used when a student who is off treatment has disabilities that do not meet the requirements of the IDEA but do limit one or more major life activity. For example, a student who has fine motor problems might need a 504 Plan to obtain accommodations such as physical therapy, a note taker, and less written homework than other students. Schools are not required to provide a written 504 Plan, but parents should request a written plan that specifically lays out all of the accommodations and educational services to be provided to the student. The approved plan should be signed by school personnel and parents.

> My 14-year-old daughter has some difficulties in school related to organization and memory (e.g., remembering to turn in homework on time). She got her first 504 Plan in second grade that provided a tutor for two hours for every day of school that she missed. It carried over to middle school, and they sent a special ed teacher who

came by the house once a week to check on assignments, which was a big help. In middle school, I found out that they kept her in from recess once for not turning in an assignment, so we modified the 504 Plan to say that she would not be punished or marked down as long as she took all tests and turned in all assignments by the end of each semester. That way, if she forgot something, she could turn it in late and still get credit. In high school, we've had been a bit more trouble in implementing the 504 Plan. So, she's going to have a neuropsych exam so we can figure out her strengths and challenges and work with the school to get her any accommodations she needs to succeed.

Individuals with Disabilities Education Act (IDEA)

The cornerstone of all federal special education laws in the United States is the IDEA. This law, first passed in 1990, has been amended several times—most recently in 2009. It covers children and their families from birth to age 3, preschoolers, and students up to age 22 who have not received a high school diploma. Under the IDEA:

- All children, regardless of disability, are entitled to a free and appropriate public education and necessary related services provided in the least restrictive environment.

- Children are entitled to a fair evaluation to determine their need for special education services.

- Parents of a child with disabilities participate in the planning and decision-making for their child's special education.

- Parents can challenge decisions made by the school system, and disputes will be resolved by an impartial third party.

> *Our son has multiple late effects from his chemotherapy, radiation, and stem cell transplant. The school system was great about providing physical therapy, occupational therapy, and speech therapy. However, they wanted to put him in a special needs school, but I wanted him to have support in the classroom. They said they had no staff, so I put an ad in the newspaper at a university graduate school near his school. We found a second-year grad student in special ed to help him in the classroom. The school district refused to hire her, so we appealed and had a hearing. We won. The aide is wonderful and helps him stay on task, understand instructions, and keep organized. I'm an effective, but exhausted, advocate.*

Several online sources provide reliable information about learning disabilities and parental rights under the IDEA and Section 504. Reputable websites include Wrightslaw (*www.wrightslaw.com*), National Center for Learning Disabilities (*www.ncld.org*), and LD Online (*www.ldonline.org*).

Referral for services. The first step to getting educational support is to submit by hand or mail a written hard copy "referral for services" letter (not an email). A parent or a child's teacher can make a request for special education testing. Don't ask for a referral verbally; testing and services must be requested in writing. Obtain a written, dated acknowledgement of the school's receipt of the request, because school staff are legally required to hold a meeting within 30 days of receiving the request.

> My son had problems as soon as he entered kindergarten while on treatment. He couldn't hold a pencil, and he developed difficulties with math and reading. By second grade, I asked the school for extra help, and they tested him. They did an IEP and gave him special attention in small remedial groups. The school system also provided weekly physical therapy, which really helped him.

The next steps in the special education process are evaluation, eligibility, development of an IEP, annual review, and 3-year assessment. You will need to become an advocate for your child as your family goes through the steps to determine the placement, modifications, and services to which your child is entitled.

> We have had an excellent experience with the school district throughout preschool and now in kindergarten. We went to them with the first neuropsychological results, which were dismal. They suggested a special developmental preschool and occupational therapy. Both helped him enormously. He had an evaluation for special education services done and now has a full-time aide in kindergarten. He is getting the help he needs.

Evaluation. Once the referral is made, an evaluation is needed to determine whether the child qualifies for services as a student with a disability. Usually, a team composed of a general education teacher, special education teacher, district representative, and others (e.g., school nurse) attend the first meeting. It helps immensely to have the liaison from the hospital present to make sure the IEP team fully understands the child's illness, treatment, and impairments. The evaluation most often includes educational, medical, social, and psychological information.

All young children treated for leukemia should have a thorough neuropsychological evaluation. This is best administered by pediatric neuropsychologists experienced in testing children with cancer. This evaluation is usually done by the hospital where the child is being treated, not by the school. The results should be shared with the school system, which must consider the findings but may also conduct its own assessment. If parents disagree with the findings from the school's evaluation, they have the legal right to request an independent educational evaluation by a third-party practitioner, which is paid for by the school district.

Children may also be evaluated to determine the need for specific therapies or services in identified areas (called "related services"). Examples of related services are physical therapy, occupational therapy, adaptive physical education, and assistive technology.

Initially, the school was reluctant to test Gina because they thought she was too young (6 years old). But she had been getting occupational therapy at the hospital for two years, and I wanted the school to take over. I brought in articles and spoke to the teacher, principal, nurse, and counselor. Gina had a dynamite teacher who really listened, and she helped get permission to have Gina tested. Her tests showed her to be very strong in some areas, and very weak in others. Together, we put together an IEP, which we have updated every spring. Originally, she received weekly occupational therapy and daily help from the special education teacher. She's now in fourth grade and is doing so well that she no longer needs occupational therapy; she only gets extra help during study hall.

From the time the parents agree to the evaluation, school districts have 60 days to complete the evaluation and present the findings. Parents attend a meeting with the IEP team to discuss the evaluation results and make a decision about whether a child is eligible for services. Students can be included in this meeting, although younger children most often are not.

Eligibility for special education. The IDEA requires that students meet two requirements to be eligible for special education services: 1) The child must have one (or more) of the 14 disabilities listed in the law; and 2) because of the disability, the child needs special education services to access the general education program. The 14 eligibility categories for special education are:

- Autism
- Deaf/blindness
- Deafness
- Developmental delay
- Emotional disturbance
- Hearing impairment
- Intellectual disability
- Multiple disabilities
- Orthopedic impairment
- Other health impairment (OHI)
- Specific learning disability
- Speech or language impairment
- Traumatic brain injury (TBI)
- Visual impairment, including blindness

Most children with effects from treatment for leukemia qualify for services under the category of OHI.

Destiny (age 11) has some long-term effects from her treatment with high-dose chemotherapy, cranial radiation, and transplantation. Her learning ability (in particular, comprehension and short-term memory) has been affected. The special ed department at the school told us she was entitled to extra help because of her "other health-impaired" status. Destiny is in a general education classroom setting, but a special education teacher comes into the room several times daily to give extra help to the kids who need it. Examples of services are: helping with problem solving (especially math), giving her extra time to do work, as well as allowing her to repeat tests that she didn't perform well on. We have found this to be a great help in Destiny's education. She is now making As and Bs as well as exhibiting a more positive attitude toward school in general.

Individual Education Plan (IEP). After eligibility is determined, a meeting is called to develop an IEP. The IEP team attending this meeting includes the parents, the student's regular education teacher, a special education teacher, a representative of the school district, someone who can interpret the instructional implications of the evaluation results, the student (when appropriate), and any other person with knowledge or special expertise regarding the child.

Attending an IEP meeting can be intimidating (because school personnel most often outnumber the parents) and emotional (because it can be difficult to discuss evaluation results and extra challenges facing your child). You are entitled to bring others with you as an advocates, to take notes, or simply to observe. Bringing a friend or two provides moral support. It is also very helpful to invite the hospital liaison or a professional advocate because they understand the lingo, which can seem like a different language, and they can help you understand how schools rate and rank test results. The hospital's school liaison will also ensure that all meeting participants understand the child's current and past medical issues and that they use that information to write the IEP goals.

An advocate is usually someone who has a great deal of experience navigating through the process and how the process works. In our case, after the first meeting with the team, we knew we needed one. We didn't understand the jargon used by the school, we didn't understand why they didn't accept any of the results of the neuropsych report, and we came out of the meeting feeling like we'd been sucker punched. I know that some areas offer free advocates, though in our area there was a long wait to obtain one. Wrightslaw has a page about how to find an advocate at www.wrightslaw.com/info/advo.referrals.htm. Sometimes attorneys will work as advocates, but we chose someone who had previously been a school psychologist. She is very pleasant and very knowledgeable. Her help has been indispensable. We would have never been able to get our child qualified for services without her. I know not every school district is like ours, but with budget constraints, our district fought tooth and nail against everything.

The IEP should describe in detail the special education program and any other related services that need to be provided to meet the individual needs of your child. The IEP describes what your child is to be taught, how and when the school is to teach it, and any educational accommodations that will be made.

Students with disabilities need to learn the same things as other students: reading, writing, mathematics, history, and other subjects that help them prepare for vocational training, jobs, or college. The difference is that with an IEP in place, many specialized services—small classes, classroom aide, resource room, physical therapy, and instruction by special education teachers—are used.

The IEP has five parts:

1. **Present level of performance:** This section describes your child's present level of social, behavioral, and physical functioning, academic performance, learning style, and medical history.

2. **Goals and objectives:** This section lists skills and behaviors that your child is expected to master in a specific time period and how progress will be assessed. These goals should not be vague like "John will learn to write a report," but rather, "John will prepare and present an oral book report with two general education students by May 1." Each goal should answer the following questions: Who? What? How? Where? When? How often? When will the service start and end?

3. **Related services:** Many specialized services can be mandated in the IEP, including the following:

   • Physical therapy and adaptive physical education

   • Occupational therapy

   • Social skills training

   • Mental health services

   • Assistive technology assessment and training

   • Functional behavior assessment and behavior intervention plans

   • Transportation to and from school and therapy sessions

For each of these services, the IEP should list the frequency, duration, start date, end date, and whether the services will be provided in a group or individual setting, for example, "Jane will receive individual physical therapy twice a week, for 60 minutes a session, from September through December, when her needs will be reevaluated."

4. **Placement:** The term placement refers to the least restrictive setting in which the IEP goals and objectives can be met. For example, one student may be in the general education classroom all day with an aide present, and another might leave the classroom

for part of each day to receive specialized instruction in a resource room. The IEP should state the amount of time (minutes or hours) the child will be in the general education program and the frequency and duration of any special services.

5. **Evaluating the IEP:** Meetings with all members of the IEP team should be held periodically to review your child's progress toward attaining the short- and long-term goals and objectives of the IEP. To determine whether the IEP is working for your child, an annual IEP meeting is required, but parents can request more meetings, if needed, to address any concerns.

Once signed by the school and the parents, the IEP becomes a legal document that the school is required to implement as written.

> *I recommend that no parent ever sign the IEP documents until they have had a chance to take them home and reread them a couple of times. We had an advocate, who would take the pages and comb through them. I don't remember ever having an IEP that didn't have at least one error in it. Sometimes it was easily fixed (like they mixed up the percentage of time in general ed classroom and special ed classroom) but sometimes we really wondered if the "error" was on purpose—like we agreed in the meeting to 30 minutes of reading assistance with a reading specialist three times a week and the IEP indicated 20 minutes per session. Had we signed the documents without review, we would have lost 30 minutes a week of specialized assistance.*

If at any time communication deteriorates and you feel your child's IEP is inadequate or not being followed, here are several facts you need to know:

- The IEP cannot be changed without parental consent.

- If parents disagree about the content of the IEP, they can withdraw consent and request (in writing) a meeting to draft a new IEP; or they can consent only to the portions of the IEP with which they agree.

- Parents can request that the disagreement be settled by an independent hearing officer in an administrative law proceeding called a due process hearing. School districts generally are represented by a lawyer at such hearings, and parents are usually best served in such proceedings by hiring a lawyer or educational advocate.

- An IEP is a legal document that schools are legally required to comply with. However, if a school does not comply with an IEP, there is no governmental agency parents can call upon to enforce it—the only enforcement mechanism is a due process hearing.

> *The IEP process was more difficult, and more psychologically damaging, than my daughter's cancer treatment. Although we provided a detailed report of her neuropsychological evaluation that included specific recommendations for the type of reading instruction proven to work with children with her deficits, the school said it did not use those nationally recognized interventions. She was subjected to testing at the beginning and end of each school year, but different types of tests were used each*

time, so we could never make an apples-to-apples comparison of results. After four years, I placed her in a private school for students with learning disabilities, where she is flourishing. To this day, she dissolves into tears if pulled out of class for educational testing without prior notice, but she has no problem going back for checkups at the hospital where she was treated for cancer.

The IEP should reflect those programs and services uniquely appropriate for the student's needs. Advocates, disability organizations, your child's medical team, teachers, and therapists can assist in figuring out which options best suit your child, but you know your child best.

This year (third grade) has been a nightmare. My son has an IEP that focuses on problems with short-term memory, concentration, writing, and reading comprehension. The teacher, even though she is special ed qualified, has been rigid and used lots of timed tests. She told me in one conference that she thought my son's behavior problems were because he was "spoiled." The IEP required that she send a note home with my son if he has a seizure, and she has never done it. I learned that the IEP is only as valuable as the teacher who is applying it.

Hundreds of accommodations are available through an IEP. Here are a few examples:

- Preferential seating
- Study groups with discussion for learning/memory
- Recording of classes for reinforcement
- Books on tape or CD
- A copy of notes from a peer to improve listening in class and reduce the need for writing
- A copy of a teacher's planning notes prior to instruction
- Shortened in-class and homework assignments
- Use of a computer for written assignments
- Keyboard training (kindergartners are not too young to learn)
- Use of graphic organizers
- Use of a calculator
- Extended time for tests
- Oral rather than written tests
- An assignment check-off system
- Breakdown of large assignments into a series of smaller steps
- Extra time to travel between classes
- Accessible locker

To learn about other accommodations, visit *www.wrightslaw.com/info/fape.accoms.mods.pdf.*

Transition services. Students with an IEP receive transition planning, starting by the time the child is 16 (or younger if determined by the IEP team or required by state law). Your child's IEP should outline actions that will be taken to prepare your child to transition from high school to college, vocational training, supported employment, or adult services. High schools may have a post high school program that teaches special education kids job and life skills. In some districts, post high school is a separate school, in others it is held in a special section of the high school.

High schools in the United States may have a Department of Rehabilitative Services (DRS) vocational counselor on staff to help students with disabilities plan for life after high school, or the school can connect the student with the DRS as part of the student's transition services. The DRS can provide:

- Career guidance and counseling

- Diagnostic evaluations

- Supported employment and training

The transition IEP should include specific goals and ways to attain them (e.g., coursework, training, employment counseling), including who will provide these services. For more information about transition planning, visit *www.wrightslaw.com/info/trans.index.htm.*

IDEA Part C—Early intervention services. Part C of the IDEA mandates early intervention services for infants and toddlers (from birth up to age 3) with disabilities, and, in some cases, children at risk for developmental delays. These services are administered either by the school district or the state health department. In these cases, services are usually provided in the family home. You can find out which agency to contact by asking the hospital social worker or calling the special education director for your school district.

The law requires services not only for eligible infants and toddlers, but for their families, as well. Therefore, an Individual Family Service Plan (IFSP) is developed. This plan includes:

- A description of the child's physical, cognitive, language, speech, psychosocial, and other developmental levels

- Goals and objectives for the family and child

- The description, frequency, and delivery of services to be provided, such as speech, occupational, and physical therapy; health and medical services; and family training and counseling

- A caseworker who locates and coordinates all necessary services
- Steps to support transition to other programs and services

By age 3, children are transitioned to the school district for assessment of the need for special education services. If the child is eligible, the school district provides early childhood special education services. For more information, *visit www.parentcenterhub. org/repository/preschoolers.*

	IDEA	Section 504
Type of law	A federal education law	A civil rights law
Who is covered	Students ages 3–22 in primary or secondary school whose disability affects their ability to access the general education curriculum. Part C covers infants and toddlers.	Any student with a disability in an educational setting. College students, regardless of age, have rights under Section 504.
Types of disabilities	Child must have one or more of the 14 disabilities listed in the law.	Any physical or mental disability (including cancer) that substantially limits one or more major life activity.
Person in charge	Special education director	Section 504 coordinator
Evaluation of eligibility	Several assessment tools are used to determine whether the child has a qualifying disability. A written request must be submitted for an evaluation, and consent must be obtained from a parent or guardian before evaluation begins. A reevaluation is required every three years, but can be done more often, as needed.	Evaluation is conducted in the area of concern. Written consent of a parent or guardian is not required for evaluation, but notice must be provided. Yearly reevaluation or review is required.
Tools used to implement law	A written Individual Education Plan (IEP) is legally required and parents/guardians must receive and sign a copy of the final plan. If a functional behavioral analysis is conducted, a behavior intervention plan can be developed for any child with a disability who also has a behavioral issue that interferes with learning.	A 504 Plan can be developed without notice to, or participation of, the parents/guardians. A written 504 Plan may be requested, but is not required by law.
Change in placement	A meeting with the parents/guardians is required before any change in placement or services is made.	Changes in placement or services can be made without notice to parents/guardians.
Due process	School districts must provide resolution sessions and due process hearings for parents/guardians who disagree with evaluation, implementation, or placement.	School districts must provide a grievance procedure for parents/guardians who disagree with evaluation, implementation, or placement; due process hearing is not required.

Individual Healthcare Plan (IHCP)

If your child has medical issues that need to be managed at school (e.g., seizures, headaches, or medication), your child's doctor should write a letter to the principal with written orders for care. The school nurse will then develop an IHCP to ensure your child's medical needs are appropriately managed at school. The IHCP can be incorporated into either an IEP or Section 504 Plan, or it can stand alone if the child does not need an IEP or 504 Plan. However, an IHCP does not provide any procedural safeguards for the student if it is not part of an IEP or 504 Plan.

The IHCP includes a brief medical history, medications and side effects, student health goals, clear descriptions of health services that will be provided by the school, and contact numbers for emergencies. Parents and school personnel must sign the plan before it is implemented, and it should be updated every year.

> We have two plans—the IEP and the IHCP—and they are for different things. The IHCP is for Marielle's migraines (which is separate from her late cognitive effects), and the IEP is based on the cancer/late effects. We update it at the beginning of every school year. Every year, we get a letter from her pediatric neurologist that states that Marielle is under her care for severe migraines that will cause days of school to be missed and that any/all absences for migraines should be allowed for the year. Also, the letter states that no work missed must be made up and the missing work cannot be counted against her grade. We also add this to her IEP—"Student will only be graded on work turned in." The IHCP is very important if your child will miss more than five days of school in a year. Our school district starts to send out warning letters at the fifth day of absence and warns of taking the parent to court for truancy after the tenth absence (or partial absence) in a year.

Your Legal Rights (Canada)

Each Canadian province and territory has its own ministry or department of education and establishes its own laws, policies, procedures, and budgets pertaining to educational requirements and services. The Council of Ministers of Education operates on a voluntary basis to advocate for educational services, establish common goals, and improve the quality of education across the country. One of the shared goals of this group in recent years has been to improve the delivery of special education services to children across Canada.

Most provinces and territories have an evaluation process similar to the one used in the United States. Canada also employs a similar IEP process, although the specific rules vary by province. For information about special needs education in Canada, visit *www.angloinfo.com/how-to/canada/family/schooling-education/special-needs-education*.

The Terminally Ill Child and School

In the sad event that a child's health continues to deteriorate, parents and school staff members should discuss ways the school can be supportive during the child's final days or weeks. Fellow students need timely and appropriate information about their ill classmate so they can deal with her declining health and prepare for her death. The following are suggestions about how to prepare classmates and school personnel for the death of a student:

- The school staff needs to be reassured that death is not likely to suddenly occur at school.

- Staff needs to be aware that going to school is vital to the child's well-being. School staff members should welcome and support the child's need to attend school for as long as possible.

- Staff can design flexible programs for the ill student.

    Jody was lucky because he went to a private school, and there were only 16 children in his class. Whenever he could come to school, they made him welcome. Because children worked at their own pace, he never had the feeling that he was getting behind in his classwork. He really felt like he belonged there. Sometimes he could only manage to stay an hour, but he loved to go. Toward the end when he was in a wheelchair, the kids would fight over whose turn it was to push him. The teacher was wonderful, and the kids really helped him and supported him until the end.

- It is helpful to provide age-appropriate reading materials about death and dying for the ill child's classmates, siblings' classmates, teachers, and school staff, as well as opportunities for discussion.

- Extraordinary efforts should be made to keep in touch when the child can no longer attend school. Cards, banners, videos, texts, emails, telephone calls, and webcam or conference calls from the entire class or individual classmates are good ways to share thoughts and best wishes.

- Classmates can visit the hospital or child's home, if appropriate. If the child is too sick for visitors, the class can come wave at the front window and drop off cards or gifts.

- The class can send books, video games, or a basket of small gifts and cards to the hospital or home.

- The class can decorate the family's front door, mailbox, and yard when the child will be returning home from the hospital.

All of the above activities encourage empathy in classmates, as well as help them adjust to the decline and imminent death of their friend. These activities also help dying children know they have not been forgotten by teachers, friends, and classmates, even if they cannot attend school.

When the child dies, a memorial service at school gives students a chance to grieve. School counselors or psychologists should be available to talk to the classmates to allow them to express their feelings. Parents usually very much appreciate receiving stories about their child from classmates.

Our 16-year-old did incredibly well psychologically during treatment. She kept up with school (tutors at home and hospital for tenth and eleventh grade). She also took the SATs and went for a college interview (bald). She wrote a research paper that blew them over at the interview. She also helped to create a multimedia project for patient information at the hospital. She was back in school for her senior year. It was a big adjustment socially. Some kids didn't remember her; some thought she was a transfer student. She was still recovering from the side effects of chemo (lower counts, weight loss, low energy). But, she was determined to put it all behind her and made college plans. She won a full scholarship to our local university.

Chapter 21

Sources of Support

*"Be strong, be fearless, be beautiful. And believe that anything is
possible when you have the right people there to support you."*

— Misty Copeland

THE DIAGNOSIS OF CANCER CAN BE a frightening and isolating experience. Every
parent of a child with cancer has a story to tell of lost or strained relationships. Yet we
are social creatures, reliant on a web of support from family, friends, neighbors, and
religious communities. We need the presence of people who not only care for us, but
who sincerely try to understand what we are feeling.

Members of families struck by childhood cancer—parents, the child with cancer, and
siblings—often turn to hospital social workers, support groups, therapists, clergy, and
camps for support. This chapter offers information about these resources, which can
help families regain a sense of control over their lives and find wonderful new friends
who understand what they are going through.

Hospital Social Workers

Pediatric oncology social workers usually have a master's degree in social work, with
additional training in oncology and pediatrics. They serve as guides through unfamiliar
territory by mediating between staff and families, helping with emotional or financial
problems, and locating resources. Many social workers form close, long-lasting bonds
with families and continue to answer questions and provide support long after treatment ends.

> *On the day of Carl's diagnosis, we were introduced to a team that we worked with
> for the next several years. The team included a primary nurse, a primary oncologist,
> a first-year resident, a second-year resident, a third-year resident, and our social
> worker. I remember that first day the social worker told us she was there to help us
> with anything we needed, such as hospital problems, billing, insurance, emotional
> issues, or behavior issues. She said her job was to be there for us, and she was,
> whenever we needed her.*

In addition to social workers, most hospitals have child life specialists, psychiatric nurses, psychiatrists, psychiatric residents, and psychologists on staff who can help you deal with problems while your child is in the hospital. Ask your child's nurse, treating physician, or the hospital social worker to help you connect with these resources.

> We went to a children's hospital that was renowned in the pediatric cancer field. The medical treatment was excellent, but psychosocial support was nonexistent. The day after diagnosis, we were interviewed for 20 minutes by a psychiatric resident, and that was it. I never met a social worker, and the physicians were so busy they never asked anything other than medical questions. I didn't know any parents of a child with my daughter's diagnosis; I didn't know there was a local support group; I didn't know there was a summer camp for the kids. I felt totally isolated.

In-person Support Groups for Parents

Many parents of children with cancer experience deep loneliness after the first rush of visits, cards, and phone calls ends—when the rest of the world goes back to normal life. Families join support groups to lessen this isolation, share suggestions for dealing with leukemia and its treatment/side effects, and talk to others who are living through the same crisis. Coping with a life-threatening illness requires a unique perspective—the ability to focus on the grave situation at hand while balancing other aspects of daily life. In support groups, many families get help finding this emotional balance. Just meeting people who have lived through the same situation is profoundly reassuring.

> The group was a real lifeline for us, especially when Justin was so sick. We looked forward to the meetings and were there for every one. It was a real escape; it was a place to go where people were rooting for us. People from the group would always swing by the ICU to see us whenever they were bringing their own kids in for treatment. We amassed a tremendous library of children's books that the group members would drop off. The support was wonderful.

For the parents of a child with cancer, the issues that other parents in their social circles are dealing with seem light years away. But the moms and dads in the kitchen at a Ronald McDonald House or the ped-onc lounge can offer practical advice about things such as mouth sores and low blood cell counts. They understand each other's feelings and emotions, because they are sharing the same experience. It is a bond that cuts across all social, economic, cultural, and racial differences.

> My 2-year-old daughter, Gina, was diagnosed one week after I gave birth to a new baby girl. I remember early in her treatment, I was sitting with Gina on my lap, and my husband sat next to me, holding the new baby. The doctor breezed in and said in a cheerful voice, "How are you feeling?" I burst into sobs and could not stop. He said "Just a minute" and dashed out. A few minutes later a woman came in with her

8-year-old daughter who had finished treatment and looked great. She put her arms around me and talked to me. She told me that everyone feels horrible in the beginning; and it might be hard to believe, but treatment would soon become a way of life for us. She was a great comfort, and of course, she was right.

There are many different types of support groups, ranging from those with hundreds of members and formal bylaws to three moms who meet for coffee once a week. Some groups deal only with the emotional aspects of the disease, while others may focus on education, advocacy, social opportunities, or crisis intervention. Some groups are facilitated by trained mental health practitioners, while others are self-help groups led by parents. And, naturally, as some members drop out and new families join, the needs and interests of the group may shift.

Our Tuesday gatherings were an anchor for us. It was a time to meet with parents who truly understood what living with cancer meant. These parents had been in the trenches. They knew the midnight terrors, the frustrations of dealing with the medical establishment; after all, it was an alien world to most of us. They knew about chemo, hair loss, friend loss, and they knew the bittersweet side of cherishing a child more than one thought one could cherish anyone. We gathered to cry, to laugh, to whine, to comfort one another, to share shelter from a frightening world. It was a haven.

Support groups link parents in similar circumstances to share practical information, provide emotional support, give hope for the future, and truly listen and empathize. It is important to remember, however, that support group members are not infallible. One person may say something thoughtless or hurtful. Someone else may provide incorrect information. It is best to accept the support in the spirit in which it is given, but to always take any concerns or questions you have to your child's doctor or nurse practitioner.

Online Support Groups for Parents

Parents from small, isolated communities or who live a long distance from their treatment center may have a difficult time finding a local support group that fits their needs. This may also be true for single parents or parents who prefer some anonymity. For these parents, online support groups can provide the understanding that only another parent of a child with cancer can give.

The support I have gained through online discussion groups is priceless. I have received a great deal of comfort from my participation in these groups. They have enabled me to connect with families from all over the world, many of whom are fighting the exact same disease. I have often come to my computer in the middle of the night, when everyone else in the house was asleep. I can express my fears at

3:00 a.m. and know someone will always be there to reassure me with the knowledge that they have felt these things, too. That's one of the most beautiful things about these groups. Someone is always there, even in the middle of the night.

To find online discussion groups, you can search the lists on *www.acor.org or groups. google.com.* Parents or guardians of a child with cancer can join the popular Momcology discussion groups on Facebook (for any primary caregivers, not just moms) by filling out an application at *www.momcology.org.* Several national support groups are listed in Appendix C, *Books, Resources, and Support Groups.* Some online discussion groups are not moderated, but many are carefully monitored by experienced peer-support leaders.

I joined a Ph+ Facebook group—all moms. I connected with some brilliant women who were months and years ahead of us in treatment, some on the same trial. They were incredible sources of accurate information as well as emotional support. There was not a lot of data on the new treatments, but we had several smart, fearless, and tenacious members who would read every new article and clinical study document, and would call the principal investigator to get additional info. We would all share what we were learning with the group. Because TKI [tyrosine kinase inhibitor] treatment was still emerging, this group of Ph+ patients and parents was an immense help.

· · · · ·

How ironic that we subscribed to this list in a moment of panic, with a black cloud lined with despair lingering above. But now we can say we have lassoed cyberspace, and here, among new friends, we have found and we have shared love, hope, support, informative information, mutual stories, mutual questions, thoughtful and sincere answers, honesty, disagreement, pain, inspiration, friendship, humor, and enjoyment, as well as understanding. This list reflects the roller coaster of life. Activity on this list enables individuals to place that initial black cloud in their back pocket, hold sunshine in their hand, and watch hope dance above.

Support Groups for Children with Cancer

Many pediatric hospitals have ongoing support groups for children with cancer. Often these groups are run by experienced pediatric social workers or psychologists who know how to balance having fun with sharing feelings. For many children, these groups are the only place where they feel completely accepted, and where most of the other kids are bald and have to take lots of medicine. The group is a place where children or teens can say how they really feel, without worrying that they are causing their parents more pain. Many children form wonderful and lasting friendships in peer groups.

Kristin goes to the kids' support group while my wife and I attend the parents' group downstairs. She doesn't talk much about what goes on, but the facilitator keeps the parents apprised of how things are going. One very vocal 9-year-old boy has recently broken the ice with the kids. He really likes to talk about his feelings about having leukemia, and it has prompted the other children to begin to share their thoughts and reactions about the things that have happened to them. They also have lots of fun.

Some support groups accommodate the whole family—the child or teen with cancer, siblings, and parents. The youngest children can play or do crafts with trained volunteers, while older kids have a chance to talk and share, and the parents can do likewise. This makes it possible for the whole family to get to know other families on the childhood cancer journey.

Support Groups for Siblings

As part of the ongoing effort to provide family-centered care, some hospitals offer support groups to improve communication, education, and support for siblings. These groups give siblings a special place to have their voices and concerns heard and to interact with others going through the same experience.

All four of my kids have been going to the support groups for over seven years now. We have one group for the kids with cancer, which is run by a social worker. The siblings group is run by a woman who specializes in early childhood development. Both groups do a lot of art therapy, relaxation therapy, playing, and talking. They meet twice a month, and I will continue to take my children until they ask to stop. I think it has really helped all of them. We also have two teen nights out a year. All of the teenagers with cancer get together for an activity such as watching a hockey game or basketball game, or going bowling, to the movies, or out for pizza. They also see each other at our local camp for children surviving cancer (Camp Watcha-Wanna-Do) each year.

Hospital Resource Rooms

Staff members in hospital resource rooms and libraries help families find information about diseases, conditions, parenting, and hospital services, and can point out helpful websites, books, and videos. Parents can also learn about support groups, classes, and community resources.

I think I first learned from a medical librarian about www.nih.gov and Medline, where you can find current research on chemotherapy and other treatments. If your local hospital is a teaching facility, they often have all the major medical journals. We were able to get full-text versions of papers that we needed.

Patient resource rooms are wonderful places. They usually have basic information on your child's illness, listings of agencies and cancer organizations, online access, and a person available to answer questions and help get you started if you're unfamiliar with doing internet searches. It should be one of the first places families are directed to.

Individual and Family Counseling

Cancer is a major crisis for even the strongest of families. Many parents find it helpful to seek out sensitive, objective mental health professionals to explore the difficult feelings—fear, anger, depression, anxiety, resentment, guilt—that cancer brings up. Individual and family counseling can help address shifting responsibilities within the family, explore methods to improve communication, and help find ways to channel strong feelings in a healthy way.

Family dynamics undergo profound changes when a child is diagnosed with cancer. Seeking professional counseling for ways to adjust and manage is a sign of strength. When a child has cancer, problems may be too complex and family members may be too exhausted to manage on their own. Seeking professional help sends children a message that the parents care about what is happening to them and want to help face it together.

> *Choosing to get therapy isn't easy. And going to a psychologist isn't easy. The only way to really work through the emotional pain is to look closely at it. Sometimes they ask hard questions. But it has been very beneficial for me. The best part about therapy is the person you are talking to is impartial. She isn't related to you, doesn't go to church with you, doesn't live with you, and has no connection to you or your situation. A totally unbiased perspective can be helpful when it feels like you are at the bottom of the pit, with.no handholds, no ladder, but a shovel right beside you to help you dig deeper. If you decide to begin therapy, do your research. I called and asked for references from a cancer helpline and the social worker at the clinic. Then I talked to a couple of therapists before I decided which one to go with. She was willing to work with me on a payment schedule.*

One of the first questions that arises is, "Who should we talk to?" There are many individuals in the cancer community who can make referrals and valuable recommendations, such as other parents who have sought counseling, your pediatrician, and a local or hospital social worker. You can ask these people for a short list of mental health professionals who have experience working with the issues your family is struggling with, for example, traumatized children, marital problems, stress reduction, or family conflicts. Generally, the names of the most well-respected clinicians in the community will appear on several of the lists.

The whole treatment experience put an enormous strain on our marriage. My wife has always been easy to excite, whereas I've always been very laid-back. There were moments when I was afraid that it would completely fall apart. Counseling really helped. We managed to survive, and I think in many ways, it has even brought us closer together.

In making your decision, it helps to understand the various types of mental health professionals and their different levels of education and licensure. The following disciplines train individuals to offer psychological services:

- **Psychology (EdD, MA, PhD, PsyD):** Marriage and family psychotherapists have either a master's degree or a doctorate; clinical and research psychologists have a doctorate.

- **Social work (MSW, DSW, PhD):** Clinical social workers have either a master's degree or a doctorate in a program with a clinical emphasis.

- **Pastoral care (MA, MDiv, DMin, PhD, DDiv):** These laypeople or clergy have received specialized training in counseling.

- **Medicine (MD, RN, ARNP, PA):** Psychiatrists are medical doctors who completed a residency in psychiatry. Physician assistants and advanced practice nurses have the equivalent of master's level training in medicine and may have additional training in mental health. These three types of specialists are the only mental health professionals who can prescribe medications. In addition, some registered nurses (RNs) obtain postgraduate training in psychotherapy, but they cannot prescribe medications.

- **Counseling (MA):** In most states, individuals must have a master's degree and a year of internship before they can work as counselors.

You may hear all of the above professionals referred to as "counselors" or "therapists." The following designations refer to licensure by state professional boards, not academic degrees:

- **LCSW** (Licensed Clinical Social Worker)
- **LSW** (Licensed Social Worker)
- **LMFCC** (Licensed Marriage, Family, Child Counselor)
- **LPC** (Licensed Professional Counselor)
- **LMFT** (Licensed Marriage and Family Therapist)

These licensure initials usually follow those that indicate an academic degree (e.g., PhD). Most states require licensure or certification for professionals to practice independently; unlicensed professionals are allowed to practice only under the supervision of a licensed professional (typically as an "intern" or "assistant" in a clinic or licensed professional's private practice). Another way to find a suitable counselor is to contact the American Association for Marriage and Family Therapy at (703) 838-9808 or online at *www.aamft.org*. This national professional organization of licensed/certified marriage and family therapists represents more than 50,000 therapists in the United States and Canada.

A psychiatrist who is the mother of a child with cancer offers a few thoughts:

> *Counseling helps, preferably from someone who regularly deals with parents of seriously ill children. This therapy is almost always short—although there may be some pre-cancer problems complicating the cancer issues that need to be hammered out.*
>
> *Antidepressants definitely have a role in the "so your child has cancer" coping strategy. They cannot make the diagnosis go away. They can improve concentration, energy, sleep, appetite, and the ability to get pleasure in life, and hope for the future—all of which you, your child with cancer, your spouse, and your other kids need you to have! They are not a magic bullet. They take two to eight weeks to work, and you may need to change once before you get the right medication, but it can make all the difference.*
>
> *Also, nurture yourself. Take bubble baths. Buy flowers. Let people pamper you. Say yes when people offer to help. Redefine normal so things can be good again. Make time for yourself. Spend time with your spouse (even an hour to walk and talk and hold hands). Find time for your non-cancer kids, reveling in their accomplishments. Celebrate what is good about your life.*
>
> *Pick out things that you feel are important to keep up with and do them. (For me it was laundry.) Ignore things that don't matter for the time being. (For me it was tidy rooms and cooking.) Make peace with your decisions and follow them.*

To find a therapist, a good first step is to call two or three therapists who appear on several of your lists of recommendations. Following are some suggested questions to ask during your telephone interviews:

- Are you accepting new clients?
- What are your fees? Do you take insurance? Do you accept my insurance? Do you bill the insurance company directly?
- Do you charge for an initial consultation?
- What training and experience do you have working with ill or traumatized children?
- How many years have you been working with families?
- What is your approach to resolving the problems families develop from trauma? Do you use a brief or long-term approach?
- What evaluation and assessment procedures will be used to define the problem?
- How and when will treatment goals be set?

The next step is to make an appointment with one or two of the therapists you think might best address your needs. Be honest about the fact that you are talking with several therapists prior to making a decision. The purpose of the introductory meeting is to see whether you feel comfortable with the therapist. After all, credentials do not guarantee that a given therapist is a good fit for you. Compatibility, trust, and a feeling of genuine caring are essential. It is worth the effort to continue your search until you find a good match.

> *I called several therapists out of desperation about my daughter's withdrawal and violent tantrums. I made appointments with two. The first I just didn't feel comfortable with at all, but the second felt like an old friend after one hour. I have been to see her dozens of times over the years, and she has always helped me. I wasn't interested in theory; I wanted practical suggestions about how to deal with the behavior problems. My 8-year-old daughter asked why I was going to see the therapist, and I said that Hilda was a doctor, but instead of taking care of my body, she helped care for my feelings.*

· · · · ·

> *We went into family therapy because every member of my family experienced misdirected anger. When they were angry, they aimed it at me—the nice person who took care of them and loved them no matter what. But I was dissolving. I needed to learn to say "ouch," and they needed to learn other ways to handle their angry feelings.*

If your child is going to go to a therapist, he needs to be prepared, just as he would be for any appointment. Following are several parents' suggestions about how to prepare your child:

• If you are bringing your child in for therapy, explain why you think talking to an objective person might benefit him.

> *In the beginning of treatment, my son had terrible problems with going to sleep and then having nightmares, primarily about snakes. We took him to a counselor, who worked with him for several weeks and completely resolved the problem. The counselor had him befriend the snake, talk to it, and explain that it was keeping him awake. He would tell the snake, "I want you to stop bothering me because I need to go to sleep." The snake never returned.*

• Older children should be involved in the process of choosing a counselor. Younger children's likes and dislikes should be respected. If your child does not get along well with one counselor, change counselors.

• Make the experience positive (e.g., describe the therapist as "the talking doctor").

• Reassure young children that the visit is for talking, drawing, or playing games, not for anything that is painful.

• Ask the therapist to explain the rules of confidentiality to both you and your child. Do not quiz your child after a visit to the therapist.

David had a very difficult time dealing with his brother's cancer. Realizing that we were unable to provide him with the help he needed, we sought professional help for him. I think the reason he feels so comfortable with his therapist is that he is aware of the rules of confidentiality. After his sessions, I'll always ask him how it went. Sometimes he'll just grin and say it was fine, and other times he might share a little of his conversation with me. I never push or question him about it. If it is something he needs to discuss, I wait until he decides to broach the subject.

- Make sure your child does not think she is being punished; assure her that therapists help both adults and children understand and deal with feelings.
- Go yourself for individual or family counseling or to support group meetings. This allows you to both take care of yourself and be a good role model for your children.

Other types of therapy used to help children with cancer, or their siblings, include music therapy (*www.musictherapy.org*), art therapy (*www.arttherapy.org*), and dance/movement therapy (*www.adta.org*).

Clergy and Religious Community

Religion is a source of strength for many people. Some parents and children find that their faith is strengthened by the cancer ordeal, while some begin to question their beliefs. Others, who have not relied on religion in the past, may now turn to it for solace.

Most hospitals have staff chaplains who are available for counseling, religious services, prayer, and other types of spiritual support. The chaplain often visits families soon after diagnosis and is available on an on-call basis. As with all types of emotional support, approaches that work well with one family may not be helpful for others.

When our son was first diagnosed, we didn't feel as if we could discuss any of our fears with the hospital chaplain. I believe it was simply because our personalities didn't "click" well together, and we would feel more uncomfortable than anything else whenever he would visit. Several months into treatment, the hospital had a new chaplain, and we hit it off immediately. It was a joy to see him walking down the hall toward my son's room. He seemed to have a natural gift for making me feel better, even when things seemed to be crumbling around me.

Parents who were members of a church, synagogue, or mosque prior to their child's diagnosis may derive great comfort from the clergy and members of their religious community. Members of the congregation usually rally around the family, providing meals, babysitting, prayers, and support. Regular visits from clergy provide spiritual sustenance throughout the initial crisis and subsequent years of treatment.

We belong to a religious study group that has met weekly for eight years. In our group, during that time, there have been three cancer diagnoses and one of multiple sclerosis. We have all become an incredibly supportive family, and we share the burdens. I cannot begin to list the many wonderful things these people have done for us. They consistently put their lives on hold to help. They fill the freezer, clean the house, support us financially, parent our children. They do the laundry covered with vomit. They quietly appear, help, then disappear. I can call any one of them at 3:00 a.m. in the depths of despair and find comfort.

Camps

Summer camps for children with cancer, and often their siblings, are becoming increasingly popular. These camps provide an opportunity for children with cancer and their siblings to have fun, meet friends, and talk with others in the same situation. Counselors are usually cancer survivors and siblings of children with cancer, or sometimes oncology nurses and resident physicians. At these camps, children can have their concerns addressed in a safe, supportive environment that is supervised by experts. Camps provide a carefree time away from the sadness and stress at home or from the all-too-frequent hospital visits.

Of all the ways to get support, I think the camp really helps the most. You are all there together for enough time to break down the barriers. Although camp does not focus on cancer, many times we really got down to talking about how we really felt. I have been a counselor at the camp for eight summers now. Most of the campers know that I relapsed three times and I'm doing great many years later. They see the many other long-term survivors who are counselors, and it gives them what they need the most—hope. The best support is meeting survivors, because nobody else truly understands.

• • • • •

Caitlin went to camp, and this was a dream come true for her. As we pulled into the parking lot, she exhaled a deep breath and said, "I made it. I am finally normal!"

Some camps are set up to accommodate not only the child who has undergone treatment, but also their siblings and parents. Some camps offer separate weeklong camping experiences just for siblings. Appendix B, *Resource Organizations*, contains a short list of camps with contact information. To view a comprehensive list, visit *www.acor.org/ ped-onc/cfissues/camps.html*.

It's like your psyche has been hit by a truck. Some days the pain is worse than others. Some days your threshold is stronger than others, but allow yourself the help that is available to get back to stable. Take it from me—it is next to impossible to pull from a dry well. Unlike children, we can't temper tantrum ourselves out of our

feelings, we can't rant and scream and stomp our feet at the unfairness of it all. We can't just sit in momma's arms and have a hug and feel better. We have to handle it with an attitude and the responsibility that is expected of being adult. And we have to be a nurse, teacher, mom, emotional measuring stick for our kids, care for the marriage, pay the bills, and, oh yeah, don't forget about ourselves—all at the same time. It's just far too much. Say "Yes" to yourself, and your needs—get help when you need it. Other things that I found helpful were:

- *Saying "No," "No, thank you," and "I'll take that into consideration when I make my decision"*

- *Saying "Yes," "Yes, please, that would be a great help," and "Sure, if you could drop off a lasagna and pick up some milk on your way over that would be great"*

- *Writing in a journal*

- *Taking a retreat weekend*

- *Playing cards with the girls*

- *Counseling (on occasion with priest, psychologist, social worker)*

- *Having movie night with my sisters (usually a comedy—you are allowed to laugh)*

- *Treating myself to an inside-and-out car wash*

- *Allowing myself to "cry in my cornflakes," then getting up, splashing some cold water on my face, and getting on with the day*

- *Enjoying a glass of wine, a candle, and Andrea Bocelli*

- *Gardening*

- *Having coffee with a friend*

- *Helping someone else who is in worse shape than I am*

- *Talking with other cancer kid moms about cancer kid family stuff*

- *Talking with non-cancer kid moms about non-cancer family stuff (the kids bickering, too much housework, the latest magazine, and what the women in it are wearing)*

- *Declaring the next five minutes as "get the crazies out" time, and tickling, dancing silly, and playing "make me laugh" (you know you're losing it when you do this, and no one else is home)*

- *Going out with my husband (even if I had to drag him, we always enjoyed the evening in spite of ourselves)*

And anything else I deemed necessary to help me get through it.

Chapter 22

Nutrition

*"Let your food be your medicine and
your medicine be your food."*

— Hippocrates

NOW, MORE THAN EVER, it is important for your sick child to eat balanced, healthful, and energy-packed meals. Yet the reality is that the eating habits of children with leukemia often go haywire. Although your child's body needs added energy to metabolize medications and repair the damage to healthy cells caused by treatment, those same treatments can wreak havoc on your child's appetite and taste sensations.

This chapter discusses eating problems, explains good nutrition, suggests ways to pack extra calories into small servings, and offers tips about how to make food more appealing to children with leukemia. In addition, parents share what their children really ate while being treated for leukemia.

How Treatment Affects Eating

Eating is tremendously affected by chemotherapy, radiation, and stem cell transplants. Listed below are several common side effects of treatment that often prevent good eating. Other side effects that impact eating—nausea, vomiting, diarrhea, constipation, and mouth and throat sores—are covered in detail in Chapter 14, *Common Side Effects of Treatment*.

Loss of appetite

Loss of appetite is one of the most common problems associated with cancer treatment. If your child loses more than 10 to 15% of her body weight, she may need to be fed intravenously or by nasogastric tube. Sometimes this can be avoided if parents learn how to increase calories in small amounts of food. In addition to simple loss of appetite, your child may have a side effect of chemotherapy called early filling. This means the child has a sense of being full after only a few bites of food. If your child is suffering from early filling and only eats when he feels hungry, he may begin losing weight and become malnourished.

My son looked like a skeleton several months into his protocol. I used to dress him in "camouflage" clothes—several layers thick. This kept him warm and prevented stares.

Increased appetite and weight gain

When children are given high doses of steroids such as prednisone or dexamethasone, they develop voracious appetites. They are hungry all the time, develop food obsessions, and frequently wake parents up during the night begging for another meal.

> *Early in her treatment, when Carrie Beth was taking dexamethasone, she would start hitting me in the face in the middle of the night demanding food. I learned to have a bag of snacks and a bottle sitting next to the bed, so I could just hand them over and go back to sleep.*

A moon face with chubby cheeks and a rotund belly are classic features of a child on high-dose steroids. Much of the extra weight is fluid, which steroids cause the body to retain. There are two important points for parents to remember about treatment with steroids. First, when the steroids stop, the extra fluid is excreted and weight drops. Second, your child's appetite may go from voracious to poor after the steroids stop, so it is unwise to limit food when your child is taking steroids. Instead, try to make the most of this brief time of good appetite to encourage consumption of a variety of nutritious foods. A well-balanced diet now will help your child withstand the rigors of the treatments ahead.

> *My daughter didn't sleep when she was on steroids, and she gained a lot of weight. She'd sit in bed and demand, all day and all night long, "toast with butter spread on it like icing on a cake." So, I gave it to her. When she was off the steroids, she'd rapidly lose the weight and she'd look skeletal. Both extremes were really hard on all of us emotionally.*

If you are concerned about the weight gain, consult your child's oncologist. If the fluid retention is extreme, the doctor may have you restrict your child's salt intake.

Lactose intolerance

Lactose intolerance is when the body cannot absorb the sugar (lactose) contained in milk and other dairy products. Antibiotics and chemotherapy can each cause lactose intolerance in some children. The part of children's intestines that breaks down lactose stops functioning properly, resulting in gas, abdominal pain, bloating, cramping, and diarrhea when dairy products are ingested. If your child develops lactose intolerance, it is important to talk to a nutritionist to learn about low-lactose diets and alternate sources of protein and calcium. The following are suggestions for parents of children with lactose intolerance:

- Add special enzyme tablets or drops to dairy products to make them more digestible. Some of these products are over-the-counter additives, but others require a prescription. Discuss these products with the oncologist before giving them to your child.

- Children who cannot tolerate the lactose in cow's milk often can manage acidophilus milk, soy milk, rice milk, coconut milk, almond milk, goat's milk, or lactose-free milk. These are easier to digest and come in a variety of flavors.

- Remember that milk is a common ingredient in other foods, such as bread, candy, processed meats, and salad dressings. Read ingredient lists carefully.

- If your child cannot tolerate any dairy products, add calcium to his diet by serving canned salmon, sardines, spinach and other green leafy vegetables, or calcium-fortified fruit juices. Consult your child's oncologist and nutritionist about calcium supplements. Many children like the taste of a chewy calcium supplement called Viactiv®, which is available at most drug stores.

> My daughter is severely lactose intolerant, but she can eat hard, aged cheeses and vegan dairy products. I make her grilled cheese sandwiches with Swiss or vegan cheeses, spread her bagels with vegan cream cheese, and put vegan sour cream on her tacos. If you go to speciality markets, they often have a large selection of vegan products that taste the same as, or similar to, the milk-based product.

Altered taste and smell

One common reason children on treatment do not eat is because, for them, food has no taste or tastes bad. If food tastes bland to your child, try serving spicy cuisines, such as Italian, Mexican, or Greek foods. Chemotherapy can causes foods, particularly red meats, to taste bitter and metallic. If that happens, avoid using metal pots, pans, and utensils, which can magnify the metallic taste. Serve your child's food with plastic knives, forks, and spoons. You can also replace red meat with tofu, pork, chicken, turkey, eggs, and dairy products.

What Kids Should Eat

A healthy diet includes enough calories to ensure a normal rate of growth, fuel the body's efforts to repair and replace healthy cells, and provide the energy the body needs to break down the various chemotherapy drugs and excrete their byproducts. While chemotherapy is being given, maintaining weight is a higher priority than a balanced diet.

When the body becomes malnourished, body fat and muscle decrease. This leads to weakness, lack of energy, weight loss, a decreased ability to digest food, and less ability to fight infection. These health issues sometimes require a reduction in the dose of chemotherapy drugs.

The U.S. government recently changed dietary guidelines (see Figure 22-1). To keep your child's body well-nourished, foods from all six basic food groups are needed: (1) protein, (2) dairy, (3) grains, (4) fruits, (5) vegetables, and (6) fats and sweets. Children on chemotherapy benefit from eating a lot of fats, which add needed calories.

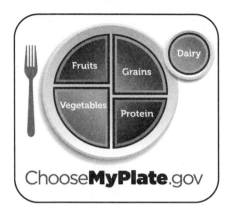

Figure 22-1: My Plate Dietary Guidelines

Examples of foods contained in each group are listed below, with a small child's serving size in parentheses beside each food. Consult a nutritionist to figure out the number of servings that is best for your child.

Proteins

Meat (1 ounce)	Eggs (1)
Fish (1 ounce)	Peanut butter (2 tbsp.)
Poultry (1 ounce)	Dried beans, cooked (½ cup)
Cheese (1 ounce)	Dried peas, cooked (½ cup)

Some typical 1-ounce servings of proteins are: a 1-inch meatball, a 1-inch cube of meat, or one slice of bologna.

Dairy products

Milk (½ cup)	Tofu (½ cup)
Cheese (1 ounce)	Custard (½ cup)
Ice cream (½ cup)	Yogurt (½ cup)

Dairy products provide calcium, vitamin D, and protein, which are necessary for bone growth and strength.

Grains

Bread (½ slice)	Cereal (½ cup)
Oatmeal (½ cup)	Granola (½ cup)
Cream of wheat (½ cup)	Cooked pasta (½ cup)
Graham crackers (1 square)	Brown rice (½ cup)

Try to use only products made with whole grains and limited sugar to get more nutrients per serving. One sandwich made with two slices of whole wheat bread provides four servings of this food group.

Fruits

Fresh fruit (1 medium piece)	Dried fruits (¼ cup)
Canned fruit (¼ cup)	100% fruit juice (½ cup)

Fruits can be camouflaged by puréeing them with ice cream or sherbet in the blender to make a tasty milkshake or smoothie, or by adding them to cookie and muffin recipes.

Vegetables

Raw vegetables (¼ cup)	Cooked vegetables (¼ cup)

If your child does not want vegetables, they can be grated or puréed and added to soups or spaghetti sauce. If you own a juicer, add a vegetable to fruits being juiced. There are also many brownie, cake, bread, and muffin recipes that use vegetables that cannot be tasted, such as zucchini bread, brownies with spinach or avocado, carrot cake, and veggie muffins.

Fats and sweets

Butter or oil	Nuts
Mayonnaise	Whipped cream
Peanut butter	Avocado
Meat fat (in gravy)	Olives
Ice cream	Chocolate

Although the guidelines call for fats to be used sparingly, higher consumption of fats is needed for children being treated for cancer. Experiment to find the fats your child enjoys eating and serve them often.

Making Eating Fun and Nutritious

In some homes, mealtimes turn into battlegrounds, with worried parents resorting to threats or bribery to get their child to eat. Parents rarely win these battles—eventually they give in, exhausted and frustrated, and serve the sick child whatever she will eat (often to the dismay of the siblings who still have to eat their vegetables). The next several sections are full of ways parents made mealtimes both fun and nutritious.

How to make eating more appealing

Many children are finicky eaters at the best of times. Cancer and its treatment can make eating especially difficult. Here are some general tips for making eating more appealing for your child:

- Give your child small portions throughout the day rather than three large meals. Feed your child whenever she is hungry.

- Make mealtimes pleasant and leisurely.

- Rearrange eating schedules to serve the main meal at the time of day when your child feels best. If she wakes up feeling well most days, make a high-protein, high-calorie breakfast.

- Do not punish your child for not eating.

> In the beginning of treatment, we decided that my son had to eat what the rest of the family was having. If he didn't eat that, he got no more food. He usually just didn't eat. Some mornings, I had trouble waking him up. He was limp and would have his eyes rolled back in his head. He was tested and diagnosed with hypoglycemia (low blood sugar). The doctor told us to give him whatever foods he was willing to eat and to make sure he ate something right before bed, even if it was ice cream or cookies and milk.

- Set a good example by eating a large variety of nutritious foods.

- Have nutritious snacks available at all times. Carry them in the car, to all appointments, and in backpacks for school.

- Serve fluids between meals, rather than with meals, to keep your child from feeling full after only a few bites of food.

- Limit the amount of less nutritious foods in the house. Potato chips, corn chips, soda, and sweets will fill your child up with empty calories.

- If your child is interested, include her in making a grocery list, shopping for favorite foods, and making meals.

How to make mealtimes fun

Here are some suggestions for making mealtime more fun:

- Try to take the emphasis off the need to eat food "because it's good for you." Focus instead on enjoying each other's company while sharing a meal. Encourage good conversation, tell stories and jokes, and perhaps light some candles.

- Make one night a week "restaurant night." Use a nice tablecloth and candles, allow the children to order from a menu, and pretend the family is out for a night on the town.

- Because any change in setting can encourage eating, consider having a picnic on the floor sometimes. Order pizza or other takeout, spread a tablecloth on the floor, and have an in-home picnic. One parent even sent lunch out to the treehouse.

  My son enjoyed eating in different places around the house and seemed to eat more when he was having fun. I sometimes fed the kids on their own picnic table outdoors in good weather, and at the same picnic table in the garage during the winter. They were thrilled to wear their coats and hats to eat. Occasionally I would let them eat off TV trays while watching a favorite program or tape.

- Some children seem to eat more if food is attractively arranged on the plate or is decorated in humorous ways. Preschoolers enjoy putting a smiley face on a casserole using strips of cheese, nuts, or raisins. Sandwiches can be cut into funny shapes using knives or cookie cutters.

  My daughter liked to have food decorated. For example, we would make pancakes look like a clown face by using blueberries for eyes, a strawberry for a nose, orange slices for ears, etc. She also enjoyed eating brightly colored food, so we would add a drop of food coloring to applesauce, yogurt, or whatever appealed to her.

How to serve more protein

Because many children cannot tolerate eating meat while on chemotherapy, below are ideas for increasing protein consumption:

- Add 1 cup of dried milk powder to a quart of whole milk, then blend and chill. Use this extra-strength milk for drinking and cooking.

- Use extra-strength milk (above), whole milk, evaporated milk, or cream instead of water to make hot cereal, cocoa, soup, gravy, custards, or puddings.

- Add powdered milk to casseroles, meat loaf, cream soups, custards, and puddings.

- Add chopped meat to scrambled eggs, soups, and vegetables.

- Add chopped, hard-boiled eggs to soups, salads, sauces, and casseroles.

- Add grated cheese to pizza, vegetables, salads, sauces, omelets, mashed potatoes, meat loaf, and casseroles.

- Serve bagels, English muffins, hamburgers, or hot dogs with a slice of cheese melted on top.
- Spread peanut butter on toast, crackers, and sandwiches. Dip fruit or raw vegetables into peanut butter for a quick snack.
- Spread peanut butter or cream cheese onto celery sticks.
- Serve nuts for snacks, and mix nuts into salads and soups.
- Put ice cream or whipped cream on top of pie, pudding, or fruit.
- Use dried beans and peas to make soups, dips, and casseroles.
- Use tofu (bean curd) in stir-fried vegetable dishes.
- Add wheat germ to hamburgers, meat loaf, breads, muffins, pancakes, waffles, and vegetables, and use it as a topping for casseroles.

Ways to boost calories

Many parents have ingrained habits about serving only low-fat meals and snacks. While your child is on chemotherapy, your mission is to find ways to add as many calories as possible to your child's food. Here are some suggestions:

- Add butter to hot cereal, eggs, pasta, rice, cooked vegetables, mashed potatoes, and soups.
- Use melted butter as a dip for raw vegetables and cooked seafood such as shrimp, crab, and lobster.
- Use sour cream to top meats, baked potatoes, and soups.
- Add mayonnaise or sour cream when making hamburgers or meat loaf.
- Make milkshakes, puddings, and custards with cream instead of milk.
- Serve your child whole milk (not 2% or skim milk).
- Make dips with cheese, avocado, butter, beans, or sour cream.
- Sauté vegetables in butter.
- Serve bread hot so it will absorb more butter.
- Add mayonnaise or butter to sandwiches.
- Spread bagels, muffins, or crackers with cream cheese and jelly or honey.
- Make hot chocolate with cream and add marshmallows.
- Add granola to cookie, bread, and muffin batters. Sprinkle granola on ice cream, pudding, and yogurt.
- Serve meat and vegetables with sauces made with cream and pan drippings.
- Add dried fruits to recipes for cookies, breads, and muffins.
- Serve ice cream or milkshakes made with real cream.

Nutritious snacks

Try to always bring a bag of nutritious snacks whenever you leave home with your child. This allows you to feed him whenever he is hungry and avoid stopping for non-nutritious junk food. Examples of healthful snacks include:

- Apples or applesauce
- Baby food
- Granola bars with no added sugar
- Celery sticks filled with cream cheese or peanut butter
- Cookies made with wheat germ, oatmeal, granola, fruits, or nuts
- Crackers with cheese, peanut butter, or tuna salad
- Dried fruit such as apples, raisins, apricots, or prunes
- Fresh fruit
- Granola mixed with dried fruit and nuts
- Muffins
- Nuts
- Peanut butter on crackers or whole wheat bread
- Protein bars
- Vegetables such as carrot sticks or broccoli florets

Snacks that you can carry in a small cooler with ice packs include:

- Yogurt, regular or frozen
- Cheese
- Chocolate milk
- Cottage cheese
- Hard-boiled and deviled eggs
- Pudding made with whole milk or cream
- Juice made from 100% fruit
- Fruit smoothies made with frozen fruit, sherbet, or ice cream

What Kids Really Eat

This chapter has listed ideas for increasing calories and making food more appealing. What follows are accounts of what several kids really ate while on chemotherapy. You will notice how varied the list is, so experiment to see what your child will eat. Remember that children's tastes and aversions may change throughout treatment.

Judd craved chicken chow mein and fried rice takeout from a Chinese restaurant. He also loved Spaghetti-Os® and hot dogs.

· · · · ·

I let Preston eat whatever tasted good to him, which was usually lots of potatoes and eggs. He liked spicy food (especially Mexican).

· · · · ·

Katy typically only ate one food for days or weeks at a stretch. One time, she ate pesto sauce (made from olive oil, garlic, Parmesan cheese, and basil leaves) on pasta for every meal for weeks. She also went through a spicy barbecue sauce phase, in which she wouldn't eat any food unless it was completely immersed in sauce. She ate no fruits, vegetables (except potatoes), or meat for the entire period of treatment. She ate only puréed baby food when she was really sick.

· · · · ·

In the beginning, when Meagan lost so much weight, we snuck Polycose® (a powdered nutritional supplement) into everything. She finally got stuck on cans of mixed nuts. They are high calorie and were instrumental in putting back on the weight. She also craved capers and would eat them by the tablespoonful.

· · · · ·

All Brent asks for are "peanut butter and jelly sandwiches, cut in fours, no crusts, with Fritos®." The only fruit he has eaten for three years is an occasional banana, and he eats no vegetables. He always ate everything before his diagnosis at age 6.

· · · · ·

The doctor told me to keep Kim on a low-salt, low-folic-acid diet. She wouldn't eat anything, so he eventually said he didn't care what she ate, as long as she ate. She liked Spaghetti-Os®, Chick-fil-A® nuggets, Chick-fil-A® soup, and McDonald's® sausage and pancakes.

· · · · ·

All Carl ate was dry cereal, dry waffles, oatmeal, and bacon. He ate no other meat or vegetables throughout treatment, but did drink milk. I thought that he would never be healthy, but he's 15 now (diagnosed when 2), eats little junk food, never gets sick, and looks great.

· · · · ·

On prednisone, Rachel ate only hot dogs, bologna, scrambled eggs with cheese, and potato chips. She would eat until she literally threw up. Now, two years off treatment, she is gradually expanding her repertoire. She only drinks milk (no water, juice, or soda), eats no sweets, and prefers all salty foods. I really have no idea whether it is learned behavior or a result of the cancer treatment.

· · · · ·

Prior to diagnosis, I was militant about serving organic, whole-grain, non-processed food. My son received a fruit or vegetable at every meal. After diagnosis, my dietary goals for Nico were centered on avoiding an NG tube. I just wanted him to keep eating. I always have healthy food in the house to offer. But he had overwhelming cravings while taking steroids. He fixated on one thing and ate only that one thing for days on end. During steroid pulses, my son would request "a box" of chicken nuggets and would eat 22 at one sitting. This last steroid pulse, he went through six boxes of breakfast sausages. I bought the organic chicken sausage, but I am not fooling myself into thinking this was healthy. We have enough trauma in our lives without fighting over food. I am not interested in adding that layer of conflict onto everything else. If I can get him to eat something nutritious, then great; otherwise, I indulge his dietary wants in the healthiest way possible (and it is not always possible).

· · · · ·

I guess Carrie Beth is the exception that proves the rule. She is on maintenance and has an excellent appetite. She eats fruits, vegetables, and lots of meat.

Dietitian/Nutritionist

It can be very helpful to consult with the hospital dietician/nutritionist to get more information and ideas about how to add more protein, calories, and vitamins/minerals to your child's diet. You can also consult with a private registered dietitian nutritionist (RDN) who has experience helping children with cancer. The Academy of Nutrition and Dietetics (*www.eatright.org*) is the country's largest group representing registered nutrition professionals; you can search for an RDN in your area on its website.

My 14-year-old daughter, Gabby, made it through transplant with no supplemental feedings. Before the transplant, she loaded up on healthy food; then when the mucositis hit, we worked with the dieticians and focused on what she could eat. She was also helped by appetite stimulants like Marinol®. I kept the fridge stocked with anything she was craving so when she was willing to eat, she didn't have to wait. I also created a goal chart that listed daily activities like taking the mouth sore medicine that tasted terrible, eating snacks, going for a walk, etc. She felt empowered when she checked off these activities every day. When she had done all of the tasks for a week, she got a big stuffed turtle from the gift shop that she really wanted. She was inpatient for less than three weeks.

Six-year-old Flynn is in maintenance for ALL. We participated in a nutrition research project for kids that was a great relief. I had become depressed in the kitchen as the ALL ruined our family meal times. Flynn developed issues around food; he had a fear of new foods and every meal time was a sad battle. But thanks to an intervention at the hospital, all that has since changed. Flynn eats a wide variety of foods, is less afraid to try new foods, eats fresh vegetables, and our meal times are back to normal. I'm so grateful for every meal we eat together as a family.

Vitamin Supplements

The nutritional needs of kids with cancer are higher than other children's, yet kids on treatment often eat less food. In addition, damage to the digestive system from chemotherapy alters the body's ability to absorb the nutrients in the food your child does manage to eat. As a result, vitamin supplements are usually necessary.

I gave my teenage daughter supplements of vitamins and some minerals. I also increased her vitamin intake by using the juicer every day. She always drank a big glass of fruit or vegetable juice, and I really think it helped her do as well as she has.

Vitamin supplements should only be given after consultation with your child's oncologist and nutritionist. Overuse of some vitamins, folic acid for example, can make your child's chemotherapy less effective. But providing other vitamins can make the difference between a pale and listless child and one with bright eyes and more energy.

Halfway through treatment, my daughter just looked awful. Her new hair began to thin out and break easily and her skin felt papery. I had been giving her a multivitamin and mineral tablet every day because her appetite was so poor, but it didn't seem to be enough. I talked to her doctor, then began to give her more of the antioxidant vitamins: betacarotene, E, and C. I bought the C in powder form, which effervesced when mixed with juice. She really liked her "bubble drinks." The betacarotene and E she swallowed along with the rest of her pills. Within a few weeks her hair stopped falling out, her skin stopped peeling, and she felt better.

Parent Advice

Several parents whose children have finished treatment offer the following tips about how to handle the inevitable eating problems of children on therapy.

Doctors sometimes reassure parents by saying, "His appetite will return to normal." Don't be surprised if this does not happen until long after the most intensive parts of treatment are completed.

Let your child control what type of food and how much he wants. In the beginning, any food is good food.

· · · · ·

Buy a juicer and use it every day. This was the only way we got any fruits or vegetables into our daughter. Make apple juice and sneak in a carrot. Sometimes we would make the juice, then blend it in the blender with ice cubes to make an iced drink, which we would serve with a straw.

· · · · ·

I solved my daughter's salt cravings by buying sea salt and letting her dip French fries in it once a week. For some reason, that satisfied her and stopped her from begging for regular table salt at every meal.

· · · · ·

One magic word: butter, butter, butter. We would make Maddie peanut butter and jelly sandwiches with a layer of butter on each side of the bread first. Milkshakes are great and Häagen Dazs® ice cream has the highest fat content. We also went to an "eat when she's hungry" mode. It was definitely more relaxing.

· · · · ·

We tried Ensure®, Sustacal®, and Carnation Instant Breakfast®. All were basically the same, with Carnation® being much more palatable. The other two have a bit of a medicinal smell and taste to them. You can add calories by throwing it in a blender with ice cream, bananas, or strawberries. My other two non-cancer kids loved this stuff. Mandy would "sip" a tiny bit but would rather eat the spicy food: bologna, Polish sausage, or tomatoes drowning in Catalina dressing. Reese's® peanut butter cups were breakfast for a long time (7 grams of protein!).

· · · · ·

There is reason for hope. My daughter ate almost nothing while on treatment. After treatment ended, she ate more food, but still no variety. She didn't turn the corner until a year off treatment, but now she is gradually trying new foods, including fruits and vegetables, again. I'm glad I never made an issue of it.

Feeding by Tube and IV

Sometimes it becomes necessary to feed children intravenously or through a gastric (G-tube) or nasogastric (NG) tube. Because intravenous (IV) feeding and feeding by tube may require additional hospitalization, it helps to understand the benefits. As appetite and weight decrease, the child's ability to tolerate and recover from chemotherapy lessens. The child becomes progressively weaker and her resistance to infection decreases. To prevent this scenario, most protocols require tube or IV feeding after 10% of body weight is lost. The two types of supplemental feeding are described below.

Total parenteral nutrition (TPN)

TPN, also known as hyperalimentation, is a form of IV feeding used to prevent or treat malnutrition in children who cannot eat enough to meet their nutritional needs. Below are some of the many reasons why your child may require TPN:

- Severe mouth and throat sores that prevent swallowing
- Severe nausea and vomiting
- Severe diarrhea
- Inability to chew or swallow normally
- Loss of more than 10% of body weight

TPN ensures that your child receives all the protein, carbohydrates, fats, vitamins, and minerals she needs. TPN is given through a central venous catheter, but children receiving TPN can also eat solids and drink fluids.

> My daughter needed TPN for two weeks after her stem cell transplant. They told us ahead of time that it would be necessary, and they were right. She got terrible sores throughout her GI tract and couldn't drink or eat. They just hooked the TPN bag up to her Broviac®. After a couple of weeks, she started gingerly sipping small amounts of water and apple juice. For some reason, I just didn't worry about her eating. I assumed that when she could eat, she would. She was a robust eater before her illness, so I thought that would help. Before we left for home, she asked for a hospital pizza (yuck!) and ate a few bites. Her eating at home quickly went back to normal, although it took some time to regain the weight she lost.

In most cases, TPN is started in the hospital. Each day the concentrations of glucose, protein, and fat will be increased, and doctors will assess your child's tolerance for the mixture. Generally, TPN is given 8 to 12 hours per day, depending on your child's situation. The infusion may be delivered over the hours that work best for your family. For example, if your child attends school, overnight infusions will probably work best.

You can request a small portable infusion pump and backpack from a home care company so your child can go about his daily activities as usual. Your child's oncologist may need to write a letter to your insurance company to verify your child's malnutrition so this therapy will be covered.

Enteral nutrition

The doctor may recommend enteral feeding if your child requires supplemental nutrition and her bowel and intestines are still functioning well. Enteral feedings are preferred over IV, whenever possible. Enteral nutrition is feeding via a tube placed through the nose and into the stomach (NG tube) or via a tube surgically placed directly into the stomach through the abdominal wall (G-tube). Nutritionally complete liquid formulas are delivered through the tube. Infrequent side effects of enteral nutrition are irritated throat, nausea, diarrhea, or constipation.

> *Rachel (age 14) used a backpack to carry a G-tube pump and her bag of Ensure®
> with her when she went out. When chemo was over, she worked for about a month
> with a psychiatrist who used hypnotherapy to get her to start eating normally again.
> After about three months, she was eating everything she used to. The tube was
> removed, and the hole closed on its own.*

· · · · ·

> *My daughter found it almost impossible to eat. She said that apart from her stomach
> feeling sick, everything tasted bad, and she didn't want to put that food in her mouth
> because the taste made her feel worse. As an adult you can say to yourself, this is for
> my own good, and force yourself to eat, but not kids. When she had to get a naso-
> gastric (NG) tube after she'd lost a third of her body weight, I felt nearly as bad as
> when she was first diagnosed. I believed that because she wasn't eating she had given
> up the will to live. I was a mess! The ward social worker gently pointed out to me
> that it was not my daughter's choice about whether to eat or not—it was entirely the
> fault of the chemo. When she got the NG tube, it was wonderful! She was able to get
> nutrition without forcing herself to eat when she really couldn't. And sure enough,
> once we got over the hurdle of that part of the treatment, she slowly regained her
> appetite again and we were able to wean her off the NG feeds. Four years later, she
> is still a very fussy eater—but I can live with that.*

> *I feel good nutrition is very important to good health, but the reality of the situation
> with our child was that he hated anything nutritious when he was on chemotherapy.
> I could doctor it up, add the best toppings, make it look terrific, season it just right,
> and it would still be rejected. So I decided that since my son wasn't allowed to make
> any decisions in regard to the pills, treatments, tests, or hospital stays, he wouldn't
> be forced to eat everything nutritious if he didn't want to. Whether this was a right
> or wrong decision, I don't know. I just know that I served him a lot of processed foods
> during those years, and he's a healthy and happy boy 10 years later. After he was
> finished with chemotherapy, however, we did require that he eat healthier foods.*

Chapter 23

Insurance, Record-keeping, and Financial Assistance

*"Prosperity is not without many fears and distastes;
and adversity is not without comfort and hopes."*

— Francis Bacon

UNDERSTANDING YOUR INSURANCE POLICY can make the difference between managing to keep your finances stable and bankruptcy. Many families find themselves fending off collection agencies while they are trying to save their child's life. Another trial for parents is keeping track of paper work—both medical and financial. But having accurate records can help prevent medical errors and reduce insurance overbillings. Having easy access to medical reports and properly organizing bills can also mean less time spent in conflicts with insurance companies and collection agencies.

This chapter describes how to understand your insurance policy and ways to work with the insurance company to cover bills. It also offers some suggestions about keeping both medical and financial records. Finally, it covers ways to find financial assistance.

Coping with Insurance

Finding one's way through the insurance maze can be a difficult task. However, understanding the benefits and claims procedures can help you get the bills paid without undue stress. The following sections outline some steps to help prevent problems with insurance.

Understand your policy

As soon as possible after diagnosis, read your entire insurance policy. Make a list of any questions you have about terms or benefits.

- Learn who the "participating providers" are under the plan and what happens if you see a non-participating provider. It is possible you will be penalized financially or that your claims may be denied if you go outside the network.

- Determine whether your physician needs to document specific requirements to obtain coverage for expensive or extended services.

  With our insurance, neuropsychological tests, outpatient occupational therapy, speech therapy, and physical therapy are covered, but the phrasing must be that it is a "medical necessity" due to diagnosis and treatments.

- Find out what your insurance copays are for different levels of service (e.g., office visit, outpatient surgery, outpatient testing, hospitalization, emergency room visits).

- Find out what your outpatient prescription drug benefits are for generic and non-generic drugs.

- Find out what your deductible is.

- Find out whether there is a point at which coverage increases to 100%.

- Determine whether there is a lifetime limit on benefits.

- Find out when a second opinion is required.

- Learn when you have to precertify a hospitalization or specialty consultation. Many insurance companies require precertification, even for emergencies.

  I realized that my daughter had been treated for over four months, and I had never called the insurance company. When I read the manual, I was horrified to find out that I had not pre-notified them about three scheduled hospitalizations. There was a $200 penalty for each lapse. I called in tears, and they only charged me for one mistake, not all three.

- Determine whether your policy has benefits for counseling. If so, find out how many visits are covered and how much of the cost is covered.

- Find out the names of approved providers for home infusion supplies (e.g., IV medications, central venous catheter supplies, and home nutrition) and home nursing care. These are often separate companies. Find out the policy coverage for these services.

  We changed to a new pediatrician, and he asked me if I thought it would be easier on my son to have visiting nurses come to our home to do the chemotherapy injections and some blood work. Since my son had very low counts, it made a lot of sense not to have to go out. It also lessened his fears to be able to stay at home and have the same nurse come to do the procedures. It was a pleasant surprise to find these services covered by our insurance.

Find a contact person

As soon as possible after diagnosis, call your insurance company and ask who will be handling your claims. Explain that there will be years of bills with frequent hospitalizations, and it would be helpful to deal with the same person each time. Your insurance company may assign your child's account to a case manager who will help you under-stand and use of your policy benefits. Try to develop a cooperative relationship with your case manager, because she can really make your life easier. Also, your employer may have a benefits specialist who can operate as a liaison with the insurer.

My employee benefits representative was Bobbi. She was just wonderful. The hospi-tal would send her copies of the bills at the same time they sent mine. Since I found so many errors, she would hold the bills a week until I called to tell her that they were correct before she paid them. She was very pleasant to deal with.

Negotiate

Do not be afraid to negotiate with the insurance company over benefits. Often, your case manager may be able to redefine a service your child needs to allow it to be covered.

Our insurance company covered 100% of maintenance drugs only if the patients needed them for the rest of their lives. Christine's maintenance drugs were only needed for two years but were extremely expensive. I asked my contact person for help, and she petitioned the decision-making board. They granted us an exemption and covered the entire cost of all her maintenance drugs.

• • • • •

Some of us have employer-paid health insurance benefits. If we are not comfortable with the level of service that the insurance contractor is providing (particularly when it comes to not resolving a bill for months or even years), that's an employee satisfaction and compensation issue. Remember, those of us with employer-paid health insurance get this instead of additional cash. Non-cash compensation has significant advantages for the employer. Sometimes, with a little luck, the right pre-sentation, and the facts, we can persuade our employer to help resolve the issue that is causing all the grief.

Appeal a denial

Policy holders have the right to appeal a denial by their insurance company. The follow-ing are ways to appeal a denial of payment.

• Keep original documents in your files and send photocopies to the insurance com-pany with a letter outlining why the claim should be covered. Make sure to request a written reply and keep a copy of the letter for your records.

We were making inquiries into hospice care, feeling it was time to explore that option. I found out that the only pediatric hospice provider in the state of Georgia was not on the preferred provider list. Our insurance company would pay for ben-efits, but at a reduced rate; not a good thing since the lifetime maximum for hospice *care was $7,500. I felt like my only options were reduced pediatric care or full benefits using adult services. I wrote a letter of appeal stating that medically and ethically, neither of these were good choices. Well, we got a better outcome than I asked for. Not only will they cover the pediatric provider, but they have waived the lifetime maximum!*

- Contact your elected representative to the U.S. Congress. All Senators and members of the House of Representatives have staff members who help constituents with problems. You can also contact your state insurance board with concerns and complaints.

  When I ran into insurance company problems, I wrote a letter to the insurance company detailing the facts, the decisions the insurance company made, and a logical explanation about why the procedure needed to happen. I also noted in the letter that a copy was going to our state insurance commissioner, and I sent both letters by certified mail. Within two days, the insurance company all of a sudden decided to cover the procedure. I later found out that the insurance commissioner's office started an investigation against them. Letters help, especially when sent by certified mail.

- If none of the above steps resolves the dispute, take your claim to small claims court (which does not require you to hire an attorney). You can also find an attorney who will represent you for free (called pro bono), or hire an attorney skilled in insurance matters to sue the insurance company.

It may not feel comfortable being so persistent, but sometimes it is needed to ensure you get the support to which you and your child are entitled.

When I finally got an advocate assigned for my child within our insurance company, I fretted to her one day that every single claim was initially rejected. She replied that the agents were trained to reject certain types of claims the first two times they were submitted as a cost-saving strategy. She said, "Very few subscribers are tenacious enough to come back three times, so we save millions of dollars each year just because they give up."

Keeping Medical Records

Some parents consider that they have two sets of books, the hospital's and their own. If the hospital loses their child's chart or misplaces lab results, the parents will still have a copy. If their child's records include hundreds of pages in an electronic chart, the parents can have a simple system that makes it easy to spot trends and retrieve dosage information. The following are suggested items that parents can record:

- Dates and results of all lab work
- Dates of chemotherapy, drugs given, and doses

- All changes in dosages of medicine
- Any side effects from drugs
- Any fevers or illnesses
- Dates of all scheduled and unscheduled hospitalizations
- Dates of all medical appointments and name(s) of the doctor(s) seen
- Dates for any procedures performed
- Dates of radiation therapy, including total dose delivered, and areas treated
- Dates of diagnosis, completion of therapy, and recurrences (if any)

Keeping daily records of your child's health for months or years is hard work. But remember that your child may be seen by pediatricians, oncologists, residents, radiation therapists, lab technicians, nutritionists, psychologists, social workers, and physical therapists. Your records can help keep it all straight and help pull all the information together. Your records also will help you remember questions to ask, prevent mistakes, and notice trends.

The following sections describe several record-keeping methods parents have used successfully.

Journal

Keeping a journal in a notebook works very well for some families. Parents make entries every day about all pertinent medical information and often include personal information, such as their own feelings or memorable things their child said or did. Journals are easy to carry back and forth to the clinic, and journal entries can be written while waiting for appointments. One disadvantage is that journals can be misplaced.

> Stephan's oncologist is kind of hard to communicate with. I learned early on to keep a journal of Stephan's appointments, drugs given, side effects, and blood counts. That way if I ever had to call the doctor I would have it right in front of me. I also recorded Stephan's temperature when his counts were low to keep track of infections.

Many institutions give families a notebook that contains information about their child's cancer and treatment plan. Often, these notebooks have blank pages for recording blood cell counts. Free treatment journals are available from the Alex's Lemonade Stand Foundation at *www.alexslemonade.org/childhood-cancer-treatment-journal*.

> Record-keeping—very important! My father came to the hospital soon after diagnosis and brought a three-ring binder and a three-hole punch. I would punch lab reports, protocols, consent forms, drug information sheets, etc., and keep them in my binder. A mother at the clinic showed me her weekly calendar book, and I adopted

her idea for recording blood counts and medications. Frequently the clinic's records disagreed with mine as to medications and where we were on the protocol. I was very glad that I kept good records.

Calendar

Many parents report great success with the calendar system. They buy a new calendar each year and hang it in a convenient place, such as next to where you store the pills. You can record counts on the calendar while talking on the phone to the nurse or lab technician and take the calendar with you to all appointments. Other family members use an online calendar which they can view on any of their electronic devices.

Each year I purchase a new calendar with large spaces on it. I write all lab results, any symptoms or side effects, colds, fevers, and anything else that happens. I bring it with me to the clinic each visit, as it helps immensely when trying to relate some events or watch trends. I also use it like a mini-journal, recording our activities and quotes from Meagan. Now that she's off treatment, I'm superstitious enough to still bring it to our monthly checkups.

· · · · ·

I wrote the counts on a calendar or on little pieces of paper that got lost. But, to be honest, I didn't keep the medical records very well. I'm upset with myself when I think of it now.

· · · · ·

The first place where my son was treated gave us a really helpful calendar that listed the drugs and doses for each day. I could just check things off when I gave them. When he relapsed the second time, we went to a different institution, enrolled in a clinical trial, and I got the full trial document. Then I could just look up what was supposed to happen and when.

Blood cell count charts

Many hospitals supply folders containing photocopied sheets for record-keeping. Typically, they have spaces for the date, white blood cell count, absolute neutrophil count, hematocrit, platelet level, chemotherapy given, and side effects.

My record-keeping system was given to me by the hospital on the first day. We were given a notebook with information about the illness and treatment. Also included were charts that we could use to keep all the information about my child's blood work, progress, reactions to drugs, etc. While we were at the hospital, we were able to get the information off one of the computers on our floor each afternoon. My notebook holds records and notes for three years. Perhaps I was being compulsive

*with my record-keeping, but it made me feel that I was part of the team working on
bringing my boy back to health.*

Tape or digital recorder

For parents who keep track of more information than a calendar can hold, and who find
writing in a journal too time consuming, using a voice recording device works well.
Small recording machines are inexpensive and can be carried in a pocket or purse. Most
smartphones also can record. Digital recordings can be downloaded to a flash drive or
computer for storage. If you want to transcribe the recordings to a written record, there
are programs such as Dragon Speak® that you can train to understand your voice, and
that can be used to change your spoken words into a written document.

> *I started keeping a journal in the hospital, but I was just too upset and exhausted to
> write in it faithfully. A good friend who was a writer told me to use a tape recorder.
> It was a great idea and saved a lot of time. I could say everything that had happened
> in just a few minutes every day. I kept a separate notebook just for blood counts so I
> could check them at a glance.*

Computer

For some parents, saving all medical records on a computer is a good option. Parents
can print out bar graphs of the blood counts in relation to chemotherapy and quickly
spot trends. You can also keep a running narrative of your thoughts, feelings, and concerns during your child's treatment. As with all other computer records, keep a backup
copy on a flash drive, external hard drive, or mobile cloud storage.

> *At our hospital, the summary of counts for a given child can be formatted to print
> out as a "trend review," with each date printed out on the left side of the page and
> the various lab values in columns down the page. The system permits printouts from
> the very first blood draw if that is desired. Periodically, on slow days, I'll ask if I can
> have a trend review. Then I put it in my binder of records.*

Keeping Financial Records

You will not need a calendar or journal for financial records, just a big, well-organized
file cabinet. It is essential to keep track of bills and payments. Dealing with financial
records is a major headache for many parents, but keeping good records can prevent
financial catastrophe. The following are ideas about how to organize financial records:

- Have hanging files for hospital bills, doctor bills, all other medical bills, insurance
  explanation of benefits (EOBs), prescription receipts, tax-deductible receipts (e.g.,
  tolls, parking, motels, meals), and correspondence.

- Whenever you open an envelope related to your child's medical care, file the contents immediately. Don't leave it on the desk or throw it in a drawer.
- Keep a notebook with a running log of all tax-deductible medical expenses, including the service, charge, bill paid, date paid, and credit card receipt or check number.
- Do not pay a bill unless you have checked over each item listed to make sure the charge is correct.
- Start new files every year.

> To be honest, the paper trail really gets me down. I can only deal with the stacks every few months. I open things and make sure the insurance company is doing its part, and then I try to sort through and pay our part.
>
> • • • • •
>
> I started out organized, and I'm glad I did because the hospital billing was confusing and full of errors. I cleared out a file cabinet and put in folders for each type of bill and insurance papers. I filed each bill chronologically so I could always find the one I needed. I made copies of all letters sent to the insurance company and hospital billing department. I wrote on the back of each EOB any phone calls I had to make about that bill. I wrote down the date of the call, the name of the person I spoke to, and what she said. It saved us a lot of grief and money.

Deductible Medical Expenses

It is estimated that families of children with cancer spend 25% or more of their income on items not covered by insurance. Examples of these expenses are gas, car repairs, motels, food away from home, health insurance deductibles and copays, prescriptions, and dental work. Many of these items can be deducted from federal income tax. Often parents are too fatigued to go through stacks of bills at the end of the year to calculate their deductions. If a monthly total is kept in a notebook or on your computer, then all that needs to be done at tax time is to add up the monthly totals.

The Internal Revenue Service (IRS) generally allows you to deduct any reasonable cost for procedures or expenses that are deemed by a doctor to be medically necessary. You may also deduct certain other expenses with proper documentation; some of the costs that are currently deductible include wheelchairs, wigs, acupuncture, psychotherapy and counseling, health maintenance organization (HMO) fees, special education or tutoring costs for sick children, meals at the hospital, parking at the hospital, travel to and from medical appointments, and transportation and lodging costs while your child is in the hospital.

To find out what can be deducted while your child is undergoing treatment, get IRS Publication 502 for the relevant tax year. You can download this publication from the IRS website at *www.irs.gov* or make a copy from a master form at your local library (ask a reference librarian where the IRS forms are kept).

Canadian families can deduct many of the same medical expenses as U.S. families. To find out what can be deducted in Canada, visit the Revenue Canada website at *www. cra-arc.gc.ca* and type in the search term "deductible medical expenses."

If you keep a calendar, an easy way to track tax-deductible items is to glue an envelope to the inside cover. Whenever you incur an expense that may be tax deductible (e.g., parking at the hospital), put the receipt in the envelope and file it when you get home.

Dealing with Hospital Billing

Unfortunately, problems with billing are common for parents of children with cancer. Here are two typical experiences:

Insurance was an absolute nightmare. It almost gave me a nervous breakdown. After all we go through with our children, to have to deal with the messed-up hospital billing was just too much. We would stack the bills up and try to go through them every two or three months. Our insurance was supposed to pay 100%, but the billing was so confusing that they refused to cover some things because it wasn't clear what they were being billed for. The hospital frequently double billed, especially for prescriptions. We just stopped getting our prescriptions there. We would call the hospital billing department to try to get the mess straightened out, but the billing department was just as confused as we were. They kept sending our account to collections. We did everything in our power to get it straight, but we never did.

• • • • •

We had two distinctly different experiences at the two institutions we dealt with. The university hospital where my daughter received her radiation gave me a folder the first day. It included, among other things, a sheet from a financial counselor giving all the information needed for preventing and solving billing problems. I never needed to call her because the hospital billing was clear, prompt, and organized. The children's hospital where my daughter was a frequent inpatient and clinic patient was another story altogether. They billed from three different departments, put charges from the same visit on different bills, frequently over-billed, continuously made errors, and constantly threatened to send the account to collections. I never spoke to the same billing clerk twice. It was a never-ending grind and a constant frustration.

It is impossible to prevent billing errors, but it is necessary to deal with them. Here are step-by-step suggestions for solving problems:

- Keep all records filed in an organized fashion.

- Check every bill from the hospital to make sure there are no charges for treatments not given or errors such as double billing.

  > During maintenance, my daughter went to the clinic every three months. She had identical treatments every visit—port accessed, vincristine given, physical exam, and intrathecal methotrexate given via spinal tap. Each bill was different, differing by hundreds of dollars, for identical visits! There were errors on each bill, including numerous charges for IV Benadryl® that she never received. I would get the errors removed, then they would reappear on the next bill.

- Check to see whether the hospital has financial counselors. If so, make contact early in your child's hospitalization. Counselors provide services in many areas, including help with understanding the hospital's billing system, understanding explanations of benefits, managing hospital/insurance correspondence, dealing with Medicaid, working out a payment plan, designing a ledger system for tracking insurance claims, and resolving disputes.

- If you find a billing error, immediately call the hospital billing department. Write down the date, the name of the person you talk to, and the plan of action.

  > I often couldn't even get through to the billing representative; I was just put on hold forever. Then I tried to discuss the problems with the director of billing, but she was never in. After about 20 phone calls, I finally said to her secretary, "You know, I have a desperately sick child here, and I've been as patient and polite as I can. What else can I do?" She said, "Honey, get irate. It works every time." I told her to put me through to somebody, anybody, and I would. She connected me to the person who mediates disputes, I got irate, and we went through all the bills line by line.

- If the error is not corrected on your next bill, call and talk to the billing supervisor. Explain the steps you have already taken and how you would like the problem fixed.

  > The hospital billing was so bad, and I had to call so often, that I developed a telephone relationship with the supervisor. I always tried to be upbeat, we laughed a lot, and it worked out. She stopped investigating every problem and would just delete the erroneous charge.

- If the problem is still not corrected, write a brief letter to the billing supervisor explaining the steps you have taken and requesting immediate action. Keep a copy of each letter that you write and all written responses.

- Every time you receive an explanation of benefits (EOB) from your insurance company, compare it to the hospital bill. Track down discrepancies.

My system for insurance record keeping was to keep all of the EOBs and bills from the hospital and check them against each other by date of service. If they matched, we paid our part. I also kept an Excel spreadsheet by year that had columns for date bill received, date of service, amount charged, date EOB received, date paid, and check number. At the end of every year, I'd send it to our accountant to review for tax purposes. I also kept files for papers (EOBs and bills). My advice to parents is to not pay until you are sure what you owe. Every time the hospital sent our case to collections, I'd be able to say, "What's the date of service and the charge?" and then I'd look at my spreadsheet and say that we didn't get that bill or it was paid on a certain date and I could supply the check number.

- If you are inundated with a constant stream of bills and there are major discrepancies between the hospital charges and what is being paid for by your insurance, ask both the hospital billing department and your insurance company, in writing, to audit the account. Insist on a line-by-line explanation for each charge.

Within five months of my daughter's diagnosis, the billing was so messed up that I despaired of ever getting it straight. When the hospital threatened to send the account to a collection agency, I took action. I sent certified letters to the hospital and the insurance company demanding an audit. When both audits arrived, they were $9,000 apart. I met with our insurance representative, and she called the hospital, and we had a three-way showdown. We straightened it out that time, but every bill that I received for the duration of treatment had one or more errors, always in the hospital's favor.

- If you are too tired or overwhelmed to deal with the bills, ask a family member or friend to help. That person could come every other week, open and file all bills and insurance papers, make phone calls, write all necessary letters, and even scan your records into your computer for storage.

- Do not let billing problems accumulate. Your account may end up at a collection agency, which can quickly become a nightmare.

Our insurance was constantly months behind in paying our bills to the children's hospital. The hospital sent our account to collections, despite my assurances that I was doing everything I could to get the insurance to pay. We were hounded on the phone constantly by the collection people, often until we were in tears. We finally just took out a second mortgage and paid off the hospital, but now I don't know if we will be reimbursed by insurance.

Not all stories are so grim. People who are in a single payer healthcare system, in some managed care systems, or on public assistance may never see bills. Many people with insurance encounter no problems throughout their child's treatment.

Our insurance paid 80% of everything, no questions asked, and always paid us within a month. People shouldn't have to worry about finances or their insurance program at a difficult time like this.

• • • • •

We have a low income, so we are on the state plan. They give us coupons for each child, and we just hand over a coupon at each visit. I have never seen a bill.

Sources of Financial Assistance

Sources of financial assistance vary from state to state and town to town. To begin tracking down possible options, ask the hospital social worker for assistance. In addition, some hospitals have community outreach nurses or case workers who may point out potential sources of assistance.

Hospital policy

If you are unable to pay your hospital bills, do not sell your house or let your account go to collections. Ask the hospital social worker to set up an appointment for you with the appropriate person to discuss the hospital policy for financial assistance. Many hospitals write off a percentage of the cost of care if the patient is uninsured or underinsured. You can also talk to the hospital about setting up a monthly payment plan.

Supplemental Security Income (SSI)

SSI is an entitlement program of the U.S. government that is based on family income and administered by the Social Security Administration. Recipients must be disabled and have a low family income and few assets. Children with cancer qualify as disabled for this program, making some of them eligible for a monthly financial payment if the family income and assets are low enough. To learn more or to apply, visit *www.ssa.gov/ssi*.

> *Our Katie was approved for SSI right away. It did take a large amount of preparation with the required paperwork. I researched and when I found a roadblock, I asked the Social Security people what I needed to overcome these obstacles. In our case, we had too much money in the bank, so we "spent down" by prepaying bills. I made sure I had all our birth certificates, that Katie's medical records were complete, etc. Since I found this so cumbersome, you can't imagine how happy I was when our income and Katie's health excluded us from SSI and we became self-sufficient again. That said, I sure was glad it was there when needed.*

If you need legal help appealing a denial for SSI, there is a professional organization of attorneys and paralegals called the National Organization for Social Security Claimants'

Representatives (NOSSCR). You can contact NOSSCR by phone at (800) 431-2804 or online at *www.nosscr.org* for a referral to a member in your geographic location.

Medicaid

Medicaid is a program that pays for medical services needed by citizens with low incomes. Medicaid is administered by state governments, and the federal government pays a portion of the entitlement. Rules about eligibility vary, but families with private insurance sometimes are eligible if huge hospital bills are only partially covered by their insurance policy. Some states cover children younger than age 21 if they are hospitalized for more than 30 days, regardless of parental income. In addition to medical bills, Medicaid sometimes also pays for transportation and prescriptions. More information is available at *www.medicaid.gov.*

Free medicine programs

Children with cancer, and survivors of cancer, often need expensive medications, and sometimes families cannot afford them. Most major U.S. drug companies have patient-assistance programs, and you can apply to obtain free or low-cost prescription drugs. Although each company has its own criteria for qualification, in general, you must:

- Be a U.S. citizen or legal resident
- Have a prescription for the medication you are applying to get
- Have no prescription drug coverage for the medication
- Meet income requirements

You may qualify even if you have health insurance, if it does not cover the medication prescribed for your child. For expensive medications, the income cut-off may be high, so it is worth investigating whether you qualify. Several organizations that can help you find and apply to patient-assistance programs are listed in Appendix B, *Resource Organizations*. Because the application process takes time and includes obtaining information from your child's doctor(s), plan ahead so you don't run out of medication.

> *Our insurance does not cover the growth hormone that my daughter needs. Her physician cannot believe that our insurance company denied coverage for a survivor with a history of radiation to the brain and multiple late effects to the endocrine system, but that's our situation. The medication is incredibly expensive. We applied to a patient-assistance program and were thrilled to find out that we qualified if our adjusted gross income was less than $100,000 a year. The application process the first year was hard and took a few months, but now we just fill in a form and send in our tax return every year, and she is requalified. We get a shipment of growth hormone every three months and keep it in the fridge.*

Although the cost of in-hospital treatment in Canada is covered by provincial governments, families have to pay for some medications. For families without private insurance, this often creates financial hardship. In many instances, the Department of Social Services can help pay for medications. The qualifications vary in each province and the decision is based on financial need. Canadian parents should contact their provincial Department of Social Services for further information.

State-sponsored supplemental insurance

Most states have supplemental insurance programs for families with children who are living with chronic conditions. These programs often help cover services, prescriptions, and co-payments that your primary insurance will not pay for. You can get more information about the specific programs in your state from your hospital social worker or by calling your state's department that regulates insurance (e.g., State Insurance Commission).

> In our state, besides my husband's insurance, we also have what is called Children's Special Health Care Services (CSHCS). It is a secondary insurance that pays for what our primary insurance doesn't—co-pays and prescriptions, trips back and forth to the hospital, doctor appointment and prescription co-pays, our stay at the Ronald McDonald House. Any expenses related to treatment that our primary insurance won't cover, this will. The amount you pay for this coverage is based on family income. It has been a lifesaver for us.

Service organizations

Numerous service organizations help families in need, providing aid such as transportation, wigs, special wheelchairs, and food. Often, all a family has to do is describe its plight, and good Samaritans appear. Some service organizations in your community may be: American Legion; Elks Club; fraternal organizations such as the Masons, Jaycees, Kiwanis Club, Knights of Columbus, Lions, and Rotary; United Way; and religious groups of all denominations. In addition, local philanthropic organizations exist in many communities. To locate them, call your local health department, ask to speak with a social worker, and ask for help.

Organized fundraising

Many communities rally around a child with cancer by organizing a fundraiser. Help is given in various ways, ranging from donation jars in local stores to an organized drive using all the local media. There are many pitfalls to avoid in fundraising, and great care must be taken to protect the sick child's privacy to the fullest extent possible. There have been some unfortunate scams in which generous people donated to funds for sick children who did not exist. If you decide to try fundraising, it is best to obtain legal assistance and to establish a trust fund for the express purpose of paying the child's medical expenses.

If your child is on or seeking Social Security or Medicaid, funds must be held in a special needs trust and paid directly to providers. If the family receives money from fundraisers, or the child's Social Security number is used to open the bank account, the child can lose funding from both Social Security and Medicaid.

Miscellaneous Insurance Issues

Loss of insurance coverage can be a nightmare. If you lose your job, change jobs, or move while your child is on treatment, speak to your employer's benefits manager promptly. You can continue insurance coverage with your previous employer through a Consolidated Omnibus Budget Reconciliation Act (COBRA) plan until you are certain your new insurance coverage is in effect, or you can look for coverage under the Affordable Care Act (ACA). Although using COBRA may impose some financial strain on your family for several months, it will ensure your child's coverage without interruption.

> *We just switched to an ACA plan from COBRA, as did a friend of mine with cancer. I am saving $300 per month and she is saving $400. ACA covers preexisting conditions, and you can get a special tax credit that is not available with COBRA if your income level is within certain limits.*

Speak to your employer about whether participation in a Section 125 Plan (sometimes called a cafeteria plan, flexible spending account, or health savings account) is an option at your place of employment. These plans generally allow you to have your employer withhold pre-tax dollars from your pay for expenses such as childcare costs and non-reimbursed medical expenses. However, you will need to fill out reimbursement forms and submit them by year's end, otherwise you might lose the money.

> *We were blessed that we had great insurance and that both of our employers were wonderful to us. My husband came home from an overseas deployment the day our son was diagnosed. They let him stay stateside to help and told him to do what his family needed. I had to quit my job, but my employer recommended that I use the rest of my FMLA time (I only used some of it when our daughter was born several months earlier) before resigning. That also gave me a paycheck until the end of the year, and I received my yearly bonus before resigning. We've been able to live modestly and focus on our kids. We know so many families that struggle financially and even go bankrupt, so we feel very lucky.*

Chapter 24

End of Treatment and Beyond

*"The best formula for longevity:
have a chronic disease, and cure it."*

— Oliver Wendell Holmes

THE LAST DAY OF TREATMENT is a time of both celebration and fear. Families are thrilled that the days of pills and procedures have ended, but some fear a future without drugs to keep the disease away. Concerns about relapse are an almost universal worry at the end of treatment; but for the majority of families, the months and years roll by without recurrence of the leukemia.

However, while many children and teens quickly return to excellent physical and mental health, others have lingering or permanent effects from the treatment. This chapter covers the emotional and physical aspects of ending treatment and the need for excellent medical follow up.

Emotions

Parents should anticipate that, after many months or years spent watching their child go through the rigors of treatment, they may have lost the feeling of a normal life. They may have relapse scares and may frequently need to call the doctor to describe the symptoms and be reassured.

> *Every time Sean sneezed, I was there with a thermometer. I was constantly on the lookout for "bad germs." It took about a year before I was finally able to relax and stop feeling so paranoid.*

> · · · · ·

> *When we got back home after the transplant, I cried for a month. The boys went back to a routine and played together all the time, but I didn't know what to do. My spouse and I had left work, left our home, left our friends, lost most of our income, and we were the only T-cell family when we were in the hospital. We didn't have a*

big family and were treated far from home, so my husband and I were on our own. It was lonely and hard. I was an emotional mess when we finally got home and had the time to let our situation really sink in. It's hard to sift through the pieces of my life and try to figure out what our future will be like from now on. I have learned to live one day at a time, and during treatment it was often one hour at a time.

With diagnosis came an acute awareness that life can be cruel and unpredictable. Many parents feel safe during treatment and feel that therapy is keeping the cancer from coming back. The end of treatment leaves many parents and children feeling exposed and vulnerable. When treatment ends, parents must find a way to live with uncertainty—to find a balance between hope and reasonable worry.

Several months after my son ended treatment, I was driving down the street, and I started to worry that Sam seemed excessively tired lately. I started to feel my throat constricting, and tears sprang to my eyes. I had to pull over because I literally couldn't breathe. I had to force myself to calm down, breathe slowly, and realize that I was just having a normal attack of being petrified that he would relapse.

· · · · ·

I had a lot of anticipatory worry—it started about six months before ending treatment. By the last day of treatment, I had been worrying for months, so it was just a relief to quit.

· · · · ·

We were thrilled when treatment ended. I knew many people who felt that celebrating would jinx them; they just didn't feel safe. Well, I felt that we had won a big battle—getting through treatment—and we were going to celebrate that. If, heaven forbid, in the future we had another battle to fight, we'd deal with it. But on the last day of treatment, we were delighted.

Last Treatment

The last day of treatment for a child in remission from leukemia generally includes a diagnostic spinal tap, a bone marrow aspiration, a complete blood count (CBC) and chemistry screen, a thorough physical exam, and a discussion with the oncologist or nurse practitioner (NP). The oncologist or NP should review the treatment given, outline the schedule for future blood tests and exams, and sensitively discuss with the family the potential for long-term side effects. After the procedures, the family will usually wait to hear the preliminary report about the bone marrow aspiration, as true relief does not come until they know that no leukemic blasts are present.

A treatment summary should be provided to you, which will include diagnosis; chemotherapy drugs given and total amounts; radiation given, location, and total dose;

surgeries; pertinent past medical history; family history; and recommendations for continued follow up into adulthood.

> *The nurses at our clinic really made a big deal on the last day of treatment. They brought out a cake and balloons, and sang "Going off Chemo" to the tune of "Happy Birthday to You." They made Gina a banner and bought her a present. I sat in a corner and cried, because I was scared to death of the future. A nurse came over, hugged me, and said, "This must be so hard; we're taking away your security blanket." She was exactly right.*

· · · · ·

> *When treatment was finally over, we felt like we had been cut adrift at sea. Suddenly, our hospital safety net was gone. This was the day that we had been waiting for—and now we were terrified.*

Catheter Removal

Children and teens usually cannot wait to have the catheter removed, as it symbolizes that treatment has truly ended. Venous catheters are usually removed soon after treatment ends.

> *During Elizabeth's last treatment, her doctor told me he was going to schedule her for surgery to remove her central line. I was so ecstatic! To me, Elizabeth wasn't really in remission as long as the central line was still there. I know it was irrational, but part of me felt as if there were cancer cells dangling at the end of that central line. If we didn't get it out right away, Elizabeth would still have cancer. I wanted it out "right now."*

Removal of an external catheter is an outpatient procedure done in the operating room, an interventional radiology room, or a sedation unit. The child is sedated, and the catheter is removed within minutes.

Implanted catheters such as the PORT-A-CATH® are removed surgically in the operating room. Children are usually given general anesthesia, and the operation takes less than half an hour. Only one incision is made, generally just above the port at the same place as the scar from the implantation surgery. The sutures holding the port to the underlying muscle are cut, and the port with tubing is pulled out. The small incision is then stitched and bandaged. When the child begins to awaken, he is brought to the recovery room where his parents can join him. The family then waits until the surgeon approves their departure. Often, the wait is short, because as soon as the child is awake enough to take a small drink or eat a popsicle, he is released. However, if your child becomes nauseated from the anesthesia, the wait can be several hours; he will not be released until he is feeling better.

Brent had a very easy time with his port-removal surgery. We scheduled him to be the first patient early in the morning, so there was no delay getting in. Then the anesthesiologist asked him what flavor of gas he wanted, which he liked. They brought him out to us while he was still groggy, and he woke up feeling goofy and happy. We went home soon thereafter. It felt more like the ending than did the last day of treatment.

· · · · ·

I remember when Andrew had his port out. As he was coming out of his anesthesia fog I leaned over to him and said rather tearfully, "Andrew, you did it; you're all done." He took his small hand and placed it at the site where that port sat for two years, felt its absence, and smiled. It was one of the best moments of my life.

Ceremonies

Some families enjoy having ceremonies to celebrate the end of cancer treatment. For younger children who have spent much of their lives taking pills and having procedures, ceremonies really help them grasp that treatment is truly over. Here are ideas from many families about how to commemorate this important occasion:

- Take "last day of treatment" pictures of the hospital and staff.
- Take a picture of your child taking her last pill.
- Give trophies to your child and siblings.

    We had a big party during which my husband, Scott, stood up and called for everyone's attention. He gave a talk about how proud we were of Jeremy and handed him a trophy. It had the victory angel on top and was engraved with "Jeremy, we are so proud of you and your victory. Love, Mom and Dad." We gave a trophy to his brother, Jason, for being the world's most supportive brother.

- Ask the clinic to present your child with a certificate or ring the "chemo over" bell.
- Go on a trip or vacation to celebrate.

    All of the parents of children with leukemia in our community have become very close. When 9-year-old Brent finished his treatment, I called to congratulate him. He was so excited telling me about it, but then his voice started to shake and he cried when he told me, "My two aunts gave me a card with money inside to go to a motel with a pool for the weekend. They gave it to me because I had leukemia. Can you believe that?"

- Throw a big party for friends and family.

Erica ended treatment in December, and we threw a big party at our church. We called it a "Celebration of Life." We invited all of the families that we had become so close to through the support group. We especially wanted the families who had lost their children to cancer, and they all came. My normally even-tempered husband gave a talk about Club Goodtimes (the support group) and how it was a club that no one ever wanted to join. When he talked about the many wonderful people we met there, his voice shook with emotion. Then the preacher prayed for the children who weren't with us. We ate a huge cake, and the children were entertained by a clown. It was both moving and fun.

• • • • •

We invited all of our friends and family to the park for "Tay's beating leukemia party." We had red and white balloons that we wrote on that said, "Healthy red cells" and "Healthy white cells." We also had black balloons that were "bad cells" that the kids sat on and popped. We had a round piñata that said "Leukemia" on it and one of the international symbols for "NO" drawn through it. The kids "beat" leukemia with a stick, and candy came pouring out. We all had a good time. It was a well-attended party. We grilled outside, drank sodas, ate watermelon, played a little volleyball, and just had a great time.

• Throw a big party at school.

Joseph finished treatment when he was in kindergarten. The kids had gone through almost an entire year with him. They had known all about his treatments and frequent hospitalizations. It seemed appropriate to have an "all done with treatment" celebration. We even had his two best friends who go to different schools come over to join us; his big brother, Nate, came down from his class to share in the fun.

It was a very joyous occasion, and we made it as much like a birthday party as we could. I brought cupcakes and juice and we played games. A friend who leads the story hour at our children's bookstore came and did some songs and stories with the kids; I even sent each classmate home with a treat bag. At the end, right before time to go home, Joseph pulled out several cans of his favorite hospital discovery, and the kids took turns blasting a shower of Silly String® on everyone else! We all clapped and cheered, and Joseph's wonderful teacher and I had a chance to have a good celebratory cry while the kids put on their things to go home. Clean-up wasn't too darn bad, and it meant a lot to all of us.

There's still a tiny remnant of green Silly String® on one of the fluorescent light fixtures, and my big second-grader likes to go down and admire it when he visits his old kindergarten teacher.

• If your child has been seeing a counselor, schedule a visit to talk about the accomplishment.
• Have friends and family send congratulations cards.

My daughter Lauren, who has Down syndrome, has been through treatment twice. Her last relapse chemo is three days from today. She adores school, just lights up when there, and this disease has stolen more than three years of school from her. One blessing is that several classmates are peer mentors. They have visited her and kept in touch for years. One is even coming home from college to take Lauren out to dinner on her last day of treatment and another one is taking her out to dinner the next night.

- If consistent with your beliefs, have a religious ceremony of thanksgiving.

  I preached the sermon at church after Kristin ended treatment. It was the first Sunday of Lent, and I related our experience to that. Other than that, we didn't celebrate, because it's still not over. We still have to be vigilant. Ending treatment was a big milestone, but it paled in comparison to having the line pulled. We all have so much more freedom: no more flushing lines, changing bandages, or wrapping up for baths and swimming.

Some parents do not feel comfortable celebrating the end of treatment. One mother described her feelings this way:

Finishing treatment was very difficult. I thought that I would feel like celebrating and cheering—but all I felt was fear. Treatment was over, but cancer was still a part of our lives. I think we will always live with the fear of relapse. It has taken me some time to come to grips with that reality.

As you have read so often in this book, every child, brother, sister, parent, and relative reacts differently to treatment—and to the end of treatment. The differences do not matter. What is important is that you feel free to express your feelings, whatever they may be. You may feel joyful, relieved, fearful, or terrified, but the end of treatment is emotionally charged for every member of the family.

What is Normal?

After years of treatment, families grapple with the idea of returning to normal. Unfortunately, most parents no longer really know what "normal" is. Parents realize that returning to the carefree pre-leukemia days is unrealistic, that life has changed. The constant interaction with medical personnel is ending, and a new phase is beginning in which routines do not revolve around caring for a sick child, giving medicines, coping with hospitalizations, and keeping clinic appointments. Although it is true that the blissful ignorance of the days prior to cancer are gone forever, a different life—one often enriched by friends and experiences from the cancer years—begins.

We're a year off treatment, and I really don't think about relapse very often. I do occasionally find myself studying her to see if she looks pale, or I worry when she seems tired or her behavior is bad. Usually, I'm feeling safer. But honestly, I don't think any of us will ever go back to the days when we just assumed that our kids would grow up, that the parents would die first; that sense of security is probably gone forever.

•　•　•　•　•

Shawn is six months off treatment, and he's just like a flower beginning to bloom. He's so happy, and I try to be happy with him. I try very hard to put worries about the future out of my mind, because I feel that those thoughts will rob me of just being able to enjoy Shawn.

•　•　•　•　•

Chemo is such a horrible thing for your child to endure, but at least you are actively fighting the beast; so, when it ends you feel a bit like you're flying without a net. You get so used to this bizarre new "normal" of treatments and blood tests and doctor visits, and then suddenly you stop, but you don't get the old normal back.

I think it's probably best to approach the end of treatment as a chance to see your child get his healthy color and energy back, and an opportunity to create and explore a new "normal" for your family that is richer and more meaningful than the one you left behind. It's also really nice to finally have the chance to reconnect with your spouse (and other children) and heal all the relationships that have taken a beating during the stressful treatment period.

As for me, for perhaps a year after Joseph's treatment, I existed in a dazed mix of emotions and thoughts. I was fearful of relapse, thrilled that Joseph had survived the cancer and the treatment, concerned about what late effects lay around the corner, all tempered with a warm and thankful feeling that I knew I would never, EVER take my kids or my good life for granted anymore, or sweat the small stuff the way I used to. There were days I felt like I didn't want to crawl out from under the bed, and other days I couldn't stop singing and being silly. I think off treatment is a lot like on treatment—you just have to take it one day at a time.

"Normal" is a moving target—different for every person and family. No one can tell you what your normal will be. Normal is whatever keeps the family moving forward together to face their individual and collective futures.

When Abby was on treatment, I spent a lot of time reading and asking questions. Our treatment community was always positive about treatment and survivorship. I knew from the online support group I belonged to that the "big comfy couch" of survivorship might have some lumps. However, I expected somehow that they would be physical and wasn't prepared for the aftermath of medical trauma exposure. Abby and our family struggled emotionally to move forward. I personally felt different;

having entered "cancer land" in my early 30s, I then awoke at 38, shaking my head wondering, "Who the hell am I?" My husband and I entered marriage counseling—there was much forgiveness to be asked for and given on both sides. Seven years later I still contemplate cancer land and its lasting impact on all of us.

· · · · ·

Well, we finally did it. We took a deep breath, a heavy sigh, and we packed up the medical supplies. While this step may seem insignificant for some, those who have dealt with a chronic/life-threatening illness in their family know that the disposal of your arsenal of medical supplies is a symbolic rite of passage. It can only mean two things: your loved one has passed on, or you simply don't need the supplies anymore. We thank God every day that we ended up with the latter reason.

Katy's medical "tower" was stored in our hallway and included various bins and drawers full of central line supplies, a mini IV pump, masks and gloves, hypodermics, and sharps containers. It was very conspicuous. You simply couldn't miss it if you walked through the house. It was our constant reminder that we had a sick child, and was at times, for me, a crutch. I think I felt that as long as the tower was there and properly stocked and arranged, I was somehow in control of Katy's illness. I feared disposing of or putting anything away, thinking that if I did, she would most assuredly relapse and I'd need it again. No, of course that's not rational, but rationality has never been one of my strong points.

However, as the months passed, the tower gathered dust, and soon I couldn't remember the last time we'd even used any of the supplies. A few more months passed, and I began to realize what an eyesore this bunch of junk was! So, after my husband, David, brought some big boxes home from work, it was time. We did it together. Into the boxes went the tubing and syringes, masks, and dressing change kits for the kids' oncology camp. Into the garbage went everything else. It was so liberating! I can't imagine why we kept that stuff around for so long. It felt like the end of an era. And in a way, it was.

For many people, helping others is a satisfying way to reach out or bring closure to the active phase of cancer treatment. Serving others can create something enormously meaningful out of personal challenges, which is why many parents and children like to give back to the cancer community in some way. Examples of ways people have given back include the following:

- I requested that the clinic and local pediatricians refer newly diagnosed families to me if the parents wanted someone to talk with. I remembered how impossible it was to go to meetings in the first few months, and how desperately I needed to talk to someone who had already traveled the same road.

- We started a Boy Scout project to keep the toy box full at the clinic.

- My children are counselors at the camp for kids with cancer.

- We organized a walk to raise funds for the Ronald McDonald House.
- We (a group of parents of children with cancer) requested and were granted a conference with the oncology staff to share our thoughts about ways to improve pain management and communication between parents and staff. It was very well received.
- We circulated a petition among parents to request increased hospital funding for psychosocial support staff. We presented it to the director of the hematology/oncology service.
- I give platelets and blood regularly.
- We held a bone marrow drive.
- I took all of our leftover catheter line supplies to camp and gave them to a family that needed them.

The possibilities are endless. Parents and children can use whatever talents they have to help others—from designing head coverings to writing newsletters for families struggling with childhood cancer.

> *I have administered several online support groups for parents of children with cancer over the past decade. Many of these groups have over 500 participants who live all over the world. Some of the members' children have been cancer free for years, some are newly diagnosed, and some are parents of children who have died. These online communities are an important way to find comfort, support, and information. Parents who are far out from treatment remain involved in order to help those who are newly diagnosed. When my son was first diagnosed, I was so reassured that people survive the ordeal. After treatment ended, I wanted to be there to help others.*

• • • • •

> *My two daughters were both diagnosed with childhood cancer—Rayne died and Izzabella is alive. Our experiences have changed the direction of my life. Because I so understand and relate to families of ill children, I've returned to school to get trained to be an ultrasound technician and a radiation therapist. I know that fear of the unknown is the enemy of parents of sick children, and I can help dispel those fears. This is my way to give back and help other families.*

An equally healthy response to ending treatment is to put it behind you. Many families, after years of struggles, just want to move on. They don't want constant reminders of cancer and feel it's not good for children to be reminded of those hard times.

> *I realized that it was time to put it behind us when I watched my two children playing house one day. There was only one adult and one child in the family. I asked what happened to the rest of the family and they both said, "Cancer; they died." I didn't want them to have any more cancer in their lives. They had had enough. I know people who worry all the time about the cancer returning, and it is not healthy*

for them or their children. I decided to get out of the cancer mode and back to being my usual upbeat self. I feel that we are finally back to normal, and it's a good place to be.

Parents and children need to talk with one another, examine their emotions, decide what course they want to chart, and work together toward creating a healthy life after cancer.

Initial Follow-up Care

Protocols for clinical trials require follow-up appointments at specific intervals to check for the recurrence of the disease. For instance, after treatment for average-risk acute lymphoblastic leukemia (ALL), your child may need monthly physical exams and a monthly CBC for the first year off treatment, and a less frequent schedule for the following years.

Clinical trial documents outline the follow-up schedule. If your child was not on a clinical trial, find out from the oncologist what the required schedule will be and where the appointments will take place. Make sure your child understands that after treatment ends, doctor appointments and blood draws will still be needed on occasion.

Shawn is a year off treatment and I find myself letting go of the bad memories more and more. They are just fading away. What I am left with is awe, admiration, and amazement that my son handled all of the hardships of treatment and survived. He's very determined and strong-willed, and I'm so proud of him. When people say to me, "Oh, you were so strong to make it through that," I respond, "All I did was drive him to the appointments; he did the rest." This experience has really changed me and my entire family. My marriage is much better, my other sons are stronger and closer to us, and Shawn has shown us all how tough a little kid can be. We take each precious day, one at a time, and try to get the most out of it. I so appreciate life and my family.

These follow-up appointments are primarily to check for return of disease, not emergence of late effects. That's why it is so important to transition to a survivorship clinic at the appropriate time—usually two years after treatment ends or five years after diagnosis.

Long-term Follow-up Care

In the past, most survivors were sent back to their local pediatricians after follow-up for the recurrence of the leukemia was complete. But as the population of long-term survivors grew, it became apparent that these young men and women often faced complex medical, psychological, and social effects from their years of treatment. As a result, some institutions started survivorship clinics to provide a multidisciplinary team to monitor and support survivors. The nucleus of the team is usually a nurse coordinator, pediatric oncologist, pediatric nurse practitioner, social worker, and psychologist. The team also includes specialists such as endocrinologists and cardiologists.

Yearly appointments with follow-up programs usually include a review of treatments received, counseling about potential health risks (or lack thereof), and treatment-specific diagnostic tests (e.g., echocardiograms or DEXA scans). Follow-up clinics not only provide comprehensive care for survivors, they also participate in research projects that track the effectiveness of and side effects from various clinical trials. Follow-up clinics also act as advocates for survivors with schools, insurance companies, and employers.

If your institution does not provide comprehensive, long-term survivorship care, you can find a list of survivor programs at *www.ped-onc.org/treatment/surclinics*. Many survivors travel to comprehensive programs for their yearly follow-up visits.

Possible late effects

At diagnosis, parents do not know the price their child will ultimately pay for survival. Short-term effects are many, but they come and then go. Long-term effects range from none to severe. These can include learning disabilities, an impaired endocrine system, osteonecrosis, neuropathy, and an increased risk of second cancers.

It is important to know the possible risks based on the treatment your child received. You can then store this knowledge in the back of your mind. As one mother said, "I hope for the best and I deal with the rest." If your child is seen at a survivorship clinic, they will conduct assessments based on the Children's Oncology Group's follow-up guidelines (available at *www.survivorshipguidelines.org*). For detailed information about possible late effects from childhood cancer, read *Childhood Cancer Survivors: A Practical Guide to the Future,* 3rd edition, by Nancy Keene, Wendy Hobbie, and Kathy Ruccione.

Healthy choices

An essential aspect of survivorship is making healthy choices. Good health habits and regular medical care help protect survivors' health and lessen the likelihood of late effects from cancer treatment. Eating a healthy diet, staying physically active, using sunscreen, avoiding excessive alcohol consumption, maintaining a healthy weight, and not smoking all help keep survivors healthy and cancer-free. To avoid injury, it is also important that survivors wear bike or motorcycle helmets, use seat belts, and call a cab if the person driving has had too much to drink. Survivors have little or no control over their genetic make-up or the drugs they took to survive, but making healthy choices about how to live the rest of their lives gives them some control over their future.

Immunizations. If your child was diagnosed before she received all her immunizations, ask the oncologist when she should resume the regular schedule. If your child had one or more stem cell transplants, then all immunizations will probably need to be repeated.

Risks of smoking. Teens need continuing counseling about problems associated with smoking cigarettes or engaging in other high-risk behaviors. The combination of effects from treatment and smoking increases the chance of heart disease, heart attack, congestive heart failure, stroke, and cancer of the mouth, throat, and lung. An article about survivors and smoking in a youth newsletter ends with these words:

> If you've had cancer and your friends haven't, they don't face the same risks from smoking that you do. You've fought hard for your life. Don't put it out in an ashtray.

Safe sex. Every teen and young adult who has survived cancer should be counseled about safe sexual practices. Despite the prevalence of sexual messages in our culture, most teens and young adults are woefully underinformed about the facts. Even though some chemotherapy drugs may cause infertility, many babies have been born to long-term survivors of leukemia. Survivors should not assume they are infertile.

In addition, sexually transmitted diseases are of concern for anyone engaging in sexual activity. All sorts of diseases (e.g., hepatitis C, HIV/AIDS, genital herpes, genital warts, gonorrhea, human papillomavirus [HPV]) can be transmitted through sexual intercourse and oral sex. One nurse practitioner at a large follow-up clinic stated:

> I tell every teenager who comes through the door, regardless of their medical background, that I think he or she is too young to have sex, and I explain why. But then I say, in the event that you do choose to become sexually active, you always need to use a condom, and not just any condom. I tell them to only use a latex condom with a spermicide, which is the most barrier-protective. I explain that no sex is the only guarantee to avoid the many diseases out there, but a latex condom with spermicide offers the next best protection. And I really stress that this should be done whoever the partner is, and for whatever type of sex. So many teenagers think that diseases only happen to other kinds of kids.

Every survivor should have a discussion with the oncologist or nurse practitioner about when to get the HPV vaccine that prevents cervical cancer.

Treatment Summary

Once treatment and follow-up for recurrence of disease are completed, many children and young adults will no longer be cared for by pediatric oncologists who are familiar with their history. A transition back to their local pediatrician usually occurs. However, many primary care doctors—pediatricians, family practice doctors, internists, gynecologists—are not fully aware of all the different treatments used for childhood leukemia, or of the late effects they can cause.

In addition, when treatment ends, patients and parents are not always given adequate information about the risks of developing late effects in the months, years, or decades after treatment. The risks of delayed effects are real, and it is vital that survivors become informed advocates for their own health care. They need to be educated, in a supportive and responsible way, about the risk of late effects; then if a problem arises, it will be recognized early and receive prompt attention. Young adults who have survived childhood cancer need to be fully informed of their unique medical history and be able to share this information with all doctors who care for them in the future.

A few months before the end of treatment, ask the oncologist or NP to fill out a summary of your child's treatment. Some institutions have developed a unique summary that includes all the essential details of treatment and recommended risk-based follow-up care. Or your team can complete the COG treatment summary form or one available from Childhood Cancer Guides at *www.childhoodcancerguides.org/wp-content/uploads/2016/02/treatment_record.pdf*. Make several copies of the completed form, because this health history will become an indispensable part of your child's medical records for the rest of her life. The hard copy version should be kept in a safe place, and a copy should be given to each medical caregiver. You can also scan the health history and store a copy on your computer, which makes it simple to print out new copies in the future and provides a backup in case the hard copy is ever lost. When your child leaves home to begin her adult life, this treatment summary should go with her, and you should keep a copy in a safe place. If you have the history on a computer, you can easily put it onto a portable device (e.g., thumb drive, flash drive, memory stick), or on mobile cloud storage, for your child to take with her or access online.

On November 19, 1998, we arrived by ambulance at the Children's Hospital where we were given the devastating news. Words that silenced time; that paralyzed my being. "Tommy has leukemia . . . and it's not good." Tommy (17 years old) was diagnosed with T-cell ALL. His white count had risen to over 90,000 and the disease had also spread to his central nervous system. Chemotherapy had to start immediately. He began an intense protocol for the treatment of his cancer that included radiation and chemotherapy.

Through the next 3 ½ years we had many ups and many downs, too many to discuss. But during his illness, when he could, Tommy consumed his days with reading. On one chilly day in Pennsylvania, he asked me to drive him to the public library. He covered his bald head with a wool beanie and his once athletic physique was frail and weakened from the intense early months of chemotherapy and radiation. I pulled up to the front of the library, and I asked if he wanted me to go along to help.

He said, "No thanks Mom, I can do it." After twenty minutes or so, Tommy exited with a HUGE stack of books—all medical books! Tommy had found his passion for life—his true love of medicine.

One of our biggest obstacles was Tommy's diagnosis of avascular necrosis (AVN) in his hips, shoulders, and knees. The AVN caused him excruciating pain, and he could only walk with the help of crutches. Partial hip replacement surgeries were done to preserve as much of the hips as possible and core decompression surgeries were done on both shoulders and knees. Tommy's main concern was to get all the surgeries over quickly so he would not get behind in his studies, be able to take finals, and be able to walk without pain. And all the while he was still undergoing chemotherapy treatments for the leukemia. After the surgeries and much rehabilitation, I saw my 19-year-old son take his first steps without crutches for the first time in nine months. It was more emotional and exciting than when he was 10 months old taking his first steps!

Tommy graduated from college in 2004 with a major in biology and a minor in biochemistry and molecular biology. He spent two years at the National Cancer Institute as a research fellow and then went on to medical school. Following his residency, he then completed a fellowship in pediatric hematology oncology. His health is good, although he still suffers from pain due to the AVN and the damage to his joints. He recently had two total hip replacement surgeries.

Tommy has lived his life with enormous strength, determination, and grace. He never ever let his illness dictate his life. With all his fortitude, I can only imagine what his future holds as a phenomenal doctor and human being. His expertise and compassion as a pediatric oncologist has already touched so many families. And those lives he will touch along the way will only be richer for having crossed his path.

Chapter 25

Relapse

"Hold fast to dreams for if dreams die
Life is a broken winged bird that cannot fly."

— Langston Hughes

PARENTS FREQUENTLY DESCRIBE the return of their child's cancer as more devastating than the original diagnosis. They may feel betrayed, guilty, and/or angry. They worry that if the previous treatments did not work, what will? Mostly, they are afraid. And their often unspoken but most crushing fear is: What if my child dies?

If your child's cancer has returned, it is worth remembering that you now have several strengths you didn't have before. You have already done this. You know the language, and you have a relationship with the medical team. You probably have friendships with other parents of children with cancer and you know they will be there for you. You can also hope that during the time your child's cancer was in remission, researchers were able to develop newer and more effective treatments. You know that something that seems insurmountable can be endured, one day at a time.

This chapter describes signs and symptoms of relapse, what emotional responses you might experience, and how to set goals and decide on a treatment plan. It provides information about immunotherapy, which was recently approved to treat some children with leukemia who relapse or who never entered remission. In addition, several parents and survivors share stories about how they managed to cope.

Signs and Symptoms

Although relapse can happen years after treatment ends, it most commonly occurs during treatment or in the first year off treatment. In fact, most treatment centers do not consider children to be long-term survivors of leukemia until they have been off treatment for at least two years or are five years past diagnosis.

The signs and symptoms of leukemia relapse are usually some of the same telltale warnings that occurred prior to diagnosis:

• Fatigue

- Fevers
- Night sweats
- Nosebleeds
- Bruises and/or petechiae
- Pale skin
- Back, leg, or joint pain
- Loss of appetite
- Enlarged lymph nodes in the neck or groin
- Enlarged abdomen caused by a large spleen or liver
- Enlarged, painless testicle
- Changes in behavior, such as excessive irritability
- Dizziness
- Headaches

Normal childhood illnesses can cause many of these symptoms, and a tired day here or a bruise there is probably no cause for alarm. However, if your child has a persistent loss of appetite, if he is often fatigued, or if he has several symptoms, it might be wise to call the oncologist. In some cases, parents have no warning. After they bring their child in for a routine visit, they receive a totally unexpected telephone call from the doctor with the news.

> My 2-year-old son was diagnosed in 2011 with B-cell ALL that was MLL positive, and he had disease in the CNS [central nervous system], which made him very high risk. He relapsed six months into maintenance. We discovered the relapse when he developed a fever and we brought him to the ER because of the fever protocol for ports. We found out that his blood had 98% blasts and bone marrow had 60% blasts. So, the leukemia was back again. They decided to have him begin the induction phase again in hopes to get into remission and then to transplant. Four months later, he had a transplant and then two months later the leukemia was back.

The three most likely sites for leukemia relapse are the bone marrow, the central nervous system (CNS), and the testes. Bone marrow relapse is the most common form of recurrence. The use of CNS prophylaxis—intrathecal medications and sometimes radiation—has greatly decreased CNS relapses. Relapse in the testicles is also uncommon, occurring in less than 5% of boys. Leukemia sometimes recurs at other sites, such as the ovaries or eyes.

> Right before Stephan went to camp, he went in for his maintenance spinal tap. I got a bill from a different specialist, and when I asked the oncologist about it, he said that Stephan had a few white cells in his fluid that he wanted to get another opinion on.

He assured me that everything was okay, but I just had that feeling that something was about to go wrong. At his next spinal, his count was 88 in the cerebrospinal fluid. A central nervous system relapse.

• • • • •

The transplant was really hard on our son. He had miserable GVHD, multiple infections, and had to have his gall bladder removed. He missed a whole year of school. Then, right after his one-year post-transplant appointment, he relapsed in his CNS. Because he had relapsed in the CNS on front-line therapy, as soon as the headaches started, he knew he had relapsed again.

• • • • •

About 22 months after my daughter, Lauren, finished treatment for high-risk B-cell ALL (protocol for children with Down syndrome) she developed a respiratory illness and had an enlarged lymph node on her neck. We went to the clinic, and her platelets were low and her liver was a bit enlarged, but nothing out of the ordinary for someone fighting a virus. We went back two weeks later, and I just knew in my heart it was back, but I prayed that we would escape it. When both her doctor and nurse practitioner came in I could tell by their faces. They found blasts in her blood. I didn't know how to tell her, so her nurse practitioner told her while I called my husband and ex. Her nurse practitioner said my daughter was stoic until she told her that Mom is sad and is calling Daddy and Brad; that made Lauren cry. It really broke my heart.

• • • • •

My son relapsed in the left optic nerve. His only symptom was some mild pain with extreme gaze (looking all the way down, up, or to the side). After a couple weeks of this, a family practice doctor looked at him and saw nothing. An optometrist saw some swelling of the optic disc (connected with the optic nerve). That sent us to an ophthalmologist, to a radiologist for a CT scan, and back to the oncologist. So, his only symptoms were some mild pain and some swelling in the back of the eye that was hard to see. Further tests of the marrow and the cerebrospinal fluid showed no leukemia cells, so we were forced to do an optic nerve sheath biopsy, which was the only place ALL cells were found.

Emotional Responses

Parents whose children are in remission think or speak of relapse with an almost palpable dread. Just the thought can cause an eruption of the same emotions that surged in them at diagnosis. Parents, their child, and the siblings may feel a wide array of emotions after a relapse—numbness, guilt, dread, anger, fear, confusion, denial, and grief.

I am a long-term survivor (30 years old), who first was diagnosed with ALL at age 8 and subsequently relapsed three times, at ages 13, 15, and 16. The first relapse was by far the worst to deal with emotionally. It had been five years since my diagnosis, so I went in for my last spinal tap and bone marrow. I had been off treatment with good counts for two years. My mother and I didn't even wait for the test results; we went out to lunch and went shopping. Later that day, I called the clinic, and my doctor told me the bone marrow was fine, but she needed to talk to my mother. I heard my mother say, "No, no, oh no," and she started to cry. I just stood there feeling numb, knowing the news was bad. The cancer had returned to my central nervous system. But at 13, I remembered clearly what I had been through, and all I could think was that it hadn't worked. I told my parents that I wouldn't go through treatment again. My father sat me down and gave me a reality check. He explained that I would die if I didn't get treatment. He said, "If you don't do it for yourself, please do it for me and your mom." The next morning I went into the clinic and started all over again.

In addition to powerful emotions, parents often experience physical symptoms such as dizziness, nausea, fainting, and shortness of breath. They wonder how they can ask their child to endure treatment again. They wonder how they will survive it themselves. They may swing between optimism and panic.

I found that relapse was far worse than the original diagnosis. At diagnosis, after a certain period of adjustment, you think that treatment has a beginning, a middle, and an end. But relapse creates a bigger burden to accept. You begin to feel that maybe the disease is more powerful than the medicine. I found that for a while I just stopped functioning and thinking rationally. I felt like I was on a runaway freight train, hurtling toward an end that didn't look so good anymore.

Goal Setting and Treatment Planning

Goal setting is straightforward for most families after a first relapse—they look at options, choose one, and start treatment again. However, for families of children who have experienced a series of relapses and years of struggle, deciding what to do next can be very difficult. In these cases, a necessary step in making plans is discussing and deciding on your and your child's goals. In a newsletter for parents of children with cancer, Arthur Ablin, MD, Professor Emeritus of Pediatric Clinical Oncology at the University of California, San Francisco, wrote of the importance of goal setting in the decision-making process after relapse:

Before determining which treatment is to be chosen, a decision must be made to determine the goal of treatment—in other words, what is it that we are trying to achieve. This crucial first step is the basis upon which any decision concerning treatment must be made. But it is too often omitted from consideration and/or discussion, even by the most experienced. The frustrations accompanying the previous failure of treatment, the fear of the loss of the hope for cure, the pressure of urgency to find solutions, the new awareness of the possibility or probability of death, lead us all to want to consider treatments first rather than these more difficult considerations involved in establishing goals.

After a discussion of goals, your family may choose treatment, treatment with palliative care (services to improve quality of life and manage pain) added, or comfort care only.

If your family decides to pursue additional treatment, there may be more than one option available. Treatment plans for a first relapse may be specified in the standard treatment or clinical trial protocol document, or your child's oncologist may suggest a different approach. Suggestions for treatment may include more intensive chemotherapy, radiation, stem cell transplantation, immunotherapy, a clinical trial, or a combination of several treatments. You may need to consider traveling to a different treatment center to access therapies that are not available at your child's home hospital.

When our son relapsed on treatment for Ph+ ALL, then a year after his transplant, we didn't know what to do. Our docs brought our son's case to the tumor board, and I joined an online support group hoping to get some information about new drugs. I connected with six people who had the same mutation that our son did, and all of them had tried nilotinib, which worked for all of them. Meanwhile, our local oncologist told our 17-year-old son he was going to die and there were no more treatments for him. She even signed him up for hospice without discussing it with us.

I realized that no one was going to be as invested or have the same sense of urgency as his Dad and I. I learned how to navigate the www.clinicaltrials.gov website to find new open trials. Every open trial listed has the contact information for the principal investigator, who is trying to enroll patients in the trial. I made numerous phone calls to treatment centers across the country looking for immunotherapy trials our son would be eligible for. If you articulate your case in a concise way that addresses the eligibility requirements of the trial, the investigators will call you back. You have access to these scientists and doctors. You have to know your stuff but you don't have to be an MD to be your child's best advocate and leader in his or her care.

There were a lot of barriers to getting accepted into the immunotherapy trials—the wait lists were long, and we didn't think he had the time to wait. I encourage parents who finds themselves in this daunting situation to be relentless in your pursuit of the very best treatment options. At one point we contacted our Congresswoman, attorneys, the manufacturer of his CAR-T cells, and the U.S. Food and Drug Administration in an effort to get him to treatment in time. I'm certain that had we not gone to these lengths, my son would not have been enrolled in the trial and alive today.

Making a Decision about Treatment

Treatment for children who relapse is evolving. The information gleaned from second opinions or your own research may reinforce what your doctor recommended, or it might provide you with other treatment options. Either way, the information may increase your comfort level during the treatment planning process. You might want to ask your child's treatment team the following questions about the suggested treatment plan:

- Is there a standard treatment for this type of relapse?

- Are these cancer cells showing the same cytogenetics as those from the initial diagnosis? If different, what does that mean for treatment?

- What is the goal of this treatment? Remission? Comfort?

- Why do you think this treatment is the best option? What are the other choices, and why are you recommending this one?

- Have you consulted with other doctors or researchers? If so, with whom? Did you all agree on this treatment or were other options suggested?

- Are any clinical trials available here or at other institutions?

- What are the potential benefits and possible side effects of the proposed treatment?

- How long is the proposed treatment?

- If radiation is to be included, what type and dose are you recommending?

- What are the known or potential risks of the treatment?

- How often will my child need to be hospitalized?

- If the treatment is investigational, is there scientific evidence that it works for my child's type of relapse?

- If we need to transfer to another treatment center for some or all of the proposed treatment, who will help us manage that process?

- Does insurance cover this type of treatment?

> Making the decision as to what treatment to choose was much more difficult when my son relapsed. The stakes were higher. While I had faith in the skills and judgment of my son's oncologists, I could not rest easy unless I had educated myself on the options available for relapse treatment. His relapse had been suspected for weeks, so I had time to investigate possible treatment choices. His relapse site was rare, which made the usual channels less effective in our case. I started with the online NCI-PDQ and a PubMed search. I asked friends to search for me. From there I contacted a physician from a children's oncology research group and asked what type of treatment protocol they had to offer for my son's type of relapse. I learned that the options were few in terms of protocols addressing my son's type of relapse.

When we sat down with the ped oncologists, I already had some background and knew what was available in terms of treatment. When they presented their choice of protocol, I asked for and was given a copy of the protocol. Reading the rationale and background of the study they were proposing helped me to understand why this protocol was suggested. As a result, I was able to make a difficult decision and enroll my son in a protocol with confidence that he was getting the best treatment available. Since it was a very difficult and intense treatment protocol, it also helped my teenage son to understand why this was the path we were following. Once begun, neither of us had any serious doubts that we'd made the best choice. Now, almost three years later, I am still very pleased that we were able to make a fully informed decision. My son is now a healthy young man away at college. He completed relapse treatment over a year ago and is doing great. His concerns these days are about the dorm food, his next midterm, and when he can see his girlfriend.

· · · · ·

My son was diagnosed with standard risk B-cell ALL when he was 8 years old. His MRD was negative at Day 29, and he completed the entire three years and two months of treatment. Six months later, at his monthly appointment, one of his testicles was slightly larger and the oncologist said, "It's probably puberty" and she added that she would schedule an ultrasound a couple of weeks later, after Christmas. He told his dad the next day that the testicle was getting larger, so we went back to the clinic. The ultrasound was positive, the additional tests the next day showed that he had relapsed in his testes, CNS, and bone marrow. He was treated for 30 days with high dose methotrexate hoping to avoid testicular radiation, but during that time it spread to his left testicle. So, he had testicular radiation, cranial radiation, and two more years of treatment, starting when he was 12. Three months after he finished the relapse therapy, he developed bad headaches while on his eighth grade class trip, and he passed out. The spinal tap showed the ALL was raging again. So, we went to transplant because his triplet sister was a perfect match and the CART-19 immunotherapy trial had never included a child with active CNS disease, so there were just too many unknowns for us.

If your child is old enough, it is a good idea to thoroughly discuss the options with her so you understand her wishes. If older children and parents disagree about how to proceed, a hospital social worker or psychologist can help you to negotiate a joint decision. These discussions will help clarify each family member's thoughts and feelings, and they will allow the child's emotional and physical well-being to be part of the equation.

After my son relapsed, we set immediately back to work trying to determine what the best treatment option for him should be. His oncologist was very committed to making him well again. As it turned out, the best option was a phase II study drug that wasn't yet available in our area. The hospital social worker helped us with travel arrangements and accommodations, and within a day we were on a plane headed for another hospital. Meanwhile, the oncologist completed all the necessary paperwork so that by the time the next course of chemotherapy was due, it could be administered at our own hospital. It was obvious to us from the very beginning of relapse that we had a wonderful medical team that was dedicated to helping our son get well again.

Unfortunately, after two courses of chemotherapy, it was clear that the drug wasn't getting rid of the cancer. Once again, we all rolled up our sleeves and tried to find another treatment that might help him. I would gather the information and then his oncologist and I would sit and review all the data. As long as the therapy was reasonable and had the potential to help without further diminishing his quality of life, it was worth considering. One of the most comforting things that my son's oncologist ever said to me was, "I will always be in your corner."

If your family decides on comfort care, not active treatment, the next chapter contains suggestions and stories from parents who have walked that path before you. If you decide on additional treatment, do not rush into it if you or your child feel uncomfortable about the plan. There is usually time to get answers to all of your questions and to get additional opinions. Doctors make recommendations based on knowledge, experience, and consultations with other experts in the field, so don't hesitate to ask your child's oncologist why she has suggested a certain approach.

Jesse relapsed four times, and in some ways it got harder and in other ways it got easier. We knew each time that her chances for survival were fading, and that was hard. But each time we grieved and worked through the feelings, and our skills at handling relapse improved. I turned to God for comfort, and I think that helped me feel that I was standing on a rock out in the ocean, rather than thrashing around in the water. My faith gave me solace. Jesse handled the relapses better than anyone else in the family. She would calmly listen to the doctors' explanations, then she would say, "Okay, what do we have to do?" She was never angry. She was sometimes sad, but mostly accepting.

Immunotherapy

Immunotherapy is a new and exciting type of treatment for children whose leukemia does not respond to conventional treatments. Immunotherapy alters the immune system—a network of organs and cells that help protect against infection and disease. The immune system keeps track of all substances normally found in the body, and any cells identified as foreign are attacked. However, the immune system doesn't always recognize cancer cells as foreign. Immunotherapies alter the immune system so it can correctly identify and kill cancerous cells. This is done in many ways, including use of monoclonal antibodies, cancer vaccines, and immune checkpoint inhibitors. But these types of immunotherapy are used primarily for adults with cancer.

In 2017, the FDA approved a type of immunotherapy for children and teens with B-cell leukemia who relapsed or whose leukemia didn't respond to initial therapy. This treatment, called chimeric antigen receptor (CAR) T-cell therapy, involves collecting T cells, genetically altering them, and then returning them to the child's bloodstream to attack the cancerous B cells.

Process of CAR T-cell therapy

The first step in CAR T-cell therapy is collecting T cells via a process called leukapheresis. Blood is withdrawn from the body, T cells are removed, and the blood is reinfused back into the child or teen. The T cells are sent to a manufacturing facility to be genetically engineered to attack cancerous B cells. The number of reengineered cells (called CAR T cells) is then increased at the manufacturing plant. During the few weeks while this is happening, the child is usually given chemotherapy to stop disease progression. When millions of new T cells are available, they are frozen and sent to the hospital to be thawed and infused into the child or teen.

> When we were accepted into the CAR-T trial, our son had to be weaned off his GVHD [graft-versus-host disease] drugs before they could collect his T cells. This was risky, but he was 17 and was willing to take the chance in hopes of a cure. After they collected and manufactured the T cells, but before they could infuse them, our son relapsed in the CNS again. This dramatically increased the risk of the procedure. The consent was brutal because of all of the possible complications, including death. My son asked the doctor, "If I die, will you still learn something from this?" The doctor said, "You are here so we can do our best to save your life." And we decided to go ahead.

· · · · ·

> Infusion day. Magic gold was 60 cc of CAR-T cells infused through Mitchell's PICC line. After we went back to the hotel he developed a fever, so he was admitted. On Day 7, he started developing neurological symptoms—irritable, slurring words. Within 24 hours, he was unresponsive and moved up to the ICU. He was in a coma for five days. My husband and I worried about brain damage and talked about the wisdom of trying this trial. Then, we just decided to give up that burden and accept whatever happened. Two hours later, he opened his eyes and tried to talk. He started talking like a 2 year old, but gradually he improved, and within two weeks was emotionally and physically back. It was a huge success, and within two months, Mitchell was starting his senior year of high school, from which he graduated with honors (after front-line treatment, relapse, transplant, relapse, and then CAR T-cell clinical trial). He is in college, doing well, but still coping with side effects from the transplant. We were so incredibly lucky.

Side effects of CAR T-cell therapy

Three side effects may occur shortly after infusion of CAR T cells. These include:

- **Cytokine release syndrome, sometimes called the cytokine storm:** When the immune system is activated by the CAR T cells, a large number of proteins called cytokines are released, which can result in high fevers, low blood pressure, pain, or poor lung oxygenation. Less common side effects of the cytokine storm are brain swelling, delirium, confusion, or seizures. These symptoms most often occur in the first week after infusion of the T cells.

- **B-cell aplasia (few or no B cells):** The reengineered T cells kill not only cancerous B cells but also healthy B cells. Because B cells help guard against infection, IV immunoglobulin is given monthly to boost immune function. It is not yet known how long these infusions are needed.

- **Tumor lysis syndrome:** This metabolic complication occurs when a large number of cancer cells are destroyed in a short amount of time. This rare side effect can occur up to two weeks after infusion of the modified T cells.

> *The consent process was hard because the known side effects were very scary and the unknowns were even scarier. They took my 14-year-old son's T cells, did the manufacturing magic, and gave him back 10% of them on Day 1 and 30% more the following day. He had what is called the cytokine storm, but a milder version than many of the other kids had. He had a low fever, mild discomfort, and was a little confused for a few days.*

· · · · ·

> *Last Wednesday, February 17, Justin had a bone marrow biopsy and spinal tap performed on the one-year anniversary of receiving his modified T cells. The initial results were good but we had to wait until this Monday to get the official word that NO Minimal Residual Disease was found! This is the longest Justin has ever been in remission and we are thrilled! Mentally, Justin is trying to wrap his head around it all. He is doing well in school and last night signed up to take the SAT, so life marches on. As happy as I am, my joy is tempered by the struggles many of our friends in our pediatric cancer family are still enduring. Survivor guilt is very real. While I know they are happy for us, there still has to be a moment of "Damn, why didn't CAR-T work for my kid?" or "Why didn't my kid survive?" My heart aches with every relapse, my heart breaks with every death. In our own quiet way we've been supporting various charities and specific individuals and are prayerfully considering what else we can do and how best to share our resources. Please keep these children in your prayers: Logan, Patrick, Valeria, Brooke, and Adam. And comfort for Kelly as her sweet boy Kevin earned his angel wings last week.*

My 4-year-old son relapsed soon after he started maintenance for his high-risk ALL and then two months after his transplant. The doctor called my husband (he's calmer than I am) to say he had relapsed. The second relapse was the first time our son had ever seen his father cry. He told his friends, "My dad was crying. He came home to tell me my cancer was back." We'd gone from a very bad situation to a grim situation. They started weaning him off cyclosporine, and our transplant doctor came to talk with us about a Phase I immunotherapy trial in another city. It was called the CART-19 trial and it involved collecting T cells, genetically modifying the T cells to attack the cancer cells, and then infusing them back into your child. Our son was patient #21. We stayed near the hospital in an apartment for six weeks, and went to the hospital weekly for labs. Four weeks after the infusion while we were out trick-or-treating, we got a call saying, "It worked, no more leukemia." I started shouting, "His cancer is gone, his cancer is gone." The woman at the door started crying and then offered us a beer. We went home the next day. That was 3 ½ years ago and he's doing great.

It is not known how long remissions after this therapy will last in children and teens. Some of the earliest recipients are now many years out and doing well, but others relapsed yet again. Much long-term follow up is needed to learn more about the effectiveness of the treatment over time as well as the potential long-term side effects.

Summary

After you have set goals, done your research, discussed options with your treatment team, received answers to all of your questions, obtained a second opinion if desired, it is time to proceed. If you choose the comfort care option, the next chapter discusses ways that many families transitioned from active care. If you chose a new course of treatment (with or without palliative care added), your knowledge and experience may prove to be a double-edged sword. You have no illusions about the difficulties ahead because you've done it before, but you also will be strengthened by your ties with the cancer community, your familiarity with your physicians and hospital routines, and your ability to work the system to get what your child needs. Many parents shared how their child took the lead with relapse treatment. While the parents agonized, their child said simply, "Let's just do it." And they did.

Long story short—my 8-year-old son was diagnosed with standard risk ALL and completed treatment on one of the experimental arms of a Children's Oncology Group trial (an arm more intense than standard treatment). He relapsed in the testes, marrow, and CNS six months after treatment ended. He relapsed in the CNS

three months after the end of relapse treatment. He had a transplant at age 14, and nine months later he relapsed in the CNS again. At that time, three children with CNS disease had been treated on the CART-19 immunotherapy trial and were doing well. However, we also know kids who died on that trial. My son said no, he was ready to go home on hospice. I understood. He'd been through years of chemo, testicular radiation, cranial radiation, total body radiation, and a transplant. I told him that he was 15 and ultimately, it was his decision, but was he sure he wanted to stop when there was another treatment on the table, scary as it was. After talking it over, he changed his mind and agreed to the trail. It worked! He's now 18 and just graduated from high school.

Chapter 26

Death and Bereavement

*"The loss of my son has illuminated for me the true definition of love...
In this book I have tried to capture a few remembered strains of the
brief, glad music of his life. These are all I have of him now, and they
comfort me even as they break my heart."*

— Gordon Livingstone, MD
Only Spring

THE DEATH OF A CHILD CAUSES almost unendurable pain and anguish for loved ones left behind. Death from cancer comes after months or years of debilitating treatments, emotional swings, and financial stress. The family begins the years of grief already exhausted from the years of fighting cancer. It is truly every parent's worst nightmare.

In this chapter, many parents share their innermost thoughts and feelings about their decisions to transition from active treatment, involve hospice, choose death at home or in the hospital, and their experiences with grief. It made no difference whether parents had recently lost a child or whether it happened years before—tears flowed when talking about their family's experience. Because family members and friends can be strong sources of support, or casualties of the grieving process, parents describe words and actions that help. They also offer suggestions about what words and actions to avoid. Grief has as many facets as there are grieving parents; what follows are the experiences of a few.

Transitioning from Active Treatment

For children or teenagers whose disease is progressing, medical caregivers and parents discuss when to end active treatment and begin to work toward making the child comfortable for his remaining days. This is an intensely personal decision. Some families want to try every available treatment and exhaust all possible remedies. Others reach a point where they feel they have done all they can and want to transition to a time of sharing memories, expressing love, and preparing for death. What all families share is a desire to continue to guide and nurture their children, parenting them even through these most difficult circumstances, up to and through the process of death itself.

After Christie came home from the transplant center, she started to perk up and feel a bit better. But she had pretty massive problems with graft-versus-host disease, infections, fragile bones, and a very weak heart. She had a stomach abscess that they thought was causing her vomiting and eating problems, so they decided to biopsy it. They came out and said they found a cluster of tumors on her ovary, which turned out to be malignant leukemic cells. In my rational mind, I knew it was time to stop. I could imagine stopping the treatment, but I just couldn't picture life without her.

• • • • •

This has been a very difficult weekend with many tears. We have had so many wonderful years beyond what we ever thought was possible with such a good quality of life for Meg and us. In spite of everything, we have no regrets. We selfishly want every moment we can have, but we have come to the crossroad where we are asking at what cost to Meg. While we have not made the commitment to hospice yet, we are all feeling that we are not far from that place, unless there is a dramatic change in Meg soon. She has really fought hard. She made this damn cancer work really hard to slow her down. She is very, very tired and while my head understands this, my heart is breaking.

Dr. Arthur Ablin, professor emeritus of clinical pediatrics at the University of California San Francisco, wrote about the difficulties of deciding to end active treatment:

All too often, the decision to abandon the goal for cure and, reluctantly, accept the reality of the inevitable death of a child is too painful and, therefore, never made. This paralyzing pain occurs with equal frequency, perhaps, for the family and the doctor. We of the medical profession have no equal in our ability to prolong dying. We have a powerful array of mechanical, electronic, pharmaceutical, and biotechnical interventions at our command. We can keep people from dying for months and even years. Applying or withholding this armamentarium is an awesome responsibility and it requires infinite wisdom to know how to manage wisely and correctly. We can do great good by applying these tools correctly but can also do incalculable harm through over-utilization. Physicians and families alike must work together to avoid the possible pitfalls . . . When cure is beyond all of us, then the challenge is to make the rest of life as worthwhile and rich as possible. There is much to do for the terminally and critically ill child and his or her family. They have that right, and we have the privilege to be of service.

One of the more difficult tasks a parent will face is sharing the news with their child that treatments have stopped working. Children and teenagers need to be an integral part of all subsequent discussions with the healthcare team. Their thoughts and feelings are crucial during the decision-making process. Honest, thorough communication between the ill child or teen, family members, and involved professionals helps everyone work together.

The history of Jody's battle with leukemia is long, and to me, marked with his resilience, strength, and incredibly strong spirit. He was diagnosed with ALL shortly after his second birthday. He relapsed just before he turned 3, then not again until he was 5½, seven months after he went off chemotherapy treatment. He underwent a bone marrow transplant approached with the good omen of having a perfect match with both his older sister and younger brother, and thrived until another relapse at age 6½. Realistic hope for Jody's long-term survival was dashed at that time. Jody achieved another remission, which lasted for several months, then experienced a bone marrow relapse. We realized that the disease was systemic, and all conventional means of treating the leukemia were, finally, hopeless.

While the doctor was ready to present us with medical options that Thursday afternoon, we already knew our decision. It was rational: Jody should go off all chemotherapy treatment. Jody's leukemia was clearly very resistant to chemotherapy drugs. It was ethical: With no chance of further good health and high-quality living, allowing death to come naturally was surely the best choice. It was humane: Jody would be treated for pain, and we would bring him home to die in familiar surroundings with his family. And it was sad: Jody's laughter wasn't to be heard again, he wasn't to feel good again, he was to become sicker and sicker and die. The unfathomable reality of life without Jody's presence was marching to meet us without reprieve.

When it is clear that death is inevitable, parents struggle with the thought of how to discuss it with the ill child and siblings. All too often in our culture, children are perceived as having to be protected from death, as if this somehow makes their last days better. On the contrary, children, often as young as age 4, know they are dying. If the parents are trying to spare the child from knowing, a difficult situation develops. The child might pretend that everything is okay to please the parents, and the parents might try to mask their deep grief with false smiles.

When my 6-year-old son, Greg, was in the hospital in intensive relapse treatment, he would repeat over and over again, "I want to go home." When he was finally well enough to come home for a while, he kept saying, "I want to go home." In frustration, I said, "Greg, you are home; why do you keep saying that?" He looked up and quietly said, "I want to go to my heavenly home. I want to go to God." I said, "Honey, please don't say that," and, knowing how much we loved him, he replied, "Okay, Mom, I'll fight, I won't go." And he did fight hard for several more months. But he was way ahead of us in acceptance, he was at peace, and he knew it was time to let go.

Denial sometimes prevents children and parents from finishing up business—distributing belongings, telling each other how much they love one another, and saying goodbye. It also strips parents of their ability to prepare their child for the journey from life to death. Children need to know what to expect about dying. They need to know that they will be surrounded by people they love and that their parents will be holding them as they pass on. They also need to know the family's beliefs about what happens after death.

Jennifer contracted a respiratory fungal infection that resulted in her being hospitalized on a ventilator. She was given lots of morphine so she wouldn't feel air hungry. She was alert off and on for a few days. We read to her and played tapes. After one week on the respirator she took a turn for the worse. She didn't respond to me after that. Her kidneys were ceasing to function, and she started to get puffy. Her liver was deteriorating, and her painful pancreatitis had come back. After 10 days on the respirator, I couldn't bear it any longer. I lay down in her bed, took her in my arms, and kissed her at least 200 times. I talked to her for a long time and told her that we would take care of her cats, and that I was sorry that she had to suffer so much, and how beautiful Heaven is. I told her to go be with Jesus, her Grandpa, and her dog. I also told her how much we all loved her and how proud we were of her. I got off the bed to change positions, and the nurse rushed in. Her heart had suddenly stopped the second I got up. I believe she heard me and just needed to know it was okay to go. She didn't want to leave until she knew her Mommy was ready.

She had told me that she wasn't afraid to die, and this has been a great source of comfort to us. I believe she was preparing for her death, even as we hoped for her remission. Before she went to the hospital, she spent all her money, gave away some of her possessions to her sisters, and said a final goodbye to her home, cats, teachers, and friends.

When it becomes clear that further treatment will not result in a cure, parents should discuss with their beloved child or teen what his or her goals and wishes are, and use that as a guide for medical and personal choices.

After Caitlin decided she wanted no more treatments, we brought her home. She asked me to give her clothes to the poor, and her special things to her brothers. She gave them the last of her money, saying she no longer had any use for it. She had already bought them Christmas presents for the coming Christmas and had given them ahead of time. Her affairs were oh so in order. She asked my friend to make me laugh after she died. She told me that it wasn't dying she minded, because her friend who had already died had come in a dream and told her that heaven was a good place, but she did not want to leave her father and me. They were agonizing conversations, yet I am so glad that we were able to have them.

Hospice Care

In the United States, there are very active and effective hospice home care services for children but few residential hospices. Hospice organizations ease the transition from hospital to home and provide support for the entire family. Hospice personnel ensure adequate pain control, allow children to control their last days or weeks of life, and provide active bereavement support to the family after the child's death.

If the family wishes for the child to die at home, a smooth transition usually occurs from the oncology ward to home hospice care. Unfortunately, sometimes children are not referred to hospice, and the parents are left to deal with their child's last days at home with no experienced help and no clear idea of what is to come. Your nurse practitioner, case manager, or hospital social worker can refer you to, or help you find, a pediatric hospice organization in your area. Before you leave the hospital, it is wise to find out the name of a contact person at the agency who will be taking over the home care of your child.

> When Jody came home, he was assigned both a pediatric visiting nurse and a hospice nurse. On their first visits, I was handed a great deal of literature to read, including a whole notebook from hospice. I lacked both the desire and energy to read the literature and learn a whole new medical system—let alone two. I just wanted one phone number to call for help, with two or three consistent people to answer.

> In actuality, the care we received was wonderful. The primary nurse would call, offer to visit if we wanted it, assess Jody's condition over the phone, handle any questions we had, and would ask if we wanted a call the next day. She would tell us who would be calling if she was not working at the appointed time. Interestingly, the service that I found most beneficial at that time was the nurse running interference for us with the doctor. The pain medications needed to be adjusted and changed at times; advice was needed about his intake, his mouth sores, and his hand and foot inflammation. As I, along with Jody, became quieter and more removed from outside activities, even the thought of calling the clinic and being made directly aware of the bustle and demands of that world was very unappealing.

Hospice not only provides assistance in physically caring for your child, it can also provide emotional support for your child, you and your spouse, and any other children in your home. If you have questions about hospice or what support is available, you can contact Children's Hospice International online at *www.chionline.org* or by phone at (703) 684-0330.

Dying in the Hospital

Some children die in the hospital suddenly, while others slowly decline for weeks or months. If your child is slowly dying, you may have choices about where he will spend his last days. There are no right or wrong choices. Much depends on the number of people available to provide care at home and how comfortable they are doing so. Many parents ask their child where she would prefer to be. Some children and teens want to be with the nurses in a hospital environment, but others want to stay at home with parents, siblings, friends, and pets.

Parents, children, and staff should talk honestly to decide on the appropriate place for the child and then obtain the support (e.g., hospice care, private nurses in the hospital, family members) needed to make the choice a comfortable reality. Remain flexible so that as the situation changes, options remain open. If the choice is made to die in the hospital, most hospitals have a palliative care team that can help families make choices that emphasize comfort.

> *Although we had been advised that it didn't look good for Greg, we were trying one last time to get him to transplant. He was sleeping quietly in his hospital bed. He had been complaining of severe head pain, and was on a low morphine drip. The afternoon nurse woke him to take vitals, and he chatted with her. He told me, "Mom, I'm going to go back to sleep, I love you." Two hours later the night nurse tried to wake him up to give him some medicine, and she couldn't wake him. They called the doctor in from his home, and he ordered a CT scan. When the film came up to the floor, the doctor took me out in the hall and said, "He's not going to live through the night." He held up the film showing a massive cerebral infarction; Greg was bleeding into the brain. He quietly died less than an hour later. Family and staff were in total shock. Nobody expected it. But, looking back, Greg had decided he had had enough; he was ready to go. I am grateful that he didn't die on a transplant floor in a strange city. We were able to call in friends and family, and we were surrounded and supported by the wonderful nurses whom we knew so intimately. I couldn't leave him until three nurses promised to stay with him and escort him to the morgue. They are still dear friends.*

Parents of children who died in the hospital stressed the importance of clear communication. Parents need to be strong advocates for adequate pain control, and they need to clearly tell the staff their wishes for their child's end of life. For example, in most hospitals, if a child's heart stops or if he stops breathing, the staff immediately begins cardiopulmonary resuscitation (CPR) and electric shocks to the heart—this is called a "code." If the parents have decided they are ready to let their child die naturally, they need to discuss their wishes with the oncologist and ensure that an order of "No Code" is put in the chart and on the child's door. A No Code order is also called a "DNR," or "Do Not Resuscitate" order. Family members should understand that a DNR does not mean "Do not care for my child." On the contrary, the medical team will provide comfort measures, such as:

- Allowing the child to sleep during the night without interruptions for checks of temperature and blood pressure
- Providing adequate pain medications
- Allowing family and friends open visitation without restrictions as to length and time of stay and number of people in the room
- A private room

I felt bad for my daughter, because like any good child, she wanted permission, even to die. My husband had promised her that he would never give up. He kept on saying, "Fight. Fight. Don't give up, don't leave me. We'll do another transplant, we'll try different medicine. It's too early to give up." I looked at him and said, "She's not going anywhere until you tell her that it's okay." Then he told her, and she took her last breath. He still feels guilty to this day because of his promises. He just didn't understand that it was time; that she needed to know that it was okay with us.

Parents also should discuss whether they want nurses or doctors present when their child dies. Many families feel very close to the hospital staff and feel supported by their presence, while others prefer to have only family and close friends at the child's bedside. Advance planning helps to ensure that, as death approaches, the family's wishes are understood and respected.

Dying at Home

A child's death at home, and the time just before, can be a peaceful experience, depending on the extent of preparation and the quality of support available to the family.

It was scary to be taking Caitlin home to die, but she was so happy to be there. Her brother was 14 years old, six-foot-three, and he carried her everywhere she wanted to go. We let her be in charge; whomever she wanted to see would be allowed in. My parents bought her a television and a VCR, each with remotes. She'd sit in bed with a remote in each hand, glad not to have to compete with her brothers, and say, "I got the power."

The night of her death her vomiting was too bad for us to stay at home. We brought her to the hospital in our car; we fixed a bed for her in the back with me and her aunt on the floor and her dad driving. She was taken directly to the pediatric floor, where they started an IV and gave her something to stop the vomiting. My husband and I were in such denial that we had packed enough for at least a 2-week stay. No one on the staff had told us that her death was very near.

Ten days after her death we had to return to the pediatric floor with our son, and one of the doctors asked me if I had known Caitlin was dying when we came in with her. I said, "No, did you?" He replied, "Yes, because her breathing had changed." This new information hurt me deeply. It would have been good to have been told that her death was near and been given some choices about how we would like to handle it. I truly believe this could have been done quickly and as gently as all of her care had been given. I would like to have had the chance to hold Caitlin in my arms as she left our world, cradling her as closely as possible for the last time. Instead, I was hanging over the railing, holding her hand.

We decided to bring Jody home to die for several reasons. First of all, the medical profession was offering no more realistic hope. Secondly, Jody was young enough and small enough to be easily held, carried, and cared for by us. Thirdly, nothing violent or terrifying happened at home, which made us seriously debate whether to go back in the hospital with him.

I saw many life values in a new way from the experience of Jody dying at home. What comes to my mind is a sunny, breezy afternoon, September 13. Only Jody and I were home. I held him outside under the plum tree for perhaps an hour and a half or longer. I couldn't support him well and read to him at the same time, so we didn't do anything. I spoke to him some, but mostly just held him quietly. I was aware as I looked up into the sky that my normal reaction on such a day would be to want to be hiking, biking, "doing" something. A surprise recognition burst and spread gently through my consciousness: I was exactly where I wanted to be and no doing of anything could mean as much as being there with Jody.

Jody's last day, September 16, was peaceful. A spiritual healer, whom Jody had known for two years, came and spent time with him. A massage therapist/healer/ friend, who had visited him several times during the five weeks he was home, gave him a long, gentle massage. My husband, Tom, stayed home from teaching that day (by chance?). Jody lay in his arms or on my lap most of the day. The visiting home nurse came by briefly and offered to stay, but we preferred to be alone. I was holding Jody; Tom was next to me holding his feet. Jody's breathing became labored and irregular. His eyes were unblinking long before he took his last breath, then a heartbeat, then another, then silence.

Involving Siblings

Whether your child is dying at home or in the hospital, siblings should be included in the family response. Being part of things and having jobs to do help brothers and sisters remain involved, contributing members of the family. Young children can answer the door or choose music to play for the sibling. Older children can help with meals, stay with the ill child to give parents a break, answer the phone, or help make funeral arrangements. These jobs should not be "make-work"—children should truly be helping. This helps them to prepare for the death, as well as have a chance to say good-bye.

We gave our children free rein to pick out the clothes that Jesse would be buried in. They made very thoughtful choices: her favorite, very comfortable pajamas with little tea cups on them, and her teddy bear.

For teens, the presence of their siblings and friends can be very significant in the final weeks.

When Megan first came home after her last hospital stay to manage the pain, she stayed on the couch and her twin sister slept on an air mattress next to her. We carried her upstairs to her bed in their shared room in a wheelchair. She lasted two nights in her own bed, then she needed a hospital bed. The pain pump worked well most of the time, but we had to work with hospice and her pain management team to get the right level of pain control. Her older brother in Florida took off a couple of months to come home and be with her before she died. Her friends were great with her, spending a lot of time at the house. They put her makeup on her and did her hair two days before she became unconscious.

Megan worried about how her twin sister, Melissa, would cope without her. While she could still speak, Megan asked me, "For our first birthday that we're not together, will you give her this 'fearless' bracelet?" It was a leather band with metal letters spelling out fearless. "Tell her she was the fearless one." I framed it and gave it to Melissa with a card saying exactly what Megan asked her mom to share with her twin. She's studying in Rome at the moment and it's one of the few things she took with her.

The Funeral

Funerals and related rituals (e.g., memorial services, wakes, shiva, burial) are important not only as a time to say good bye and to begin to accept the reality of death, but also to provide an opportunity to recognize the relationships and impact the child or teen had on others. Funerals allow friends and family to gather together to share memories and show support for the remaining family members. A funeral is a tangible demonstration of love.

We had Greg's minister, godparents, and kindergarten teacher come to our house to help plan the service. We did not want it to be scary, because we wanted all of his young friends to come. They needed to say goodbye, too, and above all, we wanted them to be comfortable. During the service, several songs were sung, and the minister didn't stand up at a pulpit. He stood on our level with his hand on Greg's casket and talked about Greg's life. It was simple and good. On the way to the cemetery it rained lightly, and the sky was filled with three rainbows. Sadness and hope.

Children of all ages should be allowed to attend the funeral if they wish, but only after they have been prepared for what to expect. They need an explanation of what the event is for, where they will be going, and what will happen. They need to know what death is, what type of room they are going to, whether the casket will be there, whether it will be open, whether there will be flowers, who will be there, how the mourners will behave, who will stay with them, what they will be expected to say or do, how long they will be there, and what will happen after the service (e.g., burial, reception). All questions should be answered honestly and the children's feelings respected. Many siblings benefit from giving one last gift to the departed, such as writing a private note and placing it in the casket, or bringing some of their sister's favorite flowers to put in her hands.

> We celebrated our 3-year-old son Kevin's life today. The past week has been a whirlwind. All of Kevin's favorite women worked nonstop for 48 hours leading up to last night. The funeral home was beautiful. There were pictures everywhere—on pedestals, in photo albums, collages, and frames. There were children's books throughout the funeral home as well as red balloons—Kev's favorite color. We had patchwork squares out to create a memorial quilt for his younger sisters, Courtney and Katie. People wrote special messages and drawings on them to capture their feelings: "Kevin, Sending you love and kisses and one BIG scoop of mashed potatoes!"

> We also had sheets of paper to write stories and memories of Kevin to make a memorial book for the girls. Kevin's favorite things were on a memorial table: his green blankie with the hole in it, his books, his Buzz Lightyear®, his green bike, his catcher's mitt, his baseball and yellow bat, golf clubs, and more. We rented a 6' projector screen and a big screen TV to display a 20-minute video in both rooms at the funeral home. It showed Kevin's life over the past year. And it was a pretty good life too: putting candles on Grammy's cake with Matthew, gymnastics with Grampie, wrestling with Courtney, reading with Daddy, playing football with Nana, kissing Auntie JoJo and Auntie Karin, playing golf in the yard, laying on the floor laughing, telling knock knock jokes, riding bikes in the house, at the beach at the Cape.

> What does a mom do? She loves, cherishes, teaches, protects, and lets go. For one brief, shining moment, we had Kevin. For happily ever after we have our memories of him.

For families that are involved in a spiritual community, their clergy have a unique opportunity to provide support, love, and comfort to the grieving family and friends. They usually know the family well and can evoke poignant memories of the deceased child or teen during the service. Members of the clergy often have excellent counseling skills and can visit the family after the funeral to provide ongoing help during mourning.

The Role of Family and Friends

Family members and friends can be a wellspring of deep comfort and solace during grieving. Some people seem to know just when a hug is needed or when silence is most welcome. Unfortunately, in our society there are few guidelines for handling the social aspects of grief. Sometimes well-meaning people voice opinions concerning the time it is taking to "get over it" or question the parents' decision to not give away their child's clothing or other belongings. Others do not know what to say, so they are silent, pretending that life's greatest catastrophe did not occur. Many friends never again mention the deceased child's name, not knowing that this silence, as if the cherished child never existed, only adds to parents' pain. Holidays can become uncomfortable, because they bring sadness as well as joy.

To ease these difficulties, bereaved parents helped compile the following lists of what helps and what does not, in the hope that it may guide those family members and friends who deeply care, but just don't know what to do or say. Parents or family members can copy these lists to share with people who want to help. These suggestions are offered with the understanding that what works for one family may not work for another. Family members and friends should use their knowledge of the bereaved family to choose options that they think will be most helpful. If in doubt, they should ask the parents. As Mother Teresa said, "Kind words can be short and easy to say, but their echoes are truly endless."

Things that help

The long lists of things that help from Chapter 18, *Family and Friends* (e.g., keeping the household running, feeding the family, and helping with bills), are still appropriate here. The following lists are specific suggestions for support with grieving.

Helpful things to say:

- I am so sorry.
- I cannot imagine the pain you are feeling, but I am thinking about you.
- You and your family are in our thoughts and prayers.
- We would like to hold a memorial service at the school for your child if you think that it would be appropriate.
- I will never forget John's sunny smile.
- I will never forget Jane's gentle way with children and animals.

Parents also offer a list of helpful things to do:

- Go to the funeral or memorial service.

    We were overwhelmed and touched by all of the people who came to the funeral. Even people that I had not seen in years—like some of my college professors— attended. Her oncologist and nurse drove 100 miles to be there.

- Show genuine concern and caring by listening.

    What has helped me the most is for people to just listen. Finding time to remember and reminisce is sometimes very difficult and painful, yet other times I feel much pride and happiness. Friends whose children also have cancer have been the greatest help to me during my daughter's illness and after her death.

- Help the siblings.

    We had friends just call and say, "We will pick up Nick on Saturday and take him to Water World, then to our house for dinner. We were hoping he could spend the night. Will that be all right?" They did this many times, and it not only was fun for him, but gave us a chance to be alone with each other and our grief.

    · · · · ·

    The day my daughter died, a close friend—herself a bereaved parent—did something wonderful. She took over my three kids, and prepared them for the funeral. She sat down with them and they read a book entitled, Today My Sister Died, *and talked about it. She described in great detail what would happen at the funeral, and, more importantly, she prepared them for some of the not-so-helpful comments that they would hear. So, when the first person said, "You're the big sister now," they had a response. She listened to them and prepared them and it truly helped them cope.*

- Write the parents a note instead of sending a preprinted sympathy card with your signature. Include special things you remember about their child or your feelings about their child. Letters, poems, or drawings from classmates and friends allow children to share their feelings with the family of the deceased, as well as provide poignant testimonials that the family will cherish.

- Talk about the child who has died. Parents forever carry cherished memories of their child and enjoy hearing others' favorite recollections.

    Months after the funeral, we gathered family members and some close friends to share memories on tape. We did a lot of laughing as well as shed a few tears. But I will always cherish those tapes.

    · · · · ·

    I think most of all parents want their child to be remembered. It really comforts me to go to Greg's grave and find flowers, notes, or toys left by others.

- When parents express guilt over what they did or did not do, reassure them that they did everything they could. Remind them that they provided their child with the best medicine had to offer.

- Remember anniversaries. Call or send a card or flowers on the anniversary of the child's death.

- Respect the family's method of grieving.

- Give donations in the child's name to a favorite charity of the child or parents, for example, the child's school library, the local children's camp, or U.S. Children's Hospice International.

  Every year we still get a card saying that Caitlin's occupational therapist donated money to Camp Goodtimes. It makes me feel good that she is remembered so fondly and that the money will help other kids with cancer and their brothers and sisters.

- Commemorate the child's life in some tangible way. Examples of this are planting trees, shrubs, or flowers; erecting a memorial or plaque; or displaying a picture of the child.

  The spring after Matthew's death, his school contacted me and said they wanted to do something special in his honor. They planted a little leaf linden tree in front of the building and built a wonderful seat around its base. They picked this particular tree because of its wonderful fragrance, and because the leaves were shaped like little hearts. A plaque beside the tree proclaims that this is Matthew's Friendship Tree. In addition to his name and the date of his birth and death, it reads: "When you remember me, please have a smile and cherish the good times we shared. And in these memories I will live with you forever."

- Be patient. Acute grief from the loss of a child lasts a long, long time. Expectations of a rapid recovery are unrealistic and hurtful to parents.

The Compassionate Friends (see Appendix B, *Resource Organizations*) has dozens of resources to help friends and all members of the family.

What not to say

Please do not say the following to grieving parents:

- I know exactly how you feel.
- It's a blessing her suffering has ended.
- Thank goodness you are young enough to have another child.
- At least you have your other children.
- Be brave.
- Time will heal.
- God doesn't give anyone more than they can bear.
- It was God's will.
- He's in a better place now.

Every time someone approached me at the funeral home with the words, "He's gone to a better place," I felt as if I would scream. Matthew's place was with me, his mother. Seven-year-old boys need their mother. It also really angered me when people repeatedly said, "Oh, with all he suffered, you wouldn't wish him back if you could." Well, yes, I would wish my child back! I would wish him back healthy and well. To this very day I would wish my child back, even if I could hold him for just a moment or hear the sound of his laughter one more time.

- God must have needed another angel.
- You need to be strong for your other children.
- It's lucky this happened to someone as strong as you.

    People would say things to me like "You're so strong," or "I just couldn't live through what you have." It makes me want to scream. Do they mean I loved my child less than they love theirs because I have physically survived?

Even if bereaved parents have deep religious faith, it is often tested by their child's death. Parents are not comforted by well-meaning friends who assume faith is making the grief bearable; indeed, many parents find it to be infuriating.

If you are struggling to find words, just say "I'm so very, very sorry" and give lots of hugs.

What not to do

The following are suggestions from parents about what not to do:

- Don't remove anything that belonged to the child who died, unless specifically asked to by the parents.

    One family member took my son's toothbrush out of the bathroom and threw it away. I missed it immediately. She probably felt she was doing me a favor, but it made me so angry. I needed to keep things. I have his hair from the second time it fell out, because he wanted to save it, and I've kept his teeth that had to be pulled during treatment. I just need to have those things, and I resent people who insist you must clear out a child's things. Parents should be able to keep things or get rid of them— whichever is comfortable—regardless of others' opinions.

- Don't offer advice.

    Christie's room is still her room. We still refer to it as Christie's room. People just don't have the right to say you shouldn't leave that room empty: it's not empty, it's full of her life. I know that they are not trying to hurt us. It just bothers them to see that room. Sometimes it is just a reminder of death; yet, there are times when being in there and surrounded by all her things brings us closer to her and her time with us.

- Don't say anything that in any way suggests the child's medical care was inadequate.

  I can't tell you how many people said things like "If only you had gone to a different treatment facility," or "If only you had used this or that treatment." What people need most is support for what they are doing or did do.

- Don't look on the bright side or find silver linings.

  I became unexpectedly pregnant the month after my daughter died. I can't tell you how many people said things like "The circle of life is complete," or "God is taking one and giving you another," or "God is replacing her." She can never be replaced. It was horrible to hear those things, and I felt it was unfair to both the unborn baby and my daughter who died.

If you don't know how to support the family, it's always helpful to bring a meal that can go in the freezer and to share memories of the child who died.

Sibling Grief

Siblings are sometimes called the forgotten grievers, because attention is typically focused on the parents. Children and teens sometimes hesitate to express their own strong feelings in an attempt to prevent causing their parents more distress. Indeed, adult family members and friends may advise the brothers and sisters to "be strong" for their parents or to "help your parents by being good." These requests place a terribly unfair burden on children who have already endured months or years of stress and family disruption. Siblings need continual reinforcement that each of them is an irreplaceable member of the family and that the entire family has suffered a loss. They have the right, and need, to mourn openly and in their own way.

Children express grief in many ways. Some children develop physical symptoms, such as stomach aches, a loss of appetite or voracious eating, or changes in sleeping or toileting habits. Many younger children regress; they may revert to diapers or baby talk, stop walking, or stop talking. Fears and phobias, such as a fear of the dark or of being alone, are common responses to loss. Children may develop unpredictable or disruptive behaviors, such as tantrums, crying, sadness, anxiety, withdrawal, or depression. Older children and teens may appear nonchalant, angry, withdrawn, or engage in risky behaviors, such as sexual promiscuity, alcohol abuse, and drug use.

Parents should engage siblings of different ages at their appropriate developmental levels. Private time together, or individual outings with the parents, can be very helpful for siblings.

The family requires such reorganization after a child's death, and there is nowhere to look for an example. Each person in the family constellation has different feelings and different ways of grieving; there is just no way to reconcile all of this when the supposed leaders of the group are totally out of it. Not to mention the fact that both my husband and I wanted more understanding and compassion from each other than we were possibly able to give.

Some parents worry that if they start talking about their feelings, they will break down in front of the children. But the children know their parents are grieving and it hurts them to feel excluded. They are grieving, too, and if they see their parents pulling away from them, they are likely to feel that their parents don't love them as much as they loved the child they lost. Here are suggestions from families about ways to pull together while mourning:

- Let the siblings go to the funeral. They have suffered a loss; they need to say good-bye and they need support for their grief just as much as adults do.

  I grew up going to my relatives' funerals. Having those positive experiences really helped me deal with the loss of my son. There is nothing more natural than to take a child to the funeral, where they are part of families loving each other, crying together, and laughing at some of the memories. Too many people try to protect kids from death, and it does them a great disservice.

- Children and teens experience the same feelings as adults. Sharing your feelings can encourage them to identify their own. (For example, "I'm really feeling sad today. How do you feel?")
- Jointly discuss how holidays and anniversaries should be observed. Each family devises different ways to handle holidays, the child's birthday, and the anniversary of her death.

  Last year we marked our first Christmas since Matthew's death. It was so incredibly hard for me to open the boxes of decorations knowing that inside I would find treasures he had made for me over the years with his own two little hands. I cried when I found his stocking, because I didn't know what to do with it. Somehow it didn't seem right to not hang it as usual.

  I decided that I would continue to place Matthew's stocking beside David's and Kristina's. Instead of Santa filling it with treats, I asked my family to fill it for me. A few weeks before every Christmas, I ask members of my family to write a memory of Matthew on a piece of paper. The only stipulation is that it must be a happy memory. On Christmas morning, I look forward most of all to the gifts my children have made for me in school, and the memories that fill Matthew's stocking.

Parental Grief

Losing a child is one of life's most horrific and painful events. There is no right way to grieve. There is no timetable, no appropriate progression from one stage to the next, and no specific time when parents should "be over it." The death of a child shatters the very order of the universe—children are not supposed to die before their parents; it seems unnatural and incomprehensible. Losing a child, especially after such a long and grueling battle to save him or her, feels cruel and unjust. When a child dies, parents mourn not only the child, but all of the hopes, dreams, wishes, and needs relating to their child. When you lose a child, you lose part of yourself and an important part of your future. Below, parents themselves share their thoughts about grief.

I truly think that it is the worst thing in the entire world. Nothing worse can happen than losing your child. There is no reprieve. None.

• • • • •

My life is void of the very essential magic of Elena, the stories, the brightness of her being. Her giggles, her sweet kisses, her calling me cupcake and giving me the nosie "uggamuggums." She would be in fourth grade Tuesday, and instead she is dead! The school planted flowers by the memorial that they gave last year on her birthday. Yes, it was hard to shop for two instead of three of my kids. I miss the games and the playing school and the calls between her friends. I miss sitting with her on my lap; I miss touching her smooth skin, touching her curly hair, and smelling her scent. I miss looking at her long fingers. But I feel that I was blessed with her life, her love of life, her friends and passions, her angels, and her beauty. I will carry her life with honor in my heart for my lifetime.

• • • • •

I was having a very hard time grieving when a wonderful therapist I was seeing said to me, "You are beating yourself up about grieving. Think about it: When you enter marriage, what are you called? A wife. When your spouse dies, what are you called? A widow. When you don't have a home and you are living on the street, what is the name for that? A homeless person. When you lose a child, what's it called, what's the name?" I said, "I don't know." She said, "Exactly. There is not even a word in our vocabulary. That's how terrible it is. It doesn't even have a name."

• • • • •

The biggest thing I had to learn was just to cope with whatever I was feeling on that particular day. When I feel angry, I just need to let myself be angry. If I need to cry all day, I do. I still have plenty of those days. If someone calls me and wants to take me out to lunch to cheer me up, I have learned to say no when I'm not feeling like going out. I know that it hurts other people to see me cry, but I need to do that sometimes. I just miss her so much.

. . . . .

Every day when I walk out of my house I tell myself to grab the mask. I feel like I walk different than everybody and talk different than everybody and look different than everybody. It's the worst part of bereavement, the isolation caused by people who just don't know how to talk to you, when really all they need to do is listen and remember with you.

. . . . .

I found myself getting busier and busier, thinking that I could outrun the pain. I realized that I couldn't avoid the hurt; I just had to grit my teeth, cry, and live through it.

. . . . .

My daughter was our firefly; she lit the whole scene up. When she died, that spirit was gone, and there was just a hole left. We just didn't feel like a family anymore.

. . . . .

I felt like our sick daughter was the center of our universe for so long, that now I need to start feeling some responsibility for my other kids whom I've been away from for so long, both physically and emotionally. I told my husband the other night that I didn't even know if I loved the three kids anymore. I cannot feel a thing. Pinch me, I don't feel it. Hug me, I don't feel it. I'm numb.

. . . . .

It's hard to admit, but there was an element of relief when my daughter died. Not relief for myself, but for her. I was almost glad that she wouldn't face a life full of disabilities. That she wouldn't face the numerous orthopedic surgeries that would have been required to repair the damage from treatment. That she wouldn't face the pain of not having children of her own. I just felt relief that she would no longer feel any pain.

. . . . .

It's hard when people I have just met ask, "How many children do you have?" In the beginning, I always felt I had to explain that I had two but one died. Now I just say one. I don't want their sympathy, I don't want their pity, but most of all I just don't want to have to explain. After two years or so, I started to feel uncomfortable giving out my life history and then having to deal with other people's discomfort. So now I just say one, and yet it still feels like I'm betraying him every time I do it.

. . . . .

At first we didn't feel like a family anymore. Now it's better, but it's still not the family that I was used to, that I want. I still feel like the mother of four children, not three. I find it very hard to answer when someone asks me how many children I have. I also can't sign cards like I used to, with all of our names, so now I just write "from the gang." I guess that's not fair to the boys, but I just can't bear to leave her name off.

· · · · ·

I had a visual image of our family of five. When Jody died, it became this physical square thing with only mom, dad, boy, girl, and it bothered me so much.

· · · · ·

I thought this morning of how I used to listen to Jesse breathe. Now I can't hear her breathe or laugh. I can't feel her arms around me. I remember missed kisses and late-night times. I ache. Heaven seems so far away.

· · · · ·

It seems that sometimes she is still so near that during conversations I can hear her comments or answers, and yet I fear the memories might fade and I so cherish the nearness. We each wear articles of her clothes or jewelry every day. One daughter is sleeping on the floor in our room, and the other two are sleeping in her bed.

· · · · ·

The worst times were the first two Christmases. We had to grit our teeth, put our heads down, and just get through it. We had to keep moving, never stop moving. I would have ignored it altogether if I didn't have another child.

· · · · ·

Birthdays are hard for us. Greg's birthday was June 10, and his brother's is June 9. So it's pretty hard to ignore. On Greg's birthday and the anniversary of his death, we blow up balloons, one for every year he would have been alive, write messages on them with markers, and release them at his grave.

· · · · ·

It seems like just about every holiday has some difficult memory attached to it now. He was diagnosed on Easter, and then relapsed the next year on Valentine's Day. I hate them both now. Christmas is always hard. And Halloween is tough because he so loved to dress up. I see all those little ones in their costumes and I'm just flooded with pain.

· · · · ·

I keep wondering if I should have put a stop to the bone marrow transplant, because I had no peace about it. I felt such fear and dread about her platelets and liver. And what I feared happened. I still pray to have peace over making that choice. To have peace over giving a teenager the weight of deciding all that herself. I still feel so guilty and know I'd still be kissing her goodnight if we hadn't gone forward—and how I miss those kisses.

I feel like Job 3:25-26: What I feared has come upon me; What I dreaded has happened to me; I have no peace, no quietness; I have no rest but only turmoil.

• • • • •

This evening my heart was so saddened. I paced up and down in front of the mantel, pausing to look at each picture of my daughter. Something that I cannot describe catches in my chest, and I can't breathe right. I look at her face and try to will it to life for a kiss and a touch, for softly spoken endearments at night. How we love all of our children, yet one missing leaves such a stabbing pain.

• • • • •

I worry that missing one child so desperately pervades my very ability to be a good mom to my other three. I so wish to find joy again, to find things in life to smile about. I so wish my children could see me smile again. I pray that God will give me this thing, because it is beyond my finding in this world.

• • • • •

I had always heard that time heals all things. I was afraid of healing, because I didn't want to feel any farther away than I felt when he died. It's been seven years, and he still feels really close—a presence. But I still so ache to touch his body, that little back and fat tummy.

• • • • •

It's been two years, and I still feel a lot of rage. I walk down the street and see kids hanging out, smoking, doing drugs, being rude, wasting themselves, and I am filled with rage that my son—such a straight arrow, so decent, so strong—is gone.

• • • • •

I feel strongly that parents should seek out other parents who have lost children. Nobody else understands as well. Nobody else is as comfortable with it. We have our own sense of humor, and we often laugh hard about things that make other people uncomfortable.

• • • • •

That 1-year rule, when you are supposed to start feeling better, I've found to be true. Not that any of the pain is lessened, but I realized I had managed to live through a year of holidays and anniversaries. I knew it was possible to do it a second, then a third time. One year isn't magic, but it does prove to you that you can survive.

• • • • •

On the anniversary of Ryan's death we all went to the cemetery, and his girlfriend's parents planted a cherry tree at the foot of his grave. That was on a Sunday. I woke up on Monday feeling just as bad as I did the day before. All I could think was, "Oh hell, I have to go through that whole cycle again." The first year did not bring me any peace.

· · · · ·

This morning was the 4-year anniversary of my daughter's death. While I was at church I wanted to write in the intentions book, "I want my daughter back," but then I didn't because nobody would understand. I guess I'm pretty unreal in my thoughts a lot of the time.

· · · · ·

At church, we always sit with the same group of close friends who helped us through Jesse's illness and are helping us grieve her death. If they begin to sing a hymn that reminds one of us of Jesse, we all start to cry, and someone produces a box of tissues, which gets passed down the aisles. People must wonder at the group that sobs through services. But it has helped me so much to have a community of grievers, it's been a very cleansing thing. It has spread out the tears.

· · · · ·

I think parents need to know that it hurts like hell and they will feel crazy. But it is a normal craziness. If they talk to other bereaved parents, they will know that pain, guilt, rage, and craziness are how normal human beings feel when their child dies.

Bereaved parents are frequently reassured that "time will ease the pain." Most find that this is not the case. Time helps them understand the pain; the passage of time reassures them that they can adjust and they will survive. The acute pain becomes more quiescent, but it still erupts when parents go to what would have been their child's graduation, hear their child's favorite song, or just go to the grocery store. Grief is a long, difficult journey, with many ups and downs. But, with time, parents report that laughter and joy do return. They acknowledge that life will never be the same, but that it can be good again.

"I just wish that I had armfuls of time."

— Four year old with cancer
Armfuls of Time

Appendix A

Blood Tests and What They Mean

KEEPING TRACK OF THEIR CHILD'S BLOOD cell counts becomes a way of life for parents of children with leukemia. Unfortunately, misunderstandings about what certain changes in blood values mean cause unnecessary worry and fear. To help prevent these concerns, and to better enable parents to spot trends in the blood cell values of their child, this appendix explains the blood cell counts of healthy children, the blood cell counts of children being treated for leukemia, and what each blood cell count value means. It also briefly describes other blood tests commonly needed in children with leukemia.

Values for Healthy Children

Each laboratory and lab handbook has slightly different reference values for each type of blood test. There is also variation in values for children of different ages. For instance, in children ranging in age from newborn to 4 years, granulocytes are lower and lymphocytes are higher than the numbers listed below. The following table lists blood tests and blood count values for healthy children older than 4 years of age.

Blood Test Type	Values for Healthy Children
Hemoglobin (Hgb)	11.5 to 13.5 g/100 mL
Hematocrit (HCT)	34 to 40%
Red blood cell (RBC) count	3.9 to 5.3 million/cm^3
Platelets	160,000 to 380,000/mm^3
White blood cell (WBC) count	5,000 to 15,000/mm^3 or 5 to 15 K/µL
WBC differential:	
Segmented neutrophils	40 to 70%
Band neutrophils	1.5 to 8%
Basophils	<0.3%

Blood Test Type	Values for Healthy Children
Eosinophils	<0.5%
Lymphocytes	20 to 50%
Monocytes	2 to 10%
Liver function tests	
ALT (sometimes called SGPT)	0 to 48 IU/L
AST (sometimes called SGOT)	0 to 36 IU/L
Bilirubin (total)	0.3 to 1.3 mg/dL
Direct (conjugated)	0.1 to 0.4 mg/dL
Indirect (unconjugated)	0.2 to 1.88 mg/dL
Kidney function tests	
Blood urea nitrogen (BUN)	6 to 20 mg/dL
Creatinine	0.5 to 1.5 mg/dL
Electrolytes	
Glucose	70 to 115 mEq/L
Potassium	3.5 to 5.0 mEq/L
Minerals	
Calcium	8.5 to 10.5 mg/dL
Magnesium	1.5 to 2.9 mg/dL

Values for Children on Chemotherapy

Blood test results of children being treated for leukemia often fluctuate wildly. WBCs can go down to zero or be above normal. RBCs may go down periodically during treatment, necessitating transfusions of packed red cells. Platelet levels may also decrease, sometimes requiring platelet transfusions. Absolute neutrophil counts (ANC) are closely watched, as they give the oncologist an idea of the child's ability to fight infections; ANCs range from zero into the thousands. Chemotherapy can also cause changes in kidney and liver function, along with changes in electrolytes and mineral levels in the blood.

Pediatric oncologists consider all of the blood test results to get the total picture of a child's reaction to illness, treatment, or infection. Trends are more important than any single value.

Common Blood Tests

Following are descriptions of the most common blood tests given to children with leukemia. If you have any questions about your child's blood test results, ask the oncologist or nurse practitioner for a clear explanation.

Hemoglobin (Hgb)

Red blood cells contain Hgb, the molecules that carry oxygen and carbon dioxide in the blood. Measuring Hgb gives doctors an exact picture of the ability of the child's blood to carry oxygen. Children may have low Hgb levels at diagnosis and during the intensive parts of treatment. This is because chemotherapy decreases the bone marrow's ability to produce new red blood cells. Signs and symptoms of anemia—paleness, shortness of breath, fatigue—may occur if the Hgb gets very low.

Hematocrit (HCT)

The HCT is sometimes called the packed cell volume. The purpose of the HCT test is to determine the ratio of plasma (the clear liquid part of blood) to red blood cells in the blood. For this test, blood is drawn from a vein, a finger prick, or central catheter and is spun in a centrifuge to separate the red cells from the plasma. The HCT is the percentage of red blood cells in the blood. For example, if the child has an HCT of 30%, it means that 30% of the amount of blood drawn was red cells and the rest was plasma.

When a child is on chemotherapy, the bone marrow does not make many red cells and the HCT goes down. When the HCT is low, less oxygen is carried in the blood, so your child will have less energy. Your child may be given a transfusion of packed red cells if the HCT goes below 18 or 19%.

Red blood cell (RBC) count

RBCs are produced by the bone marrow continuously in healthy children and adults. These cells contain hemoglobin, which carries oxygen throughout the body. To determine the RBC count, an automated electronic device is used to count the number of red cells in a blood sample.

White blood cell (WBC) count

The total WBC count indicates the body's ability to fight infection. Treatment for leukemia kills healthy white cells as well as diseased ones. It also impairs the ability of the bone marrow to make more WBCs. To determine the WBC count, an automated electronic device counts the number of white cells in a blood sample.

WBC differential

When a child has blood drawn for a complete blood count (CBC), one section of the lab report will state the total WBC and a "differential," meaning that each type of white blood cell will be listed as a percentage of the total. For example, if the total WBC count is 1,500 mm^3, the differential might appear as in the following table.

White Blood Cell Type	Percentage of Total WBC
Segmented neutrophils (also called polys or segs)	49%
Band neutrophils (also called bands)	1%
Basophils (also called basos)	1%
Eosinophils (also called eos)	1%
Lymphocytes (also called lymphs)	38%
Monocytes (also called monos)	10%

Absolute neutrophil count (ANC)

The ANC (also called the absolute granulocyte count or AGC) is a measure of the body's ability to withstand infection. Generally, an ANC above 1,000 means the child's infection-fighting ability is near normal.

To calculate the ANC, add the percentages of neutrophils (both segmented and band) and multiply by the total WBC count. Using the example above, the ANC is 49%+ 1%= 50%, and 50% of 1,500 (.50 x 1,500) = 750, so the ANC is 750.

Platelet count

Platelets are needed to repair the body and stop bleeding by forming clots. Because platelets are produced by bone marrow, platelet counts often decrease when a child or teen is on chemotherapy. Signs of low platelet counts are bruises and bleeding from the gums or nose. Platelet transfusions are sometimes given when the platelet count is lower than 20,000 or when there is bleeding. Platelets are counted by passing a blood sample through an electronic device.

Alanine aminotransferase (ALT)

ALT is also called serum glutamic pyruvic transaminase (SGPT). When doctors talk about liver functions, they are usually referring to blood tests that measure liver damage. If chemotherapy is causing liver damage, the liver cells release an enzyme called ALT into the blood serum. ALT levels can go up into the hundreds, or even thousands, in some children on chemotherapy. Each institution and protocol has different points at which chemotherapy drug dosages are decreased or stopped to allow the child's liver to recover.

Aspartate aminotransferase (AST)

AST is also called serum glutamic oxaloacetic transaminase (SGOT). AST is an enzyme present in high concentrations in tissues with high metabolic activity, such as the liver. Severely damaged or killed cells release AST into the blood. The amount of AST in the blood is directly related to the amount of tissue damage. Therefore, if your child's liver is being damaged by chemotherapy, the AST count can rise into the thousands. Viral infections or reactions to an anesthetic can also cause an elevated AST.

Bilirubin

The liver converts hemoglobin released from damaged RBCs into bilirubin. The liver then removes bilirubin from the blood and excretes it into bile, which is a fluid released into the small intestine to aid digestion. If too much bilirubin is present in the body, it causes a yellow color in the skin and whites of the eyes that is called jaundice.

The two types of bilirubin are indirect (also called unconjugated) and direct (also called conjugated). An increase in indirect bilirubin is seen when destruction of RBCs has occurred. An increase of direct bilirubin is seen when there is a dysfunction or blockage of the liver.

Blood urea nitrogen (BUN)

The BUN blood test is used to assess kidney function. It is also used to detect liver disease, dehydration, congestive heart failure, gastrointestinal bleeding, or shock. The test measures the amount of an end product of protein metabolism, called urea nitrogen, in the blood. For children with kidney or liver damage, BUN is often at abnormal levels.

Creatinine

Creatinine is a breakdown product of protein metabolism found in the urine and the blood. In children with leukemia, creatinine is measured to assess kidney function. An elevated blood creatinine level is often seen in children whose kidneys are not working well.

Glucose

The amount of glucose (sugar) in blood changes throughout the day, depending on when, what, and how much people eat, and whether they have exercised. A normal blood sugar level two hours after eating is less than 140 mg/dL. A normal fasting (no food for eight hours) blood glucose level is between 70 and 99 mg/dL.

Potassium

Potassium is important for the proper functioning of the nerves and muscles, particularly the heartbeat. Too much or too little potassium increases the chance of irregular heartbeats. Potassium levels can be altered by chemotherapy or other treatments for children with leukemia.

Calcium and magnesium

Calcium and magnesium are minerals that can be compared to the spark plugs in your car—they spark the chemical reactions in your body needed to make it function properly. Calcium and magnesium also help to develop and maintain the strength of bones. In addition, magnesium is needed for muscle development and nerve conduction throughout the body. Some chemotherapy drugs given to children with leukemia decrease the calcium and magnesium levels in the blood.

Your Child's Pattern

Each child develops a unique pattern of blood counts during treatment, and some parents like to track the changes. You can put lab sheets in a binder or enter blood test results into a computer program that shows trends over time. Doctors consider all of the laboratory results before deciding on a course of action. They should be willing to explain their plan so you can better understand what is happening and worry less.

If your child is participating in a clinical trial and you have obtained the entire clinical trial protocol (discussed in Chapter 8, *Choosing a Treatment*), it will contain a section that clearly outlines the actions that should be taken by the pediatric oncologist if certain changes in blood cell counts occur.

Resource Organizations

THE RESOURCE ORGANIZATIONS LISTED in this appendix are starting points for finding the information or help you need. The organizations are listed in the following order:

Service Organizations (United States)

Alex's Lemonade Stand Foundation (ALSF)
www.alexslemonade.org

ALSF raises money to fund innovative research for better treatments and cures for pediatric cancer. It also offers financial assistance for travel to and from specific treatment centers and a SuperSibs program providing emotional support to siblings of kids with cancer.

Chai Lifeline/Camp Simcha
www.chailifeline.org

Chai Lifeline offers support service programs for Jewish children and their families, including medical referrals, support groups, visits to hospitalized and housebound children, financial aid, transportation, and a camp for kids with cancer.

Flashes of Hope
www.flashesofhope.org

This organization matches professional photographers with families to create powerful, uplifting photographic portraits of children fighting cancer and other life-threatening illnesses.

Gabe's Chemo Duck Program
www.chemoduck.org

Parents can use Chemo Duck in play therapy to reinforce the education a child receives from a child life specialist or nurse. Chemo Duck can be personalized with a central line, a feeding tube, chest tube, or other medical device so the child can become comfortable with them through caring for his or her duck.

The JMML Foundation
www.jmmlfoundation.org

The mission of the JMML Foundation is to cure juvenile myelomonocytic leukemia (JMML) and to improve the quality of life of JMML patients and families worldwide through research, education, advocacy, and charity.

Leukemia & Lymphoma Society (LLS)
www.lls.org

LLS provides financial assistance to families, funds research, sponsors a national education program for the public and the medical community, and publishes many booklets about cancer-related topics.

Monkey in My Chair
www.monkeyinmychair.org

Monkey in My Chair provides children with cancer a "monkey kit" that includes a big stuffed monkey that takes their place in school when they are unable to be there. The kit contains a book to help teachers explain childhood cancer and its treatment to classmates to help them gain insight and empathy.

National CML Society (NCS)
www.nationalcmlsociety.org

The NCS provides educational resources, access to chronic myelogenous leukemia (CML) specialists, and a network of people who share their personal CML experiences and successes.

Ronald McDonald House Charities (RMC)
www.rmhc.org

RMC is committed to helping families of seriously ill children by providing Ronald McDonald Houses, the Ronald McDonald Learning Program, and Ronald McDonald Family Rooms within hospitals.

Songs of Love Foundation
www.songsoflove.org

This volunteer group has more than 200 artists who produce personalized musical portraits for children with chronic or life-threatening diseases.

Service Organizations (Canada)

Childhood Cancer Canada Foundation (CCCF)
www.childhoodcancer.ca

CCCF invests in collaborative cancer research and provides support programs for families, such as a teen connector website, scholarships for survivors, and financial assistance.

Kids Cancer Care of Alberta
www.kidscancercare.ab.ca

This foundation helps Alberta children with cancer and their families by providing camps, direct service programs for children and families, research funding, hospital programs, and student scholarships.

Kids with Cancer Society (KCS)
www.kidswithcancer.ca

KCS provides programs and services to help families of children with cancer in Northern Alberta and the Northwest Territories.

Leukemia & Lymphoma Society of Canada (LLSC)
www.llscanada.org

LLSC provides financial assistance to families, funds research, sponsors a national education program for the public and the medical community, and provides information about cancer-related topics.

Service Organizations (Australia)

Cancer Australia – Children's Cancer website
http://childrenscancer.canceraustralia.gov.au

This government cancer program brings together a range of evidence-based information on children's cancers for families, health professionals, and researchers. The site includes links to support organizations and clinical trials.

CanTeen, The Australian Organization for Young People Living with Cancer
www.canteen.org.au

CanTeen provides support services for young people ages 12 to 24 through programs that include face-to-face counseling, phone support, peer mentors, and printed resources.

Challenge Foundation
www.challenge.org.au

The Challenge Foundation offers services for families of children with cancer, including camps, hospital support, respite and holiday accommodations, parent support, and family activity days.

Childhood Cancer Association
www.childhoodcancer.asn.au

This South Australian organization provides emotional, practical, and financial support to families. Programs include peer, family, and sibling support; accommodations for families from rural areas; respite support; educational assistance; and bereavement services.

Sisters of Charity Outreach Country Care Link
www.sistersofcharityoutreach.com.au/service/country-care-link

Country Care Link provides support and hospitality to people visiting Sydney for medical purposes.

Leukaemia Foundation
www.leukaemia.org.au

This organization is dedicated to the care and cure of patients and families living with leukemia, lymphoma, myeloma, and related blood disorders. The Foundation provides emotional support, education programs, information, accommodation, transport, and financial support.

Redkite
www.redkite.org.au

This organization serves children with cancer and their families through financial assistance, emotional support, and educational assistance.

Ronald McDonald House Charities Australia (RMC)
www.rmhc.org.au

RMC is committed to helping families of seriously ill children by providing Ronald McDonald Houses, the Ronald McDonald Learning Program, Ronald McDonald Family Rooms within hospitals, and the Ronald McDonald Family Retreat (free holiday accommodations).

Camps

For a comprehensive list of camps for children with cancer, visit *www.ped-onc.org/cfissues/camps.html*.

Camp Quality (Australia)
www.campquality.org.au

Camp Quality provides fun therapy for children and families of children with cancer, including camps for ill children and their siblings, family camps, fun days, pamper days for moms and daughters, and fishing weekends for fathers and sons.

Camp Simcha
www.campsimcha.org

This camp is run by the national, nonprofit Jewish organization Chai Lifeline.

Canadian Association of Pediatric Oncology Camps (CAPOC)
https://capoc.ca

CAPOC's website includes a map showing camps for children with cancer in Canada.

Children's Oncology Camping Association International
www.cocai.org

This is an umbrella organization of 130 camps for children with cancer in the United States and Canada.

Educational and Legal Support

Job Accommodation Network (JAN)
www.jan.wvu.edu

JAN facilitates the employment and retention of workers with disabilities by providing employers, people with disabilities, their family members, and other interested parties with information about job accommodations, entrepreneurship, and related subjects.

Learning Disabilities Association of America (LDA)
www.ldaamerica.org

LDA serves parents, professionals, and individuals with learning disabilities; has local chapters; and provides educational materials.

National Center for Learning Disabilities
www.ncld.org

This center offers extensive resources, referral services, educational programs about learning disabilities, and an online community for young adults with learning disabilities. It also promotes public awareness and advocates for effective legislation to help people with learning disabilities.

Center for Parent Information and Resources (CPIR)
www.parentcenterhub.org

The CPIR provides resources for parents of children with disabilities, an interactive map of parent training and information centers in the United States, as well as information about parent technical assistance centers.

Financial Help

Compass to Care
http://compasstocare.org

Compass to Care schedules and pays for travel to and lodging arrangements at a hospital more than 60 miles from a child's home. Child must be younger than 18 with a demonstrated financial need and on active treatment for cancer.

Family Reach Foundation
http://familyreach.org

Family Reach is a national nonprofit dedicated to alleviating the financial burden of cancer. Working with more than 200 hospitals and cancer centers nationwide, they provide immediate financial assistance, education, and navigation to families before they hit critical breaking points.

First Hand Foundation
www.firsthandfoundation.org

This foundation assists children who have health-related needs (e.g., medical treatment, wheelchairs, assistive technology, hearing aids) when insurance and other sources of financial resources have been exhausted.

National Children's Cancer Society (NCCS)
www.nationalchildrenscancersociety.org

NCCS serves as a financial, emotional, and educational resource for families that cannot make ends meet when their child is diagnosed with cancer. It provides transportation assistance and emergency assistance for children who have been inpatient for 30 days or more.

Free Air Services (United States)

Air Charity Network
http://aircharitynetwork.org

The network is made up of independent member organizations identified by specific geographical service areas. These organizations are groups of volunteer pilots or groups that coordinate free airline tickets or reduced-price services.

Air Care Alliance
www.aircarealliance.org

This is a nationwide association of humanitarian flying organizations that provide flights for medical treatment.

Corporate Angel Network, Inc.
www.corpangelnetwork.org

This network gives patients with cancer, bone marrow donors, and bone marrow recipients available seats on corporate aircraft to get to and from recognized cancer treatment centers. Patients must be able to walk and travel without life-support systems or medical attention. A child may be accompanied by up to two adults. There is no cost or financial-need requirement.

Miracle Flights for Kids
www.miracleflights.org

This organization purchases commercial airline tickets, uses private aircraft, and combines resources from individual donors to provide free transportation to medical treatment centers across America for low-income children.

National Patient Travel Center
www.patienttravel.org

This organization refers callers to the most appropriate and cost-effective charitable or commercial services, including volunteer pilot organizations and special airline transport programs.

Free Air Service (Canada)

Hope Air
www.hopeair.ca

Hope Air provides free air transport to Canadians in financial need who must travel from their communities to recognized facilities for medical care.

Free Air Service (Australia)

Angel Flight Australia
www.angelflight.org.au

Angel Flight coordinates free, non-emergency flights to help people dealing with bad health, poor finances, and daunting distances to medical care.

Government Agencies

National Center for Complementary and Alternative Medicine (NCCAM)
http://nccam.nih.gov

NCCAM disseminates accurate information about complementary and alternative healing practices.

Physician Data Query (PDQ)
www.cancer.gov/publications/pdq/information-summaries/pediatric-treatment

PDQ is the National Cancer Institute's computerized listing of accurate and up-to-date information for patients and health professionals about cancer treatments, research studies, and clinical trials.

U.S. Department of Justice ADA Information Line
www.ada.gov

This website offers comprehensive information about the Americans with Disabilities Act (ADA).

Insurance

Patient Advocate Foundation (PAF)
www.patientadvocate.org

PAF provides patients with arbitration, mediation, and negotiation to settle issues with access to care, medical debt, and job retention related to their illness.

Medications (low-cost or free)

Partnership for Prescription Assistance (PPA)
www.pparx.org

PPA works with 475 public and private programs that provide prescription medications free of charge to patients who do not have access to necessary medicines.

RxHope
www.rxhope.com

RxHope lists patient-assistance programs that are offered by federal, state, and charitable organizations.

NeedyMeds, Inc.
www.needymeds.org

This nonprofit organization provides free help to people who cannot afford medicine or health care.

Stem Cell Transplantation

Blood & Marrow Transplant Information Network (BMT InfoNet)
www.bmtinfonet.org

BMT InfoNet supplies high-quality, easy-to-understand information about bone marrow, peripheral blood stem cell, and cord blood transplants.

Children's Organ Transplant Association (COTA)
http://cota.org/learn-more

COTA provides fundraising assistance to families facing a life-saving organ, stem cell, or bone marrow transplant. Funds raised in a COTA campaign can be used for any expenses related to the transplant.

Help Hope Live

www.helphopelive.org

This organization provides fundraising assistance and donor awareness materials to transplant patients.

Be the Match (formerly National Marrow Donor Program)

www.bethematch.org

This group helps people find bone marrow donors and cord blood units to get the best match; supports patients through the entire transplant process; and offers free DVDs, CDs, workbooks, and written education materials in multiple languages.

National Bone Marrow Transplant Link

www.nbmtlink.org

This organization helps patients and families through the process of bone marrow/stem cell transplant, offers one-on-one phone support and a phone support group, a searchable online library, free online information, or a hard copy of information for a small charge.

Wish Fulfillment Organizations (United States)

In addition to the large organizations listed below, many smaller and local organizations grant wishes to seriously ill children. A comprehensive list of wish fulfillment organizations can be found online at *www.ped-onc.org/cfissues/maw.html*.

Children's Wish Foundation International

www.childrenswish.org

This group fulfills the wishes of children with life-threatening illnesses in the United States and Europe.

Clayton Dabney Foundation for Kids with Cancer

http://claytondabney.org

This foundation provides last wishes and financial assistance to families of terminally ill children.

The Dream Factory, Inc.

www.dreamfactoryinc.org

The Dream Factory grants the wishes of children ages 3 to 18 who are critically or chronically ill (has chapters in 30 states).

Make-a-Wish Foundation of America

www.wish.org

This foundation grants wishes to children younger than age 18 with life-threatening illnesses (has U.S. and international chapters and affiliates), regardless of financial need.

Sunshine Foundation

www.sunshinefoundation.org

The Sunshine Foundation grants wishes to chronically or terminally ill children ages 3 to 18 (no geographic boundaries).

Wish Fulfillment Organizations (Canada)

Children's Wish Foundation of Canada

www.childrenswish.ca

This foundation provides a once-in-a-lifetime experience for children ages 3 to 17 with life-threatening diseases (has chapters throughout Canada).

Make-A-Wish Canada

https://makeawish.ca

The national office and eight regional chapters of Make-A-Wish Canada grant magical wishes to children with life-threatening illnesses who are ages 3 through 17, without regard to family income.

Wish Fulfillment Organizations (Australia)

Make-A-Wish Foundation of Australia National Office

www.makeawish.org.au

Make-A-Wish grants seriously ill children in Australia their most-cherished wish.

Starlight Children›s Foundation Australia

www.starlight.org.au

This foundation brightens the lives of seriously ill and hospitalized children and their families throughout Australia by granting wishes, providing vans that travel to remote hospitals, and offering activities, entertainment, and social engagement in hospital Starlight Rooms.

Hospice and Bereavement (United States)

Children's Hospice International (CHI)
www.chionline.org

CHI provides resources and referrals for children and families of children with life-threatening conditions.

The Compassionate Friends National Office
www.compassionatefriends.org

Compassionate Friends offers understanding and friendship to bereaved families through support meetings at local chapters and telephone support (they match people with similar losses). It also publishes a newsletter for parents and one for siblings.

Hospice and Bereavement (Canada)

Canadian Network of Pediatric Hospices (CNPH)
http://cnph.ca

CNPH fosters collaboration and sharing among pediatric residential hospices in Canada.

Hospice and Bereavement (Australia)

Bear Cottage
www.bearcottage.chw.edu.au

The Bear Cottage Children's Hospice is located near Sydney. It offers both respite and palliative care to children and young people with life-limiting illnesses and their families.

The Compassionate Friends New South Wales
www.tcfnsw.org.au

Compassionate Friends assists families in the positive resolution of grief following the death of a child and provides information to help others be supportive.

Hummingbird House
http://hummingbirdhouse.org.au

Queensland's only children's hospice is in a north suburb of Brisbane. It provides respite and palliative care to children and teens with life-limiting illness, with a family-centered approach.

Palliative Care Australia (PCA)
www.palliativecare.org.au

PCA provides information, resources, and referrals.

Books, Websites, and Support Groups

A WEALTH OF INFORMATION about childhood leukemia is available in libraries and online. This appendix briefly describes how to find the information you need. It also lists books, websites, and support groups you might find helpful when seeking information or support.

How to Find Information

Libraries have a computerized database of all materials available in their various branches. If you need help learning how to use these book-locating systems, ask a librarian. You can also learn how to request a book from another branch and how to put a book on hold if it's currently checked out. Some libraries have access to a digital library service that will allow you to check out the electronic version of a book or journal and read it on your own computer or other device.

If a book is not in your library's collection, ask a reference librarian whether it can be obtained from another library via interlibrary loan. This is common practice, and you might be able to get medical texts from university or medical school libraries. Some local libraries also have online databases that list all publications available at regional libraries so you can request that a book be sent to your local library for pick up.

If you want to read medical journal articles, you can access them through your local library. The librarian can show you how to use the database to search for articles and where to find the periodicals. Public libraries usually subscribe to only the most popular medical journals, such as the *New England Journal of Medicine* and *Journal of the American Medical Association*. If you are able to visit a university or medical school library, you will find many more print medical journals available. If you do not live close to one of these libraries, ask your local librarian to help you obtain copies of the articles you want.

An astonishing amount of information is available through the internet. Libraries from all over the world can be accessed, and you can download information in minutes from huge databases such as MedLine or Cancerlit. Obtaining information from respected organizations, large medical databases, reputable journals, or large libraries is exceedingly helpful for parents of sick children. However, the huge numbers of people using the internet has spawned websites, chat rooms, and social media sites that may or may not contain accurate information. You may want to read information only from reliable sources and adopt the motto: "Let the buyer beware."

Books

Below are some print books (many are also available as ebooks) that parents of children with leukemia have found helpful. You might find there are some print books you wish to own. If they are not in stock at your local or online bookstore, ask whether they can be special-ordered for you—most bookstores are happy to do this for customers. Copies of out-of-print books can often be located through the internet from used bookstores or private sellers on sites such as Amazon.com. Ebooks are available in many different formats and from many online booksellers (e.g., *www.amazon.com, www.barnesandnoble.com*) or from local libraries.

General reading (for adults)

Cochran, Lizzie. *Singing Away: Stories of Faith, Hope & Love in the Fight Against Childhood Cancer.* (2013). True stories written by families of children with cancer.

Jampolsky, Gerald G. *Advice to Doctors and Other Big People from Kids.* (1991). This book is full of stories from children with catastrophic illnesses that remind us how perceptive and aware children of all ages are, and how necessary it is to involve them in medical decisions. Available at *www.healingcenter.org/library.html.*

Kushner, Harold. *When Bad Things Happen to Good People,* revised ed. (2004). Rabbi Kushner wrote this comforting book about how people of faith cope with catastrophic events.

National Cancer Institute. *Children with Cancer: A Guide for Parents.* (2015). This booklet describes the different types of childhood cancer, medical procedures, dealing with the diagnosis, family issues, and sources of information. To obtain a free copy, visit *www.cancer.gov/publications/patient-education/guide-for-parents.*

Sourkes, Barbara M. *Armfuls of Time: The Psychological Experience of the Child with a Life-Threatening Illness.* (1996). Written by a psychologist, this eloquent book features the voices and artwork of children with cancer. It clearly describes the psychological effects of cancer on children and explains the power of the therapeutic process.

General reading (for children)

Bourgeois, Paulette. *Franklin Goes to the Hospital.* (2011). Franklin the turtle goes to the hospital for an operation to repair his broken shell, and everyone thinks he's being very brave. But Franklin is only pretending to be fearless. He's worried that his x-rays will show just how frightened he is inside.

Crary, Elizabeth. *Dealing with Feelings. I'm Frustrated; I'm Mad; I'm Sad Series.* (1992). Fun, game-like books to teach young children how to manage feelings and solve problems.

Diaz, Jonathan and others. *True Heroes: A Treasury of Modern-day Fairy Tales Written by Best-selling Authors.* (2015). Gorgeous photographs and stories written by best-selling authors make children with cancer the heroes of their own modern-day fairy tales.

Gaynor, Kate. *The Famous Hat.* (2008). This book helps children with cancer prepare for hospitalization, chemotherapy, and hair loss.

Keene, Nancy; Romain, Trevor. *Chemo, Craziness & Comfort: My Book About Childhood Cancer.* (2002). A 200-page resource that provides practical information for children between 6 and 12 years of age and their parents. Warm and funny illustrations and easy-to-read text help children (and parents) make sense of cancer and its treatment. Available to families from *www.acco.org/books*.

Martin, Kim. *H is for Hair Fairy: An Alphabet of Encouragement and Insight for Kids (and Kids at Heart!) With Cancer.* (2005). A 32-page picture book that inspires, comforts, educates, and encourages children being treated for cancer.

Schultz, Charles. *Why, Charlie Brown, Why?* (2002). Tender story about a classmate who develops leukemia.

Skole, Gary; Skole, Jarrod. *Imagine What's Possible: Using the Power of Your Mind to Help Take Control of Your Life During Cancer.* (2011). Techniques using visualization and guided imagery to help children ages 9 to 12 cope with fear, pain, anxiety, and other challenges.

General reading (for teens)

Gravelle, Karen. *Teenagers Face to Face With Cancer.* (2000). Sixteen teenagers talk openly about their experiences with cancer—from the physical difficulties of coping with treatment to the emotional trauma, which can be as painful as the illness itself. A heartfelt, honest book that demonstrates clearly how having cancer changes young people and how strength can emerge from struggles.

Paul, Trisha. *Chronicling Childhood Cancer: A Collection of Personal Stories by Children and Teens with Cancer.* (2014). Ten children and teens describe the cancer experience in their own words and pictures.

General reading (for siblings)

National Cancer Institute. *When Your Brother or Sister Has Cancer: A Guide for Teens.* (2012). This 100-page book helps teen siblings of a child with cancer prepare for and cope with some of the challenges they face. Available free at *www.cancer.gov/ Publications/patient-education/sibling-has-cancer.*

O'Toole, Donna. *Aarvy Aardvark Finds Hope: A Read Aloud Story for People of All Ages About Loving and Losing, Friendship and Hope.* (1988). Aarvy Aardvark and his friend Ralphie Rabbit show how a family member or friend can help someone who is in distress.

Dodd, Mike. *Oliver's Story.* (2004). A 40-page illustrated book for 3- to 8-year-old siblings of children diagnosed with cancer. Parents can order a free copy in English or Spanish from *www.acco.org/books.*

Loughridge, Sally. *Daniel and His Starry Night Blanket: A Story of Illness and Sibling Love.* (2015). With lovely images and comforting words, this book explores the many emotions felt by Daniel over the course of his sister's treatment for cancer.

Hospitalization

Keene, Nancy. *Your Child in the Hospital: A Practical Guide for Parents,* 3rd ed. (2015). A pocket guide to help parents prepare their children for short- or long-term hospitalization.

Parenting

Faber, Adle; Mazlish, Elaine. *How to Talk so Kids will Listen…and Listen so Kids Will Talk.* (2002). A best-selling classic about how to effectively communicate with your child.

Nelson, Jane. *Positive Discipline.* (2006). This parenting book explains how to focus on solutions while being kind and firm.

Radiation

National Cancer Institute. *Radiation Therapy and You: Support for People with Cancer.* (2016). A 55-page booklet that explains radiation therapy, what to expect, possible side effects, and follow-up care. Available online at *www.cancer.gov/publications/ patient-education/radiation-therapy-and-you.*

School

Leukemia and Lymphoma Society. *Living & Learning with Cancer.* (2013). Booklet about returning to school and obtaining any needed accommodations. Available at *www. lls.org/content/nationalcontent/resourcecenter/freeeducationmaterials/childhoodblood-cancer/pdf/learninglivingwithcancer.pdf.*

Princeton Review. *K&W Guide to Colleges for Students with Learning Differences,* 13th ed. (2016). Excellent reference book that is available at most large libraries.

Silver, Larry. *The Misunderstood Child: Understanding and Coping with Your Child's Learning Disabilities,* 4th ed. (2006). Comprehensive discussion about positive strategies that can be implemented at home and in school to help children with learning disabilities.

Siblings

Faber, Adele; Mazlish, Elaine. *Siblings Without Rivalry: How to Help Your Children Live Together So You Can Live Too,* revised edition. (2012). Offers dozens of simple and effective methods to reduce conflict and foster a cooperative spirit.

Greves, Julie; Tenhulzen, Katy; Wilkinson, Fred. *Upside Down and Backwards: A Sibling's Journey Through Childhood Cancer.* (2014). Child life specialists and social workers from Seattle Children's Hospital describe the effect of cancer on siblings. Aimed at 9- to 12-year-old siblings.

Wozny, Sharon. *Jamie's Journey: Cancer from the Voice of a Sibling.* (2016). With comforting text and gorgeous illustrations, this book gently explores the sometimes difficult emotions that arise in siblings of children with cancer.

Survivorship

Keene, Nancy; Hobbie, Wendy; Ruccione, Kathy. *Childhood Cancer Survivors: A Practical Guide to Your Future,* 3rd ed. (2012). A user-friendly, comprehensive guide about late effects of treatment for childhood cancer. Full of stories from survivors of all types of childhood cancer. Also covers emotional issues, insurance, jobs, relationships, and ways to stay healthy.

Technical reading

Medical textbooks are very expensive. If you'd like to read one, you can usually obtain it through interlibrary loan (ask your local reference librarian).

Bleyer, Archie; Barr, Ronald. *Cancer in Adolescents and Young Adults,* 2nd ed. (2016). Medical textbook.

Institute of Medicine. *Comprehensive Cancer Care for Children and Their Families.* (2015). Summarizes needed improvements in research, treatments, and outcomes. Available as full text online or as a paperback at *www.nap.edu/catalog/21754/comprehensive-cancer-care-for-children-and-their-families-summary-of.*

Pizzo, Philip A.; Poplack, David. (editors). *Principles and Practice of Pediatric Oncology,* 7th ed. (2015). Medical textbook.

Treatment journals

Alex's Lemonade Stand Treatment Journal. (no date). Alex's Lemonade Stand Foundation provides a free treatment journal to help parents of children with cancer keep track of important information. Parents can request a free copy of the journal at *www. alexslemonade.org/childhood-cancer-treatment-journal*.

Crawford, Bonnie; Lazar, Linda. *In My World.* (1999). Journal for teens coping with life-threatening illnesses. Includes chapters called "Things Accomplished in My Life," "I've Been Thinking," and "Questions I'd Like Answered." Available by calling (866) 218-0101 or visiting *www.centering.org*.

Terminal illness and bereavement

Callanan, Maggie; Kelley, Patricia. *Final Gifts: Understanding the Special Awareness, Needs, and Communications of the Dying.* (2012). Written by two hospice nurses with decades of experience, this book helps families understand and communicate with terminally ill people. Compassionate, comforting, and insightful, it movingly teaches how to listen to and comfort the dying.

Gilbert, Laynee. *I Remember You: A Grief Journal,* 2nd ed. (2000). A journal for recording written and photographic memories during the first year of mourning. Beautiful book filled with quotes and comfort.

Kübler-Ross, Elisabeth. *On Children and Death: How Children and Their Parents Can and Do Cope With Death.* (1997). In this comforting book, Dr. Kübler-Ross offers practical help for living through the terminal period of a child's life with love and understanding. Discusses children's knowledge about death, visualization, letting go, funerals, help from friends, and spirituality.

Mitchell, Ellen, and others. *Beyond Tears: Living After Losing a Child.* (2009). Comforting book written by nine mothers who each lost a child. Includes a chapter written from the perspective of surviving siblings.

Orloff, Stacy; Huff, Susan. *Home Care for Seriously Ill Children: A Manual for Parents.* (2003). Helps parents explore the possibility of home care for the dying child. Contains practical information about what to expect, methods of pain relief, and management of medical problems. Available from Children's Hospice International by emailing *info@chionline.org* or online at *http://75.103.82.45/publication-order-form*.

Wolfelt, Alan. *Healing a Parent's Grieving Heart: 100 Practical Ideas After Your Child Dies.* (2002). A list of practical actions a parent can take to memorialize their child's life and to cope and heal in the months and years that follow.

Sibling grief (adult reading)

Grollman, Earl. *Talking About Death: A Dialogue Between Parent and Child*, 4th ed. (2011). A classic guide for helping children cope with grief. Contains a children's read-along section to explain and explore children's feelings. In very comforting language, the book teaches parents how to explain death, understand children's emotions, learn how children react to specific types of death, and know when to seek professional help.

Schaefer, Dan; Lyons, Christine. *How Do We Tell the Children? A Step-by-Step Guide for Helping Children and Teens Cope When Someone Dies*, 4th ed. (2010). If your terminally ill child has siblings, read this book. In straightforward, uncomplicated language, the authors describe how to explain the facts of death to children and teens, and show how to include children in the family support network, laying the foundation for the healing process to begin. Also includes a crisis section with quick references for what to do in a variety of situations.

White, P. Gill. *Sibling Grief: Healing After the Death of a Sister or Brother.* (2008). This book explains the emotional significance of sibling loss, drawing on clinical experience, research, and wisdom from hundreds of bereaved siblings to explain the five healing tasks involved in sibling grief.

Sibling grief (young child)

Buscaglia, Leo. *The Fall of Freddy the Leaf: A Story of Life for All Ages.* (1982). This wise yet simple story about a leaf named Freddy explains death as a necessary part of the cycle of life.

Karst, Patrice. *The Invisible String.* (2000). This gentle, sweet book explains the connections between family members and helps children cope with fear of separation and loss, whether through absence or death.

Hanson, Warren. *The Next Place.* (2002). A book of warm and peaceful images that helps young children think about the continuity and beauty of all lives, and provides comfort to teens and adults, as well.

Hickman, Martha. *Last Week My Brother Anthony Died.* (1984). A touching story of a preschooler's feelings when her infant brother dies. The family's minister (a bereaved parent himself) comforts her by comparing feelings to clouds—always there but ever changing.

Mellonie, Bryan; Ingpen, Robert. *Lifetimes: The Beautiful Way to Explain Death to Children.* (1983). Beautiful paintings and simple text explain that dying is as much a part of life as being born.

Varley, Susan. *Badger's Parting Gifts.* (1992). Badger's friends share the memories he left them and learn to accept his death.

Sibling grief (school-aged children)

Romain, Trevor. *What on Earth Do You Do When Someone Dies?* (1999). Warm, honest words and beautiful illustrations help children understand and cope with grief.

Temes, Roberta. *The Empty Place: A Child's Guide Through Grief.* (1992). Explains and describes feelings after the death of a sibling, such as the empty place in the house, at the table, and in a sibling's heart.

Sibling grief (teenagers)

Gravelle, Karen; Haskins, Charles. *Teenagers Face to Face with Bereavement.* (2000). The perspectives and experiences of 17 teenagers comprise the heart of this book, which focuses on teens coping with grief.

Grollman, Earl. *Straight Talk About Death for Teenagers: How to Cope with Losing Someone You Love.* (1993). Wonderful book that discusses denial, pain, anger, sadness, physical symptoms, and depression. Charts methods to help teens work through their feelings at their own pace.

Hyatt, Erica Goldblatt. *Grieving for the Sibling You Lost: A Teen's Guide to Coping with Grief and Finding Meaning After Loss.* (2015). Helps teens understand grief, the symptoms that accompany it, various ways to cope, creating meaning out of loss and suffering, and when and how to ask for help.

Websites

This section lists websites that are not included in Appendix B, *Resource Organizations,* but that many parents find helpful. As with any resource, check with your child's treatment team about the accuracy of any information found on websites.

Calendars and practical help

CareCalendar
www.carecalendar.org

CareCalendar is a free service to organize meals and other help for families in need. The coordinator can upload photos and status updates to these password-protected sites.

CaringBridge
www.caringbridge.org

CaringBridge allows people who are ill or injured to create a website to share medical updates and personal photos with those who care about them. This website also provides users with the ability to post a simple task calendar to let supporters help with meals and chores.

Lotsa Helping Hands
www.lotsahelpinghands.com

An online task scheduling and information-sharing website for families that need support from friends and family. The site allows the site manager to sign up new members, schedule tasks, communicate needs, and post messages and photos to members of the community.

My Med Schedule App
http://mymedschedule.com

A software application to help you keep track of medication schedules, dosages, and any other important information, with reminder timers. You can record lab results and track them over time. The app is password protected and can be used from a computer, smartphone, or other device.

Dictionary

National Cancer Institute Dictionary of Cancer Terms
www.cancer.gov/dictionary

This dictionary provides definitions of cancer terminology.

Education

Wrightslaw
www.wrightslaw.com

This site provides accurate, up-to-date information about special education laws for parents, advocates, and attorneys.

Employment and family leave

National Conference of State Legislatures
www.ncsl.org/research/labor-and-employment/state-family-and-medical-leave-laws.aspx

This site lists state family medical leave and parental leave laws for all 50 states.

U.S. Department of Labor
www.dol.gov/whd/fmla

The Wage and Hour Division of the Department of Labor provides detailed information about employees' rights under the Family and Medical Leave Act.

Fundraising

YouCaring
www.youcaring.com

YouCaring allows individuals to create a webpage to raise money for medical expenses or other pressing bills. The link to your page can be shared by email and on social media so friends, family, and community members can help to spread the word widely and donate to you directly. Several other personal fundraising sites are available, including *www.gofundme.com* and *www.crowdrise.com*. Fundraising sites charge varying fees for processing the money donated, so read the fine print very carefully.

General online medical resources

Medline Plus

www.nlm.nih.gov/medlineplus/druginformation.html

A service of the National Institutes of Health, this site provides accurate information about drugs, including precautions and side effects.

National Cancer Institute

www.cancer.gov

A huge, reliable site that provides accurate information about cancer, treatments, and clinical trials.

Pediatric Oncology Resource Center

www.ped-onc.org

Excellent source of information about pediatric cancers created and managed by a mother of a long-term survivor. Contains detailed and accurate material about diseases, treatment, family issues, activism, bereavement, and survivorship. It also provides links to other helpful cancer sites.

PubMed

www.ncbi.nlm.nih.gov/PubMed

The National Library of Medicine's free search service provides access to more than 25 million citations in MEDLINE and PREMEDLINE (with links to participating online journals) and other related databases.

Quackwatch

www.quackwatch.com

This is an international network of people who post information about health-related frauds, myths, fads, fallacies, and misconduct.

Rx List—The Internet Drug Index

www.rxlist.com/drugs/alpha_a.htm

This site provides accurate information about prescription medications and a medical dictionary.

Survivorship

Ped-Onc Resource Center Survivor Issues
www.ped-onc.org/survivors

This collection of information for families of survivors includes resources, technical and nontechnical articles, accurate information about late effects, sources of scholarships for survivors, list of survivorship clinics, and much more.

Children's Oncology Group Long-term Follow-up Guidelines
www.survivorshipguidelines.org

This downloadable document details current knowledge about the late effects of childhood cancer. The late effects are listed by treatment (chemotherapy drug or radiation dose/site) and guidelines for needed diagnostic tests are provided. It includes individual "Health Links" with information about dozens of specific late effects.

Online Support Groups

Be sure to check the accuracy of any medical information obtained from an online support group with members of your child's treatment team.

The Association of Cancer Online Resources, Inc. (ACOR)
www.acor.org

ACOR is a unique collection of 142 online cancer communities that is designed to provide timely and accurate information in a supportive environment. It hosts several pediatric cancer discussion groups, including one for parents of children with ALL.

Facebook Support Groups

Numerous groups (most require permission to join) exist on Facebook to help families of kids with cancer. A few that were active at the time this book was written are listed below.

- **ALL:** *www.facebook.com/groups/5945722681*
- **APL:** *www.facebook.com/groups/AcutePromyelocyticLeukemia*
- **Bone Marrow & Stem Cell Transplant Patient Support:** *www.facebook.com/groups/5945722681*
- **Children with CML:** *www.facebook.com/groups/207664421574*
- **JMML:** *www.facebook.com/groups/jmmlsupport*
- **Momcology:** *www.momcology.org/sitepage/support-groups*

Imerman Angels

www.imermanangels.org

Imerman Angels offers one-on-one mentoring for adolescents and young adults with cancer.

Momcology

www.momcology.org

Momcology is an international online support group for mothers and other primary caregivers of children who have been diagnosed with cancer. Participants can request to join private Momcology Facebook support groups based on diagnosis, special care issues, or geographic region. A Facebook profile is needed to participate.

Stupid Cancer

www.stupidcancer.org

This is an online resource for and by adolescents and young adults with cancer. It includes medical information, links to scholarships and grants, regional and national conferences, a talk radio podcast, and an active peer support community, including a one-on-one peer support smartphone app.

Index

All-trans retinoic acid (ATRA), 49, 50, 176, 193

Alopecia. *See* Hair loss

ALT (alanine aminotransferase), 436

Alternative treatments, 206–207

AML. *See* acute myeloid leukemia

American Academy of Pediatrics
    assent, 97
      child life programs, 101
      donating marrow, 251
      essential hospital services, 20

American Association for Marriage and Family Therapy, 347

American Board of Medical Specialties, 127

American Cancer Society
    and wigs, 217

ANC. *See* Absolute neutrophil count

Anemia, 14, 120, 435

Anesthesia, 105–107

Anesthesiologists, 106–107, 114, 235

Anger
    conflict resolution and,
    of children, 79, 269, 304
    at diagnosis, 7–8
    at healthcare team, 137
    professional therapy for, 346
    siblings, 268

Anniversaries, 422, 426

Antibiotics
    dental work and, 213
    prophylactic antibiotics, 196
    stem cell transplantation, 261
    with catheters, 156

Antinausea drugs, 197–201

Anus, protecting, 214, 220

Anxiety, 3, 77, 104, 308, 346

APL, 48, 50–51
    APL differentiation syndrome, 177

Appealing insurance claim, 371

Appetite, 353

ARA-C. *See* Cytarabine

Armfuls of Time (Sourkes), 431

Arsenic trioxide, 50, 175, 177

Asparaginase, 34, 36, 37, 39, 40, 175, 178

Aspartate aminotransferase (AST), 437

Aspirin, 182, 186, 206, 221

Assent to clinical trial, 97

Ataxia-telangiectasia, 25

Ativan (lorazepam), 198, 200

ATRA, 49, 50, 176, 193

Attending doctors, 127

Auditing hospital accounts, 379

Australia
    camps, 443
    free air service, 446
    hospice and bereavement, 450
    service organizations, 442–443
    wish fulfillment, 449

Avascular necrosis (AVN), 190, 225

B

B-cell ALL, 33–35

B-cell aplasia, 408

Bactrim, 118, 186, 196

Bed wetting, 209–211

Benadryl (diphenhydramine), 121, 198, 199

Benzene exposure, 25, 45

Bereavement. *See* Death

Bilirubin, 434, 437

Blast, defined, 15

Blended families, 286

Blood components, 13–15
    Blood transfusions, 120

Blood cell counts
    charts to track, 374
    children on treatment, values for, 434
    healthy children, values for, 433-434
    pattern, 438

Blood draws, 109

Blood patch, 114

Bloom syndrome, 25, 45

Body surface area (BSA), 170
    Bone growth test, 110

Bone marrow aspiration, 110
    at diagnosis, 3
    on last day of treatment, 386
    sedation for, 105, 111

Dilaudid (hydromorphone), 202, 203
Diphenhydramine (benadryl), 121, 198, 199
Dishonesty of parents, 308
Distraction, 105, 291
DNA, 17–20
DNR (Do Not Resuscitate) orders, 416
Doctors
    changing doctors, 138
    communicating with, 131–135
    conflict resolution, 136
    radiation oncologists, 225
    relationships with, 129
    second opinions, 135
    types of, 126–127
Dosages of chemotherapy drugs, 170
Down syndrome
    ALL, and, 25, 40–41
    AML, and, 45, 49, 51–53
Doxorubicin (adriamycin), 176, 182
Drugs
    antibiotics, 196
    antinausea drugs, 197
    chemotherapy, 169–195
    free medicine programs, 381, 447
    mistakes at hospitals, 134, 149
    pain medications, 202
Dying. *See* Death

E

Early filling, 353
Early intervention services, 336
Eating habits. *See* Nutrition
Echocardiogram, 111, 395
Education. *See* School
Elspar (asparaginase), 175, 178
EMLA cream, 204
Emotions
    children, 304–307
    ending treatment, 385
    parents, at diagnosis, 3–9
    relapse, response to, 401
    siblings, 265–271

Employment. *See* Jobs
End of treatment, 385–398
    catheter removal, 387
    ceremonies at, 388
    emotions, 385
    follow-up care, 394
    normal, returning to, 390
    treatment summary, 396
Engraftment, 250
Enteral nutrition, 367
Erwinia asparaginase, 175, 178
Erythrocytes. *See* Red blood cells
Ethyl chloride spray, 107
Etoposide (VP-16), 176, 182
Exercise
    anger, dealing with, 309
    in hospitals, 294
    physical therapy, 226
Explanation of benefits (EOBs), 375, 378
External catheters, 153–158

F

Family
    blended families, 286
    death, role at, 420
    extended family, 288
    Family and Medical Leave Act (FMLA), 282, 459
    grandparents, 288
    helpful things to do, 290
    helpful things to say, 298
    improving family life, 303
    marriage and partnerships, 283
    notifying, 83
    restructuring life, 281
    single parents, 287
Family and Medical Leave Act (FMLA), 282, 459
Fanconi anemia, 25, 45
Fatigue, 214
Fats in diet, 357, 360
Fentanyl, 106, 202

prognosis, 62
signs and symptoms, 59
treatment, 62
who gets, 59

K

Kaopectate, 213
Kytril (granisetron), 198, 199

L

Lactose intolerance, 354
L-Asparaginase. *See* Asparaginase
Learning disabilities, *See also* Special education
 Canada, legal rights in, 338
 identifying, 330
 legal rights, 327
 radiation therapy and, 218, 244
 referral for services, 329
Leucovorin, 34, 37, 38, 39, 40, 41, 51, 187
Leukapheresis, 407
Leukemia
 definition of, 13–15
 types of, 16
Leukocytes. *See* White blood cells (WBCs)
Lidocaine, 107, 108, 204, 223
Li-Fraumeni syndrome, 25, 45
Listening to children, 302
Liver
 alanine aminotransferase (ALT), 436
 aspartate aminotransferase (AST), 437
 bilirubin, 437
 serum glutamic oxaloacetic transaminase (SGOT), 437
 veno-occlusive disease (VOD), 262
LMX cream, 107
Lomotil, 213
Lorazepam (ativan), 198, 200
Licensed practical nurses (LPNs), 128
Lumbar punctures. *See* Spinal taps
Lymphocytes, 219, 433, 434, 436

M

Magic Mouthwash, 223
Magnesium citrate, 212
Maintenance phase, 34, 36, 37, 40
Marriage and partnerships, 283–286
 blended families, 286
Mask for radiation therapy, 238–239
Massage, 105, 205, 225
Match, what is, 247
Matched unrelated donor (MUD), 63, 64, 75, 250
Medicaid, 378, 381
 fundraising, and, 383
Medical expenses. *See also* Financial issues; Insurance
 fundraising websites, 459
 Section 125 plan, 383
 tax deductible, 217, 376
Medical records, 132, 372–375, 397
Medical team, 125–139
 communication with, 131
 conflict resolution, 136
 members of, 126–128
 transitioning from treatment, 394–395
Medicine, free programs, 447
Meditation, 104, 205, 225, 309
Melphalan, 63, 176, 185
Memorial services, 419
Meperidine (demerol), 202, 203
Mercaptopurine (6-MP), 34, 36, 39, 40, 176, 185
 pharmacogenetics of, 171
Mesna, 39, 179, 184, 260
Metamucil, 212
Methlyenetetrahydrofolate reductase (MTHFR), 173
Methotrexate, 176, 186
 folic acid and, 186, 206
 learning disabilities, 218
 pharmacogenetics of, 173
 spinal taps, 113
 sun sensitivity, 186, 229
Milk (lactose) intolerance, 354
Milk of magnesia, 212

P

Pain management, 103
    medications, 105
    psychological methods, 103
Parenteral nutrition, 366
Parking
    at hospital, 144
    tax deduction, 375, 376, 377
PDQ, treatment information from, 446
    ALL, 41
    AML, 48, 55
    JMML, 64
    CML, 75
PEG-asparaginase. *See* Asparaginase
Pentamidine, 196
Percocet (oxycodone), 202, 204
Peripherally inserted central catheters (PICC
    lines), 163–165
Petechiae, 14, 26, 46, 400
Pets, living with, 230, 261
Pharmacogenetics, 32, 171
Phenergan (promethazine), 198, 201
Philadelphia chromosome, 29, 30, 37–38, 70, 72
Philadelphia chromosome-like ALL, 38
Physical responses to diagnosis, 3
Physical therapy, 226, 328
    IEP, part of, 330, 333, 336
Physicians. *See* Doctors
PICC lines, 163–165
Pill-taking, 116–118, 119
Plaque buildup on teeth, 212
Plasma, 13, 109, 435
Platelets, 14, 121
    counts, 433, 436
Pneumocystis pneumonia (PCP), 196
Pneumonia, 118, 123, 196, 227
Ponatinib, 72, 74, 176, 189
PORT-A-CATH. *See* Subcutaneous ports
Potassium, 434
    diarrhea, and, 213–214
    steroids, loss of, 192

Prednisone, 176, 190
    behavior changes, 190
    increased appetite, 354
    osteonecrosis, 225
    side effects, 190, 230
    taste, 116
Preschoolers, 329, 336, 337
    distracting, 105
Primapore, 168
Procedures, 101–123
    blood draw, 109
    bone growth test, 110
    bone marrow aspiration, 110
    echocardiogram, 111, 395
    finger pokes, 111
    gastrostomy, 112
    lumbar puncture, 113
    pain management, 103
    planning for, 101
    questions to ask, 108
    sedatives and anesthetics for, 105–108
    starting an IV, 114
    subcutaneous injections, 115
    taking oral medications, 116
    taking a temperature, 119
    teens and medication, 119
    transfusions, blood, 120
    transfusions, platelets, 121
    urine specimens, 122
    x-rays, 122
Prochlorperazine (compazine), 198, 201
Promethazine (phenergan), 198, 201
Prophylactic antibiotics, 196
Propofol, 106, 236
Protocol, 88, 99
Psychologists
    family-centered care, 126
    conflict resolution and, 137, 342
    counseling with, 347
Puberty
    radiation therapy, effects on, 242, 244
    stem cell transplantation and, 263

R

S

for acute myeloid leukemia (AML), 49
alternative treatments, 206
choosing a treatment, 87–100
for chronic myelogenous leukemia (CML), 73
for juvenile myelomonocytic leukemia (JMML), 62
last day of, 385
standard treatment, 88
summary of, 386
where to receive, 20
Tretinoin, 176, 193
Tube feedings. *See* Enteral nutrition
Tumor board, 135
Tumor lysis syndrome, 408
Twins
leukemia in, 25, 45
syngeneic transplants, 75, 248
Tylenol, 174
Tyrosine kinase inhibitors (TKIs), 72

U

Umbilical cord blood stem cell transplant, 247, 249, 250
Urine specimens, 122

V

Vacation days, using, 282,
Valium, for procedures, 106
Vapocoolant sprays, 205
Varicella zoster immune globulin (VZIG), 228
Vegetables, servings of, 357
Veno-occlusive disease (VOD), 262
Versed, for procedures, 106
Vesanoid (tretinoin), 176, 193
Viactiv, 355
Vincristine, 176, 194
constipation from, 194, 211
side effects from, 195, 226, 327
Viruses, 121, 221, 227, 228, 396
stem cell transplantation and, 261
Visualization, 104, 205
Vitamin supplements, 364

Vomiting, 223
drugs to prevent, 197–201
VP-16 (etoposide), 176, 182
VZIG (varicella zoster immune globulin), 228

W

WBCs. *See* White blood cell counts (WBCs)
Weakness, 214
White blood cells (WBCs), 14–15
ALL prognosis and, 28
AML prognosis and, 49
colony-stimulating factors, and, 196
charts, keeping, 374
White blood cell differential, 219, 433, 436
Wigs, 217, 324
medical deduction on taxes, 376
Wish fulfillment organizations, 448–449
Withdrawal of children, 301, 305, 425
Worries of siblings, 266

X

X-rays, 122

Z

Zofran (ondansetron), 198, 200, 237

About the Author

Nancy Keene is the mother of a long-term survivor of high-risk acute lymphoblastic leukemia. A well-known writer and advocate for children with cancer, she has written and co-authored many books on topics ranging from childhood cancers to working with your doctor. Her work has appeared in publications such as *Reader's Digest, Journal of the American Medical Association, Exceptional Parent,* and *Coping Magazine.* She was the first chair of the Children's Cancer Group (CCG) Patient Advocacy Committee, and then the first chair of the Patient Advocacy Committee of the Children's Oncology Group (COG)—consortiums of researchers from more than 250 children's hospitals. Nancy has been interviewed on National Public Radio (NPR), frequently speaks to professional and parent groups, and has participated in online support groups for parents of children with cancer since 1996. In her spare time, she likes to read, hike with her dogs, and kayak in the waters of the Pacific Northwest.

Childhood Cancer Guides™

Questions Answered
Experiences Shared

When your life is turned upside down, your need for information is great. You have to make critical medical decisions, often with what seems like little to go on. Plus, you have to break the news to family, quiet your own fears, help your ill child and your other children, figure out how you are going to pay the bills, and sometimes get to work or put dinner on the table.

Childhood Cancer Guides provide authoritative information for the families and friends of children with cancer or survivors of childhood cancer. Our books cover all aspects of how these illnesses affect family life. In each book, there's a mix of:

- **Medical information**

  Dozens of experts on childhood cancer and survivorship contributed to these books to provide state-of-the-art information to help you weigh treatment options. Modern medicine has much to offer. When there are treatment controversies, we present differing points of view.

- **Practical information**

  After making treatment decisions, life focuses on coping with treatment and any side effects that develop. We cover day-to-day practicalities, such as those you'd hear from a helpful nurse or a knowledgeable support group.

- **Emotional support**

  It's normal to have strong reactions to a condition that threatens your child's life. It's normal that the whole family is affected. We cover issues such as the shock of diagnosis, living with uncertainty, and communicating with loved ones.

Each book contains stories from parents, children, and siblings who share, in their own words, the lessons they have learned and what truly helped them cope.

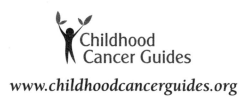

www.childhoodcancerguides.org